Primary Diagnosis and Treatment

A Manual for Clinical and Health Centre Staff
in Developing Countries

Daniel E. Fountain, M.D., M.P.H.

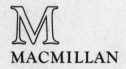

MACMILLAN

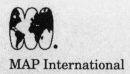

MAP International

First published 1992

Published by THE MACMILLAN PRESS LTD
London and Basingstoke
Associated companies and representatives in Accra,
Auckland, Delhi, Dublin, Gaborone, Hamburg, Harare,
Hong Kong, Kuala Lumpur, Lagos, Manzini, Melbourne,
Mexico City, Nairobi, New York, Singapore, Tokyo.

In association with
MAP International   MAP International
P.O. Box 50   East Africa Office
Brunswick, GA 31521-0050 P.O. Box 21663
USA.   Nairobi, Kenya, East Africa

ISBN 0–333–57605–5

Printed in Hong Kong

Design, layout and illustrations by Regina Vergara Art

A catalogue record for this book is available from the
British Library.

Dedication

This book is dedicated to people:
- to sick persons who want to get well.
- to all who care for sick persons by helping them get well and by showing them how to stay well.

Our hope is that this book will bring healing to many persons and health to all.

Thanks

Many people have worked hard to make this book possible:

- health care workers: doctors, nurses, health assistants, student nurses.
- sick persons who have showed us much about illnesses, about getting well, and about health.

To all of them we want to say thank you.

We also want to thank many colleagues at MAP International who have worked hard to put this book together. Our thanks go especially to:

- Regina Vergara for her long hours of illustrating and formatting.
- Dr. Sharon E. Bolin for proofreading.

Writing a book is a family task. So I want to thank my family for their encouragement and support.

Table of Contents

Chapter 9 - <u>Strategies for Signs</u>

Foreword

Recently I was asked to speak to a meeting of English doctors on the subject of what we in Europe can learn from the experience of health care in developing countries. By using the illustration, "Who provides primary health care best?" I emphasised that, to me, doctors in the developing world are not the most appropriate providers of primary health care. Doctors certainly have a place in the team providing primary health care. However, their training is more toward provision of health care in hospitals concerned with complex conditions. Primary health workers have advantages which frequently make them more appropriate as front line health workers in primary health care. First of all, they have more time to give people. Frequently they speak the same language as most of their patients. They also recognise and understand the problems, anxieties, and fears of sick persons more easily than does a doctor.

Health care professionals around the world now appreciate how much we can do to improve health by changing peoples' lifestyles and nutritional habits. Curative care has little effect on health. Primary health workers have particular responsibility in health improvement because most of these efforts in health improvement fall on their

Who provides primary health care best?

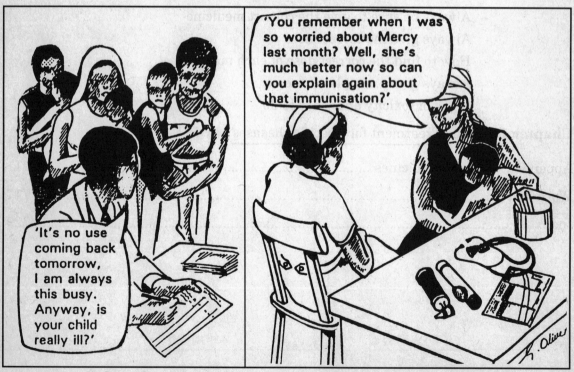

A doctor?   A primary health worker?

shoulders. However, helping people change their lifestyles and nutritional habits can be successful only when they have gained the respect and support of the patients and the community they serve. They will gain this confidence best when they manage to diagnose and treat common health problems affecting the children and adults in the community. From his long experience, Dr. Fountain offers a carefully written and well prepared book which attempts to help to do this well. This is especially important because many of them work in isolation without a doctor to help them meet the more complex health problems.

This is not a book to read and put away on a bookshelf. If you are to provide the service that people expect and you would wish to offer them, you will need to refer regularly to sections of this book.

David Morley, M.D.
Professor Emeritus
Institute of Child Health
London

About the Author

Dr. Daniel E. Fountain, a medical missionary with the American Baptist Churches of the USA, has served for more than 25 years as medical director of a large hospital and community health program in Zaire. He has trained primary health workers who are the principal source of health care for millions of people. He established one of the first rural health zones in central Africa, and has been a consultant to the government of Zaire in the training of health personnel and in community health. For the past several years, he has been a consultant with MAP International in several other countries in Africa, as well as in the United States. He has written a number of books in French for primary health workers. This book is an English edition of one used for many years in French-speaking African countries.

Preface

Good health is a valuable possession. We want to keep it. We do not want anything to take it away from us.

Disease is like a thief. A disease comes into our bodies and "steals" our health. We become ill. Our good health is gone because a disease has "stolen" it.

When a thief comes into your house, he comes secretly. He takes your possessions and goes away with them. But often he leaves behind signs of his theft: a broken window, a footprint, a mark on the door, or a torn piece of cloth.

When you call the police, they come to see what has happened. They ask you many questions. They look carefully for signs of the theft. They look for signs that will help them know who the thief is.

A disease comes into our body quietly, just like a thief comes into the house. But a disease makes signs that can show us what the disease is. We can look for these signs made by the disease. When we find them, we can often find what the disease is. Then we will know how to treat the sick person and help him get well.

The purpose of this book is to help you know how to look for the signs that diseases make in our bodies. It will tell you the questions to ask the sick person. It will show you how to examine him to look for signs of disease. It will then show you how to decide which disease is probably the cause of the person's illness. In the last part of the book you will find what to do to help the sick person get well and recover his good health.

The book has three parts. The first part is about the consultation, and it tells you how to examine a sick person. This includes children as well as adults. The consultation begins with taking the history of the illness and the previous health of the sick person. The book describes the important steps to follow in taking a good history.

Then comes the physical examination of the sick person. The book shows you how to look carefully at adults and children to find the important signs of the illness making the person sick. The book also discusses briefly the indications for doing simple laboratory procedures. Then comes a chapter on how to look at all of the information found in the history and the examinations, and then how to decide on the diagnosis.

The second part of the book is a series of more than 60 strategies to help you find the correct diagnosis. Each strategy is based on a common symptom or sign of the disease. It presents the important and common illnesses that can cause that symptom or sign. The strategy reviews the questions to ask in the history and the signs to look for in the physical and laboratory exams in order to find the cause of the symptom or sign.

Then comes a diagram or "flow chart," which will help you find the most probable cause of the person's illness. With each strategy, you can review the possible causes of each symptom or sign or a sick person. You can be sure to ask all the necessary questions and to look for all the important signs of disease. Finally, by following the arrows on the diagram, you will find the most probable cause of the illness: the diagnosis.

The third part presents in brief form the specific treatment for the common illnesses discussed in the book. The treatment shows you the medicine and care to give, important instructions to tell the sick person, and whatever education may help to prevent further attacks of the illness.

This book is like a road map. A road map shows you how to get from one city to another. You can see on the map the road you must follow to get where you want to go.

This book will show you how to go from one place to another. It will show you how to get from the signs of disease the sick person has to what he needs in order to get well. It shows you the road to follow, from the problem of the sick person: his illness, to the solution: what he needs to recover his good health.

This book is your guide book. Your work is very important for many people. You are the person who can help sick persons get well. You must know how to do this well. Therefore, read this book carefully. Learn how to take a good history and how to do a good physical examination. Learn how to think carefully and how to make a good diagnosis.

Keep this book on the table of your consulting room. Use it frequently when you examine sick persons. Use it every time you are not sure what disease is making a person sick. Use it when you are not sure what to do to help him get well. In this way, you will save many lives. You will help very many people get well. You will be a respected leader in your community.

Chapter 1
UNDERSTANDING WHAT DIAGNOSIS IS

1.1 What is "diagnosis?"

1.2 Why must we make a diagnosis?

1.3 What must we do to make a diagnosis?

1.4 What must we look for to make a diagnosis?

1.5 What steps must we follow to make a diagnosis?

1.6 How can we make the right diagnosis?

1.7 Why is it often difficult to make the right diagnosis?

1.8 How can we tell which patients are seriously ill?

1.9 How can you learn to make a good diagnosis?

1.1 What is "diagnosis?"

Patients come to us because they are ill. They do not feel well. They want us to help them get well as quickly as possible. As health workers, our job is to help our patients get well. We do this by helping them get rid of their illness.

To help each patient get well, there is one very important thing we must do first. We must find out what is making the patient ill. We must find out the disease making him ill. Then we will know what to do to make the disease go away. We will know how to help the patient get rid of the disease and therefore get well.

A disease is something that makes a person ill. For example, malaria is a disease. A very small parasite causes malaria. The malaria parasites get into the blood of a person. They make him ill. First, the parasites cause chills so that the patient feels cold and shakes all over. Then he gets a high fever and often a severe headache.

When this sick person comes to us, we try to find the disease that is making him ill. We ask the patient what he feels. We look at him carefully. We look at a drop of his blood under a microscope. We find the malaria parasites in this blood. So we know the patient has malaria. In other words, we make the diagnosis of malaria.

SUMMARY

1. A disease is what makes a person ill.
2. To make the diagnosis, we find the disease that makes our patient ill.
3. The diagnosis is the name of the disease making him ill.

Here we must make a short explanation. Our patients are men and women. They are also boys and girls. We want to make this book easy to read and to understand. So when we talk about a patient, we will call the patient "he" or "him." But what we will say about "he" or "him" will apply to women and girls as well as to men and boys.

1.2 Why must we make a diagnosis?

1.2.1 Diagnosis leads to treatment

Our patient comes to us because he feels ill. He wants us to help him get well. For the patient, the diagnosis is not very important. But getting well is very important to him. We also want him to get well. But he will get well only when his disease goes away.

Our job is to give him the treatment that will make his disease go away.

We can do this only when we know which disease he has. If we do not know which disease he has, we cannot know the right treatment to give him.

So we must first make the diagnosis. Then we can give, or prescribe, the right treatment for him.

Diagnosis ------------> Treatment

1.2.2 Wrong diagnosis - wrong treatment

Let us look again at our patient with malaria. We may think that he has another disease, such as pneumonia. We make the diagnosis of pneumonia. We then give him the treatment for pneumonia.

But he has malaria, not pneumonia. So our treatment will do him no good. His malaria will continue to make him ill.

Wrong diagnosis ------------> wrong treatment

1.2.3 Right diagnosis - right treatment

But if we make the diagnosis of malaria in our patient, we will give him the treatment for malaria. Now his malaria will go away. He will get well. So making the right diagnosis is very important.

It is like the key to a door. Only one key will go into the lock and open the door. No other key will work. Making the right diagnosis is like finding the right key to the door. It "opens the door" to the right treatment. We can then know how to help our patient get well.

Right diagnosis -------------> Right treatment

Questions for study

1. What does it mean to "make a diagnosis?"
2. A person with a high fever has malaria parasites in his blood. What is the diagnosis?
3. Why is it important to make the right diagnosis?
4. What happens if we make the wrong diagnosis?

1.3 What must we do to make a diagnosis?

How can we tell if a patient has malaria? How do we make this diagnosis?

When a patient comes to the clinic, he does not tell us he has malaria. He probably does not know what disease he has. He only knows how he feels. He will say, "I have a fever," or "I have chills," or "I have a bad headache."

Our job is to find which disease is giving him the fever, the chills, or the headache. How do we do this?

That is the purpose of this book. This book will show you how to make a diagnosis. It will explain all you must do to find the disease that is making your patient ill.

1.3.1 Our work is like that of the police

Let us compare a disease to a thief who comes into your house to steal. The thief comes quietly so that you will not see him or hear him. He breaks a door or a window to get in and out. He takes what he can find and goes away with it. Later, you discover that a thief has come into your house and stolen your things.

You call the police. The police come to see what has happened. You want them to find the thief. But even more than that, you want them to get back what the thief has stolen.

1.3.2 Asking questions

The police begin by asking you questions:

When did you discover the theft?

- Did you hear anything?
- Where did you keep the things that were taken by the thief?
- Do you have an idea who could do such a thing?

1.3.3 Examining the house

Next, the police look carefully at your house. They examine the broken door or window. They look at the place where you kept the stolen things. They try to find anything left by the thief. They look outside for footprints or other marks. They look for any sign that will help them decide who is the thief.

1.3.4 Writing a report

After this, the police write a report of all you have told them and of all they have found. They look carefully at this report and examine all the information. They make a list of all the persons they know who could possibly be the thief. They find each person and ask him many questions.

If they do their work well, they will find the thief. You hope they will also find the stolen things and get them back to you.

1.3.5 Disease is like a thief

Disease is like a thief, and your body is like your house.

1. The disease comes into your body quietly. You do not see it come or hear it enter.
2. The disease may come through a break in the skin - a wound or an insect bite.
3. It may come through the mouth in what you eat or drink.
4. It may come in the air you breathe.
5. The disease robs you of your health. It takes away your strength and your sense of feeling well. It leaves bad feelings in their place. These bad feelings may show what disease is making you ill.

1.3.6 Health workers are like the police

We health workers are like the police. Our patient comes to us because an illness has "stolen his health." He wants us to help him get his health back. But to do so we must first find the disease that has "stolen" his health. So we follow the same steps the police follow when they look for a thief.

1. Like the police, we ask many questions. We must find out when the disease came. We must learn about all the bad feelings the patient has.
2. We then examine the patient carefully to find any signs made by the disease.
3. We write down all these things in a report.
4. We think carefully about this report. We analyse all the information we have found.
5. We make a list of all the possible diseases that could be making our patient ill. We look for each of these possible diseases.
6. We must decide which is the one that has indeed made our patient ill.

SUMMARY

1. The diagnosis the police make is the name of the thief.
2. The diagnosis we make is the name of a particular disease.
3. The steps we and the police follow to make the diagnosis are very much alike.

Questions for study

1. What do the police do to find a thief?
2. What do we do to make a diagnosis?
3. What are the six steps to follow to make a diagnosis?

1.4 What must we look for to make a diagnosis?

1.4.1 Diseases cause symptoms

When a person becomes sick, he begins to have unpleasant feelings. He feels ill. He may feel pain here or there. In our example of malaria, the patient feels cold all over, then hot. He has pain in his head. These unpleasant feelings come from the malaria.

We call these unpleasant feelings **symptoms. Symptoms are the unpleasant feelings the patient has when he is ill.**

We cannot see or feel the patient's symptoms. He must tell us about them. We ask him questions about his symptoms to be sure we understand how he feels. We want to know about all of his symptoms and when each one came. Only the patient can give us this information.

1.4.2 Diseases cause signs

The patient's disease causes the symptoms. The disease can also do more. It can make changes in the body of our patient. It can affect his blood, his heart, his liver, or any other part of his body.

Physical signs

For example, malaria makes changes in the body. Malaria can change the body temperature. The temperature goes up, and we can measure this with a thermometer. We say the patient has a fever.

The malaria parasites can also destroy many red blood cells. When this happens, the blood becomes thin and less red. We call this anemia.

We can get an idea of what the blood of the patient is like by looking inside his eyelids. Inside the eyelids is a membrane. We call this the conjunctiva. Normally the conjunctiva looks red. This is because there are many narrow blood vessels there. If the patient has anemia, the conjunctiva looks pale. This is because the blood in these narrow blood vessels has become very pale. We can see this when we look inside the patient's eyelids.

Malaria also can cause the spleen to swell and become big. We can feel the big spleen when we examine the abdomen of the patient.

We call these changes **signs. Signs are the changes a disease makes in the body of the patient.**

Malaria can cause the patient to have fever, pale conjunctiva, and a big spleen. These are signs of malaria, the changes in the body caused by the malaria parasites. We can find these different signs when we examine the patient. Often the patient does not know that these signs are present. We must look for them ourselves.

We call these signs **physical signs.** This is because **we find them when we do the physical examination of the patient.**

Laboratory signs

There is another way to look for signs of disease. This is in the laboratory. We look for laboratory signs of the patient's disease. Let us look again at our example of malaria.

1. The malaria parasites get into many red blood cells. So we look at the patient's red blood cells. We put a drop of the patient's blood on a glass slide. Then we put a drop of a special stain on top of the drop of blood. Now we examine it under the microscope. In this way we can see the malaria parasites in the red blood cells. We are then certain our patient has malaria.

2. We also measure the amount of hemoglobin in the patient's blood. Hemoglobin is the red substance in the red blood cells. The malaria parasites can destroy many red blood cells. When this happens, the amount of hemoglobin will diminish and the patient will have anemia. By measuring the hemoglobin in the blood, we can tell if the patient has anemia.

So in a patient who may have malaria, we look for two laboratory signs:

1. Malaria parasites in the red blood cells, and

2. A diminished hemoglobin in his blood.

We call these signs **laboratory signs** of malaria.

Questions for study

1. What is the difference between **symptom** and **sign**?
2. What is the difference between **physical sign** and **laboratory sign**?
3. What must we do to learn about the patient's symptoms?
4. What must we do to find signs of his disease?

SUMMARY

There are three things that help us make a diagnosis:

1. The **symptoms**, the unpleasant feelings the patient has. He must tell us about his symptoms.
2. The **physical signs**. We find these when we examine the patient.
3. The **laboratory signs**. We find these when we examine his blood, urine, stool, or other body substances in the laboratory.

REMEMBER:

1. Symptoms are the bad feelings of the patient that come from the disease. He must tell us about his symptoms. We learn about his symptoms:
   - By listening to him, and
   - By asking him questions.
2. Signs are the changes in the patient's body made by the disease. We must look for these signs. We find signs:
   - By examining the patient, and
   - By doing laboratory examinations.

BEFORE YOU READ FURTHER

1. Make a list of 10 different symptoms of disease.
2. Make a list of 10 different physical signs of disease.
3. Make a list of 10 different laboratory signs of disease.
4. Discuss these lists with your fellow students. Do you all agree on these lists?
5. Think about this:
   - What symptoms will a patient with a high fever have?
   - What symptoms will a patient with anemia have?

1.4.3 Each disease causes certain symptoms and signs

Each disease affects the patient in a certain way. Each disease causes certain symptoms and certain changes in the patient's body. One disease causes certain symptoms and signs. Another disease causes other symptoms and signs. The symptoms and signs of one disease are different from those of another disease.

We have seen that malaria causes certain symptoms, certain physical signs, and certain laboratory signs. Tuberculosis causes other symptoms and signs. These are some of the symptoms of tuberculosis:

Symptoms of tuberculosis

1. Tuberculosis causes a cough.
2. The patient with tuberculosis usually coughs up sputum.
3. Often there is blood in the sputum.
4. Tuberculosis can cause pain in the chest.

Physical signs of tuberculosis

Tuberculosis also causes changes in the body of the patient, especially in the lungs. These are some of the physical signs of tuberculosis:

1. Tuberculosis changes the sound of air coming into and going out of the lungs during breathing. We can hear these changes when we listen to the patient's chest through the stethoscope.
2. Tuberculosis causes a fever. But this fever is lower than the fever of malaria. Also, this fever stays for many weeks. It usually comes in the afternoon and evening, but not in the morning.
3. Tuberculosis often makes the patient lose weight. He becomes thin. We can see that the patient has lost weight. We also can weigh him and find out how much weight he has lost.

These changes - different breath sounds, low fever for weeks, and loss of weight - are physical signs of tuberculosis.

Laboratory signs of tuberculosis

When a patient with tuberculosis coughs, he often coughs up thick secretions. We call this sputum. The sputum comes from his lungs. Often it contains the bacteria that cause tuberculosis. We call these bacteria the tubercle bacilli.

We can examine the sputum in the laboratory. We put a drop of sputum on a microscope slide and put special stains on it. We then examine it under the microscope to look for tubercle bacilli.

This is a laboratory sign of tuberculosis - tubercle bacilli in the sputum. We can make the diagnosis of tuberculosis if we find these bacilli in our patient's sputum.

Table 1 shows the symptoms and signs of malaria and tuberculosis. These symptoms and signs help you decide which disease is making the patient ill.

Table 1 - Symptoms and signs of malaria and tuberculosis			
Disease	**Symptoms**	**Physical signs**	**Lab signs**
Malaria	Chills Feeling hot Headache	Fever Pale conjunctiva Big spleen	Parasites in red blood cells Low hemoglobin

Tuberculosis	Cough
	Sputum
	Blood in the sputum
	Pain in the chest
		Changes in the
		  breath sounds
		Loss of weight
		Low fever
			Tubercle
			  bacilli in the sputum

So when a person becomes ill, we find out from him his symptoms. We also look for physical signs and laboratory signs of his disease.

If we find the symptoms and signs of malaria, we make the diagnosis of malaria. If we find the symptoms and signs of tuberculosis, we make the diagnosis of tuberculosis.

It is the symptoms and signs of disease that lead us to the diagnosis.

Symptoms + Signs ----------------> Diagnosis

Questions for study

1. What will a patient who has malaria tell you about what he feels?
2. What will you find when you examine him?
3. What will a patient who has tuberculosis tell you about what he feels?
4. What will you find when you examine him?

1.5 What steps must we follow to make a diagnosis?

To make a diagnosis, we must find out all the information we can about the patient and his illness. We must find out what the disease has done to him.

1.5.1 The history

First of all, we must find out from him how he feels, what his symptoms are. We call this first step taking the history.

The history is the story of the patient's illness. The patient tells us about his illness. We ask him questions to be sure we know how he feels. We also ask him questions about his health before he became ill. We ask questions as well about the members of his family and his close friends. We want to know about their health also.

1.5.2 The physical examination

Next we examine the patient. We look for signs of disease. These are the changes the disease has made in his body. For example, we look for fever, for a big spleen, or for changes in the sounds of breathing.

This is the physical examination. We look at the whole body of the patient to find the physical signs made by the disease.

1.5.3 Laboratory examinations

There are other signs that we can find only in the laboratory. In the physical examination of our patient, we cannot find malaria parasites in his blood. We cannot find tubercle bacilli in his sputum. To find these, we must use the microscope.

So the next step in making the diagnosis with many of our patients is to do laboratory examinations. In the lab, we examine the blood, the urine, the stool, and the sputum of our patients. We do this to look for lab signs of disease.

With these three steps - history, physical examination, and laboratory examinations - we learn much information about the patient and about his disease. This information is necessary for making the right diagnosis. But there are two more steps we must take.

1.5.4 The patient's record

We must write down all this information in the record of the patient. This is what we must write down.

1. The story of his illness - the symptoms he has and when each symptom first appeared.

2. Information about the health of the patient before he became ill.
3. Information about the health of the members of his family and of his close friends.
4. The signs of disease we found in the physical examination.
5. The laboratory signs.

1.5.5 Analysis and decision

Finally, we must look very carefully at this report. We must analyse all the information we have found. We must think about all the diseases which could possibly be causing the illness of our patient.

Then we can decide which of the possible diseases is the most probable cause of our patient's illness. This will be our diagnosis.

SUMMARY

Here, then, are the steps we must follow to make the right diagnosis:

1. Taking the history.
2. Doing the physical examination.
3. Doing the necessary laboratory examinations.
4. Writing a report of all the information we have found.
5. Analysing this information.

Then we can make the diagnosis.

Questions for study

1. There are five steps to follow to make the right diagnosis. How does each one of these steps help us to make the right diagnosis?
2. What must you write in the patient's record?

1.6 How can we make the right diagnosis?

1.6.1 Collect good information

To make the right diagnosis, we need much information about the patient's illness. This information must be **correct**. It must be **complete**. How do we get this information?

When we take the history, we try to understand as well as possible how the patient feels. For example, where does he hurt? What does the pain really feel like? This is not always easy to do. But it is very important. We also must try to find out all the symptoms the patient has.

So we ask many questions. We ask many questions about each symptom. We ask many questions about all the symptoms the patient may have.

Chapter 2 will show you how to take a good history of adult patients. Chapter 4 will show you how to take a good history of infants and children. These chapters will show you the questions to ask to find out what the patient feels and what are all the symptoms he has. Study these chapters very carefully.

We must get **correct** and **complete** information from the physical examination. We must know how to look for signs of disease in each part of the patient's body. We must also be able to tell if a sign is really present or not. For example, does a patient have a big spleen or not? Does he have changes in the breath sounds of air coming into the lungs or not?

Chapter 3 will show you how to do a good physical examination on adults. Chapter 4 will show you how to examine infants and children. You must learn how to do each examination well. You must learn how to find all the important physical signs of disease.

This is also true for laboratory signs of disease. If you do the laboratory exams yourself, be sure you know how to do each one. Be sure to do it correctly each time. If the result is wrong, you will make the wrong diagnosis. So be sure your results are correct.

Someone else may do the laboratory exams for you. But be sure he or she knows how to do them well. Be sure he or she can find the correct result.

You will read about this in chapter 5. But you will need another book to find out **how** to do each laboratory exam.

1.6.2 Think about the information

You have now found out much information about your patient's illness. You are sure the information is correct. You have written it in the patient's record.

Now think about it. Analyse this information carefully. What does each piece of information mean? What could be the cause of each symptom or sign? What disease, or diseases, could cause all the symptoms and signs you have found?

We will talk about this in chapter 6. You will see how to analyse this information. You will learn the kinds of questions to ask yourself about this information. This is very important. If you think carefully about all the information you have found, you will most likely make the right diagnosis.

1.6.3 Know the common diseases

One more thing is important. You must have a good knowledge of all the common diseases in your area. You must know the symptoms and signs each one causes. You must know what to do to make the diagnosis of each of these diseases.

For this you will need other books. You will need books on pathology - the study of diseases. These books will help you know the diseases of men and women and of infants and children. Keep these books in your clinic or health center. Read them often. Try to remember the important symptoms and signs of each disease.

SUMMARY

To make the right diagnosis you must:

1. Have a good knowledge of all the important diseases in your area.
2. Be able to take a correct and complete history.
3. Do a careful physical examination.
4. Do laboratory exams correctly.
5. Be able to analyse all this information carefully.

Questions for study

1. Why is correct information necessary to make the right diagnosis?
2. Why is it necessary to get complete information about the patient's illness?
3. What must you do with all this information?
4. Why is it important to study about all the common diseases in your area?
5. What must you know about these diseases?

1.7 Why is it often difficult to make the right diagnosis?

Making a diagnosis appears simple. Perhaps you think it is easy. Sometimes it is. Often, however, it is difficult to make the right diagnosis. There are many reasons for this.

1.7.1 Absent symptoms or signs

Sometimes a patient has a particular disease, but certain symptoms or signs are absent. This is true especially at the beginning of a disease. Some of the symptoms and signs have not come yet.

Hepatitis causes a yellow color to come into the eyes, mucous membranes, and skin. We call this "jaundice." It comes on the 4th or the 5th day of the disease. But if the patient comes to you on the 2nd day, he will not have jaundice. You will not be able to make the diagnosis of hepatitis.

Malaria usually causes a fever, but not always. A patient can have malaria even if his temperature is normal. Malaria often causes a big spleen, but not always. It can cause anemia, but not always. So a patient can have malaria even without a big spleen, anemia, or even a fever.

Tuberculosis frequently causes sputum. But it may not do this in the early stages of the disease. Often it is difficult to find tubercle bacilli in the sputum of a patient with tuberculosis. This is true especially at the beginning of the disease. The patient has tuberculosis, but we cannot find the bacilli in his sputum.

1.7.2 An incomplete history

Sometimes a patient does not give us a good history of his illness.

1. Perhaps he has forgotten some of his symptoms.
2. Perhaps he is ashamed to tell us about certain symptoms.
3. Perhaps he is unable to explain clearly how he feels. This is especially true with young children. It is also true with patients who are very seriously ill and may even be unconscious.

Therefore, the history is incomplete. Important information is missing.

1.7.3 Different diseases causing the same symptom or sign

Different diseases can cause the same symptom or sign. For example:

1. Tuberculosis makes the patient cough, but so do pneumonia, asthma, and heart failure.
2. Malaria causes a high fever, but so do pneumonia, measles, meningitis, and other infections.

Often we have difficulty in deciding which disease is the real cause of a symptom or sign. For this reason we must take a **complete** history and do a **complete** physical examination and laboratory exams. We must look for all the symptoms and signs caused by the disease.

1.7.4 No symptoms

A patient can be ill but have no symptoms. He feels well even though he has a disease. For example:

1. Diabetes can be present and cause no symptoms. We find it only when we examine the urine or the blood of the patient.

2. A patient can have high blood pressure but not feel ill. We find his disease only when we take his blood pressure.

1.7.5 No signs

In other cases, a patient can feel ill and have many symptoms. But we are unable to find any signs of disease. This is especially true with nervous or mental diseases. These diseases are often difficult to diagnose. The patient knows he is ill. But we can find no signs of disease.

1.7.6 A poor history or a poor examination

At other times we fail to take a good history. Or else we do an incomplete physical examination.

1. Perhaps we forgot to ask certain questions.
2. Perhaps we failed to look for certain signs of disease.
3. Perhaps there are many patients to see and we are in a hurry.

So we take a poor history. Or we do not do a careful physical examination. Because of this, certain information is missing. So we cannot make the right diagnosis.

1.7.7 Incorrect laboratory examinations

An incorrect laboratory examination can lead to the wrong diagnosis. For example, the patient has tubercle bacilli in his sputum. But we did not find them. So we do not make the diagnosis of tuberculosis.

1.7.8 No diagnosis possible

Sometimes we cannot make a diagnosis. Perhaps we can find no definite signs of a specific disease. Perhaps we cannot be sure which of two or more diseases the patient really has. Or perhaps the patient needs special exams we cannot do, such as an X-ray, or more complicated blood tests.

What is important in this case is to do the right thing with the patient. If the patient does not seem very ill, we give treatment for his symptoms. But in other cases, the patient may seem quite ill. Then we must send the patient to hospital. We will talk much more about this in chapter 6. We will also talk about how to know which patients must go to hospital.

SUMMARY

Making the right diagnosis can be difficult. Much time and work are necessary.

1. You must spend enough time to take a good history and to do a good physical examination.
2. You must do careful laboratory examinations. Or you must be sure that the person doing the laboratory exams does them well.
3. You must have a good knowledge of all the common diseases you will see.
4. You must know what questions to ask and what signs of disease to look for.
5. You must be willing to work long and hard and to do a good job.

The recovery of your patients depends on all of this.

Questions for study

1. What eight problems can give difficulty in making the right diagnosis?
2. What can you do to avoid each of these eight problems?
3. What must you do if you cannot make a diagnosis?

1.8 How can we tell which patients are seriously ill?

Often we must examine many patients in a day. We will be able to spend only a little time with each patient. This is because there are too many patients. So we must make a decision. We must decide which patients need a lot of our time and which ones need only a little of our time.

A patient who is seriously ill or who has a complicated illness probably needs a lot of our time. There will be many questions to ask in the history. We must do a careful and complete physical examination. Perhaps we must also do some laboratory exams. With this patient we must take the time necessary to obtain all the information we need to make a good diagnosis.

Other patients will have simple illnesses that are not serious, such as a small wound, a cold, a small infection. We take the history quickly. We can see quickly what the signs are. We may need only two or three minutes to examine and treat such patients. Then we will have more time for the patients who are seriously ill. How can we decide which patients have serious illnesses?

1.8.1 Signs of serious illness

Some experience is necessary to decide which patients are seriously ill. Here are certain things which indicate that a patient has a serious illness.

1. He looks very ill.
2. He has one or more severe symptoms, such as severe pain, a bad cough, or frequent diarrhea.
3. He has been ill for a long time.
4. Because of the illness he is unable to work, or to eat, or to sleep.
5. He has one or more signs of serious illness, such as a high fever, convulsions, bleeding, dehydration. or much loss of weight.

1.8.2 Signs of a simple illness

Here are indications that the disease is simple and not serious.

1. The patient does not seem ill. He is relaxed, talks easily, and is calm.
2. The disease is in just one small part of the body - a small wound, a boil, conjunctivitis. A small wound of the eye or the hand, however, can be very serious.
3. The patient has no severe symptoms and no signs of serious disease.
4. The illness does not affect the patient's work, eating, sleeping, or other normal activities.

Always remember that a disease which looks simple may indeed be serious. Remember also that a simple disease can sometimes become serious. So try to take enough time with each patient to make the right diagnosis and to give good treatment. Try also to avoid wasting time on a simple illness. If you take too much time on a simple illness, you will not have enough time for patients who are seriously ill.

Questions for study

1. Why is it important to decide which patients have a serious illness?
2. To decide who has a serious illness and who has only a simple illness, what must you look for?

We have now made the diagnosis. That is fine. But that is only part of our job. The other part is to give good treatment to all of our patients. Giving good treatment often takes much time. It can take more time than making the right diagnosis. So we must use our time wisely.

We must spend enough time to take a good history. We must do a complete physical examination. We need time to write the necessary information on the patient's record. And we will need time to analyse this and to decide on the diagnosis. We must also have enough time to give the necessary treatment and instructions to each patient. You will find the treatment and the instructions for each different disease in Part Three of this book.

REMEMBER:

1. Different diseases cause different symptoms and signs.
2. Each diagnostic step is important. Do it well.
3. Making the right diagnosis may be hard work.
4. Give much time to patients who are seriously ill. Give less time to patients who are not seriously ill.
5. Learn to tell the difference between serious illnesses and simple illnesses.

1.9 How can you learn to make a good diagnosis?

Get a good notebook. As you read this book, make notes of what you learn. Write down the important things in each paragraph and in each section. Think about them carefully. Be sure you understand each important thing. If you do not, ask about it.

Take your notebook and this book to class. Write down notes of what your teacher says. Often he or she will explain ideas which you did not understand before. There may be new ideas which you will need to write down.

There are many questions in this book. Write the answers to each question in your notebook. You will find the answers to some of the questions in what is written in this book. For other questions, the answers are not in this book. To answer them, you must think. Think about the important things you have already learned. These things will help you answer these questions.

Discuss these questions and your answers with your fellow students. There may be some questions that you and they will not be able to understand. Ask your teacher or your doctor about these things. Write in your notebook what he or she tells you.

Put into practice what you learn from this book. The next chapter talks about taking the history. Take good histories from your patients. Remember what questions to ask to find out about their symptoms and their health.

Other chapters talk about examining adults and about examining children. So examine them as you read. Learn how to do everything the book describes.

Practice on your fellow students. One of them can pretend he or she is ill. You can take the history of the "illness." Then you can pretend to be ill. Your fellow student can ask you about your "illness."

Examine each other. As you examine each other, you will learn what is normal. This will help you recognize the signs of disease when you examine your patients.

Write in your notebook what you learn from this practice. You will examine adults with different diseases. You will find important signs of disease in some of your patients. Write these in your notebook.

For example, you examine a patient who has a big liver. Write down the patient's name, age, and sex. Write down his symptoms. Write down all the signs you find when you examine him. How big is his liver? What does it feel like? Does he have other signs of disease, like jaundice, or fluid in the abdomen? All of this will help you remember what liver disease is like. It will also help you learn to examine your patients well.

Questions for study

1. What is all the information you need to make a diagnosis?
2. How can you be sure you have gotten good information?
3. What must you do with this information to make the right diagnosis?
4. How can this book help you learn how to make a good diagnosis?
5. How can a notebook help you? What must you write in it?
6. How can your fellow students help you learn how to make a good diagnosis?
7. How can your work in class help you?
8. How can your work with patients help you?

There is one further point we must consider. Young children and adults are different. Making a diagnosis in a baby is not the same as making a diagnosis in an adult. When we examine a child, we must do some things differently both in taking the history and in doing the physical examination.

Babies and young children are unable to speak. They cannot tell you how they feel. So you will take the history from the mother or father or from another person.

The bodies of babies and adults are different also. Diseases can cause certain changes in babies and other changes in adults. Tuberculosis in babies and children is different from tuberculosis in adults. Malaria, pneumonia, heart disease, and other diseases are different in children from these diseases in adults.

So in this book we have separated the examination of adults from that of children.

Chapter 2
TAKING THE HISTORY

2.1 What is the "history?"

2.2 Why is history-taking important?

2.3 Why must history-taking be complete and in order?

2.4 How do you gain the confidence of the patient?

2.5 What do you look for in the history?

2.6 How can you learn to take a good history?

2.1 What is the "history?"

The history is the story of the patient's illness. It tells you how the illness began and when it began. It is the story of all the symptoms and when each symptom began. It tells you how the illness has developed.

The history tells you how the illness has affected the patient. It also tells you what the patient has done about the illness up to this moment.

The history should tell you also about the health of other members of the patient's family and his close friends. It should likewise tell you about the patient's health before this illness began. Finally, the history should tell you about the living conditions of the patient, where and how he lives.

2.2 Why is history-taking important?

Taking the history is the most important part of the examination of the patient. The physical examination and the laboratory examinations are also important. But taking the history is more important. This is because the history gives you much information about the illness. The other examinations give you less information about the illness.

In many patients, the history alone will give you a good idea of the diagnosis. It will indicate which disease is probably causing the patient's illness.

However, you must always do the physical examination and often do certain laboratory examinations. These examinations will give you information about the signs of the disease. But taking the history gives you the most information about the illness.

2.3 Why must history-taking be complete and in order?

2.3.1 Be complete

To make a good diagnosis, you need to know all you can about the patient's illness. So you must ask the patient about every aspect of the illness. This is especially true if the patient seems to be seriously ill.

If the history is incomplete, important information will be missing. As a result, you will probably be unable to make the right diagnosis. So learn to take a complete history.

2.3.2 Follow the right order

To take a complete history, you must do it in order. Start always at the beginning. Follow each step in order, asking questions about each aspect of the illness.

If you do not follow a good order, you will forget certain things. The history will be incomplete. Important information will be missing. And you will often miss the right diagnosis.

2.3.3 Urgent history

There are times when you must take a history very quickly. The patient is very seriously ill. So you cannot take the time to ask about everything. This is not common, but it does happen. In this case, this is what you must do.

1. Ask the most important questions.
2. Look for the most important signs.
3. Start giving urgent treatment.
4. Then come back later to get the rest of the history.

SUMMARY

Taking a good history is very important.

1. Always take a complete history.
2. Always follow the right order.
3. In urgent cases, get the important history first. Then start treatment. After this, get the rest of the history.

Questions for study

1. What are all the things you can learn from the patient's history?
2. How does the history help you make the right diagnosis?
3. Why must you take a complete history?
4. What can happen if you do not follow the right order in taking the history?
5. In an urgent case, how can you take a complete history?

2.4 How do you gain the confidence of the patient?

Always start by greeting the patient. Unless the condition of the patient is urgent, shake his hand. Find out his name, where he comes from, and something about his family. Make him feel as comfortable as possible. Show him that you are interested in him and that you want to help him.

A smile is a very good way to win the confidence of the patient. The smile costs you nothing. But it is of great value.

Getting the confidence of the patient is essential. Only then will he be able to talk to you without fear. He will be able to tell you all that you need to know about his illness.

2.5 What do you look for in the history?

2.5.1 The patient's story

Start the history by asking the patient what is wrong.

- What is bothering you?
- How do you feel sick?
- Why did you come to the clinic or to the health center?

Let the patient talk. Let him tell you about his illness. Do not interrupt him. Wait until he is finished before starting to ask questions.

Some patients will tell you a lot. Others will talk only briefly. Be patient. Listen carefully to what the patient says. Then begin to ask questions about the different aspects of the illness. Ask questions also about the health of the patient before he became ill. Ask about his family. There are eleven important things to ask about in the history.

2.5.2 The important symptoms

The patient may have only one important symptom, such as pain, or vomiting, or a cough. Or he may have several different symptoms. Ask him what symptom, or symptoms, bothers him the most. Make a note of this symptom, or these symptoms. We call this the presenting symptom (or symptoms). This will help you very much to think about the diagnosis.

Find out all you can about each symptom. Ask the patient to describe it to you carefully. You must understand as clearly as possible just how the patient feels.

This can be difficult, but it is very important. It is difficult because a symptom may feel like one thing to one patient and like something else to another patient. Let us look at some of the important symptoms.

Pain

1. What is the pain like? Ask the patient to describe it to you. It may be:

- Sharp pain, like a knife blade.
- Dull pain, like a headache.
- Throbbing pain, like a toothache. This usually means an infection in the deeper tissues or in a bone.

- Intermittent pain or colic. This pain comes and goes. It is like the pain of giving birth to a baby. This intermittent pain or colic comes in diseases of the intestines, the pelvic organs, or the urinary tract.

2. Where is the pain? Ask the patient to show you exactly where he is hurting. Tell him to point to the place where he feels the pain. Sometimes the pain is in just one place and does not move. Sometimes the pain moves from one place to another. Sometimes the pain is in one place but then reaches out to another part of the body, like the back, a leg, or an arm. We call this kind of pain "radiating pain."

3. When pain is in the abdomen, find out exactly where it is. The organs in the abdomen give pain in certain places:

- The liver: in the right upper region or "quadrant."

- The stomach and spleen: the left upper region or "quadrant."

- The stomach and pancreas: the upper middle region, or "epigastric" region.

- The small intestine: around the navel or umbilicus.

- The kidney: the flank.

- The large intestine, the pelvic organs, and the bladder: the lower abdomen.

Find out if the pain is on the right side, the left side, in the middle, or all over.

4. When does the pain come? The pain may be present all the time and not change. Or the pain may come or change because of certain activities or functions of the body. So ask what helps the pain. Ask what makes the pain worse.

- Pain on breathing deeply or coughing: from the lungs or the pleura.

- Pain in the chest when the patient does work, like walking up a hill: from a disease of the heart, the lungs, or the blood.

- Pain before, during, or after a meal: often from a disease of the stomach, the intestines, or the liver.

- Pain during or after passing a stool: from a disease of the large intestine or the anus.

- Pain before, during, or after urination: from a disease of the bladder, the urethra, or the vagina.

- Pain before, during, or after the menstrual period: from the female genital organs.

- Pain related to certain movements: from a disease of the bones, joints or muscles.

Learn well the kinds of pain that come during different diseases. Find out all you can about the patient's pain. This will give you an idea about which disease the patient may have. For example,

- A patient has chest pain when he coughs or breathes deeply. He may have pneumonia.

- A patient has severe pain in the right lower quadrant for a few hours. He may have appendicitis.

- A patient has pain that comes and goes all across the abdomen. He may have an obstruction of the intestines.

Now ask questions about other symptoms that can come with these diseases. Look for signs of these diseases in the physical exam.

REMEMBER:

Different diseases cause different kinds of pain.

Fever

Fever is really a sign of disease. But usually some symptoms go with it. So the patient often knows he has a fever.

1. A high fever that goes up quickly causes chills with shaking.
2. A low fever makes the patient feel cold, but it does not cause chills.
3. Later on the patient will feel hot and then have much sweating, especially at night.

So ask the patient about chills, feeling cold, feeling hot, and sweating. Find out when these symptoms of fever come.

- In the morning.
- During the afternoon.
- At night.
- Every day.
- Every other day.
- Only on some days.

Some infections, like typhoid fever or meningitis, cause a continuous fever that stays high for days. One kind of malaria causes a fever every other day. Another kind of malaria causes a fever that goes up and down every day. Others infections, such as a deep abscess or a kidney infection, cause an intermittent fever that goes up and down. Learn the kind of fever that goes with each different infection.

REMEMBER:

Different diseases cause different kinds of fever.

Cough

1. When does the patient cough?
   - All the time?
   - Only at night?
   - Only after smoking?
2. Is there pain with the cough? This can mean an infection in the lungs or pleura, or a fracture of a rib. In these cases there will often be pain when the patient breathes deeply.
3. Does the patient cough up sputum? If so, what is it like?
   - Clear, like saliva.
   - Thick and white, or yellow, or green. This can come with pneumonia or with tuberculosis.
   - With blood. See the strategy on page 277.
   - With a bad odor. This is a sign of a lung abscess.

If possible, look at the patient's sputum yourself. See the strategy for cough on page 260.

Vomiting

1. When does the patient vomit?
   - All the time?
   - Only in the morning?
   - Only after eating?
2. Ask what the patient vomits. If possible, see what he vomits:
   - Clear fluid
   - Food. If he often vomits his food, he may have a blockage or obstruction in his stomach. Certain foods or medicines also may cause vomiting.
   - Blood. This is a sign of a very serious disease, usually of the stomach or liver.
   - Green or brown fluid. He may have an obstruction of the intestine.
   - Brown fluid that smells like fecal matter. The patient most certainly has an obstruction of the intestine.

See the strategies for vomiting on pages 306 and 314.

Diarrhea

1. Find out how often the patient has a stool:
   - Once a day.
   - Many times a day. How many?
2. Ask how much stool comes out each time : a lot? or only a little?
3. Ask if there is pain with each movement.
4. Find out what the stools are like. If possible, look at the stools yourself.
   - Liquid fecal matter: comes in many infections with fever.
   - Much water with little or no fecal matter: severe dysentery or malnutrition.
   - Stools with blood or pus: one of the dysenteries.
   - Pure blood: an intestinal hemorrhage.

See the strategies for diarrhea on pages 326 and 330.

Convulsions

1. Find out what the convulsions are like.
   - Do they affect the whole body?
   - Do they affect only one part of the body? What part?
   - Does the patient lose consciousness?
   - Does the patient pass urine or stool during the convulsion?
2. Find out when the convulsions come, and how often.
3. Ask if they come only when there is a fever.
4. Has there been an accident, or a blow to the head?

See the strategies on convulsions on pages 422 and 428.

SUMMARY

You must learn as much as you can about these important symptoms. Ask the patient to describe them to you as clearly as possible. Often a good description of these symptoms will give you a very good idea of the diagnosis.

Questions for study

1. In a patient who has pain, what are all of the things you must find out about his pain?
2. You yourself have certainly had pain at some time. Try to remember what each episode of pain was like. Write a description of each episode of pain.
3. Think of several diseases that cause fever. What is the fever like in each of these diseases?
4. You yourself have certainly had fever. How did the fever make you feel?
5. Diarrhea is different in different diseases. Why is this so? What must you find out about the patient's stools?
6. Sputum is different in different diseases. Why is this so?
7. Persons who are ill often vomit. What are some of the reasons that they vomit? What must you find out about what they vomit? Why?
8. What do you need to know about a patient's convulsions?

2.5.3 The start of the illness

When did the illness start?

This is an important question. Find out how many hours, days, weeks, months or years ago the illness started. The patient may be unable to tell you exactly. But try to find out if it is a matter of months, or only of a few days.

An acute illness is an illness that lasts only from a few hours up to a month. A chronic illness lasts more than a month. Finding out how long the patient has been ill can help you make the diagnosis. Look at these examples.

1. A patient who has a cough for just 3 days does not have tuberculosis. Tuberculosis is a chronic disease, and the cough lasts for weeks or months.

2. A patient with severe pain in the neck for one day may have meningitis. If the pain has been present for weeks or months, it comes probably from a disease of the muscles or the bones.

REMEMBER:

Acute means short. Chronic means long.

How did the illness start?

1. Did it start slowly? This is a sign of a chronic disease.
2. Did it start quickly? This is a sign of an acute disease.

It is important to know how the illness started. For example, a patient has pain in the lower right region of the abdomen. This could be appendicitis, or it could simply be intestinal worms.

- Appendicitis: starts very quickly and becomes very serious in a few hours.
- Intestinal worms: the pain starts slowly and may stay for several months.

2.5.4 The development of the illness

As a disease develops, the symptoms and signs change. New symptoms come. Perhaps other symptoms go away. Find out, therefore, the order in which the symptoms came.

1. Which one, or ones, came first?
2. Which ones came next?
3. How soon afterwards did they come?
4. Have some symptoms already gone away?

Ask the patient to think carefully about this. Ask him to try to remember the order in which the symptoms came. This is important. This will often make clear what disease is causing the patient's illness. So take time to find out the development of the disease from the beginning to the end.

2.5.5 Possible causes of the illness

Did anything happen to cause the illness? This is an important question. Sometimes the answer to this question will give you the diagnosis of the disease. For example:

1. A man has a feeling of burning in the epigastric region for three days. The burning started right after he drank much wine. So he may have gastritis caused by an excess of wine.
2. A woman has had pain in the abdomen for a day or for a few days. Ask her what she ate or what she drank before the pain started. Perhaps the pain came because of something she ate or drank.
3. A man has had pain in the back for one month. The pain began when he lifted a heavy load. So he probably has an injury of the bones or muscles in the back.

4. A woman has pain in the left leg. The pain began just after she fell down. She probably has an injury to the muscles or bones of the leg.

5. A man has a severe headache for the last three months. It began after a long difficult discussion about a serious family problem. The headache probably comes from the anger or fear caused by this family problem.

6. When a patient has pain in the abdomen, ask about what he ate or drank at the beginning of the illness.

7. When a patient has pain in the back or in the extremities, always ask if he fell, had an injury, or did some unusual activity.

8. In patients with headaches or other nervous symptoms, ask about problems at home, in the family, or at work.

Questions about events of this kind can help you very much. Often the patient has forgotten the event. Or he does not think that the event is important in his illness. Therefore, he does not tell you about it.

So you must ask specific questions about these things. Soon you will have more experience about this. You will know what sort of events or circumstances to ask about.

2.5.6 Is the illness serious?

Many patients think they are very ill. Often, however, the illness is not serious. Ask the patient how his illness has affected his life.

1. Is he able to work normally?

2. Does he eat well?

3. Does he sleep well?

If the patient continues to work, to eat, to sleep well, and to do his other activities normally, probably the illness is not serious. But if the illness keeps him from doing these things, the illness may be serious.

2.5.7 Treatment already received for this illness

Often the patient has already received treatment for this illness from another clinic, hospital, or health center. Always ask about this. If he has already received treatment, find out what treatment he has received. This may help you in making the diagnosis.

1. A patient tells you that he receives insulin regularly. So he probably has diabetes.

2. Another patient has received treatment for tuberculosis. So look carefully for signs of tuberculosis.

Sometimes previous treatment can change the signs and symptoms of a disease. For example, a father and mother bring you their baby who has signs of meningitis. The baby has no fever when he arrives, but meningitis almost always gives a fever. Ask the parents if the baby has received treatment somewhere else. Perhaps a health worker in another health center has just given the baby penicillin and aspirin. So that is why the baby has no fever at the moment. But if the baby does indeed have meningitis, the fever will soon come back. This is because the baby has not received sufficient treatment.

The answer to this question about previous treatment may also help you in prescribing your treatment. If a patient has received treatment previously, ask him if it helped him or not.

Perhaps the treatment helped him, but he still has the illness. In this case, he will need more of the same treatment. Perhaps the treatment did not help him. Then he will need a different treatment.

This is important especially for infections like sexually transmitted diseases, tuberculosis, and other chronic infections. A patient may have received an antibiotic which did not help him. Do not give him this same antibiotic again. Give him a different one.

Ask the patient if he has received treatment from a traditional healer. If so, find out what treatment he received. Ask if the treatment made his illness better. Try to find out what cause or causes the traditional healer found for this illness.

A long treatment by a traditional healer indicates that the illness has been present for a long time. It also indicates that the illness may be serious. It may indicate that there are important social and emotional elements in the illness. So ask carefully about this.

Certain medicines can be dangerous. They can cause problems like an intoxication which will need treatment. Ask the patient about all of the medicines that he has received. Ask about herbs or any other medicines he has received from a traditional healer. Ask about medicines or treatments that he has given to himself.

2.5.8 Attacks of this same illness in the past

Certain diseases can come back many times. Asthma, gastritis, diseases of the liver, the heart, and other organs can come again and again. Perhaps the patient has already had an illness like this one in the past months or years. Ask about it. Find out, if possible, what the diagnosis was, what treatment the patient received, and if the treatment helped him.

Sometimes the patient already knows what disease he has. Perhaps he knows he has asthma, or diabetes, or gastritis. But be careful. Sometimes the previous diagnosis is not correct. Or perhaps the patient is not telling you the truth. Therefore, find out as much as you can about the previous illness. Then compare it with the present illness.

Knowing about previous illnesses can help you make the right diagnosis. For example, a woman comes to the clinic with severe pain in the right lower region of the abdomen. The pain started yesterday. You think that she may have appendicitis.

But ask her if she has had this same pain before. Perhaps she has had pain like this during the past months at the time of her monthly menstrual periods.

Compare her present pain with the pain of the previous months. If this pain is like the pain of the previous months, she probably has dysmenorrhea, or a disease in her pelvic organs. She probably does not have appendicitis.

2.5.9 The symptom review by systems

Each organ, when it is ill, causes certain definite symptoms. Cough, for example, comes usually from a disease of the heart or of the lungs. Vomiting comes usually from a disease of the stomach, the liver, or the intestines. Diarrhea is frequently a symptom of an intestinal disease.

In your efforts to make a diagnosis, try to determine which organ, or which system of organs, is affected by the disease. The symptoms of the patient usually indicate which organ or system is ill. If the disease affects the lungs, like pneumonia or asthma, the patient will have symptoms of lung disease. If the stomach is ill, the patient will have stomach symptoms.

Therefore, you must find out from your patient which symptoms are present. Find out which symptoms are absent. This will indicate to you which organ or system is ill. It will also give you a good idea as to which disease is making the patient ill.

To do this well, you must know the symptoms which come from each organ or from each system of organs. Learn these symptoms by heart.

For example, if the patient has a cough, think about the heart and the lungs. Then ask the patient about other symptoms of the heart and the lungs. See if the patient has any of these other symptoms.

We call this the symptom review by systems. It is a list of all the symptoms that come from each organ and system. Learn this list well. Then you will be able to ask quickly about all of these symptoms. You will not forget any of them.

General symptoms

1. Weakness.
2. Loss of weight.
3. Fever, which may give chills, feelings of being cold or hot, and sweating.
4. Pain, or "aching," in many parts of the body.

Symptoms of the heart - cardiac symptoms

1. Cough. A cough without sputum is a dry cough. A cough with sputum is a productive cough.
2. Sputum. The sputum from heart disease is often clear, like saliva. It may have a lot of foam in it. Sometimes there is blood in the sputum. This makes the sputum red-brown, like water with rust in it.
3. Trouble breathing. We call this dyspnea. In diseases of the heart, there are three kinds of dyspnea.
   - Dyspnea of effort: trouble breathing which comes when the patient does some physical activity, like walking up a hill.
   - Dyspnea at rest: trouble breathing even when the patient is sitting or lying down and resting.
   - Orthopnea: trouble breathing when the patient lies down flat. He must then sit up or stand up in order to breathe.
4. Pain in the chest, often in the middle, sometimes all around the chest. This pain usually comes when the patient does some work or other physical activity.
5. Pain or heaviness in the upper right region of the abdomen. This pain comes from the liver. In diseases of the heart, blood fills the liver very full. This causes pain.
6. Swelling of the feet, legs, and sometimes of the lower abdomen. We call this edema.
7. Frequent urination during the night. We call this nocturia. The patient must urinate two, three, or sometimes more times during the night.

Symptoms of the lungs - pulmonary symptoms

1. Cough, sometimes dry, sometimes productive of sputum.

2. Sputum. Find out what the sputum is like:
   - Clear.
   - With white, yellow, or green pus.
   - With blood.
   - With a bad odor.

3. Pain in the chest. Often this pain comes with coughing or with breathing deeply.

4. Trouble breathing, or dyspnea. This is usually dyspnea of effort. But it may be dyspnea at rest. Some diseases of the lungs can even cause orthopnea, such as asthma or severe pneumonia.

5. Wheezing. This is noisy breathing which comes because the patient has difficulty pushing air out of the lungs. We call it dyspnea of expiration. It comes in asthma, and sometimes with heart disease.

You will notice that cough, sputum, pain in the chest, dyspnea of effort, and sometimes dyspnea of expiration can come both from diseases of the heart and from diseases of the lungs. When a patient has one or more of these symptoms, you must examine him carefully to find out which organ is ill.

REMEMBER:

Diseases of the heart and of the lungs can cause similar symptoms.

Symptoms of the stomach and intestines - digestive symptoms

1. Pain in the abdomen. Often this pain in associated with eating. It comes before, during, or after each meal.

2. A feeling of burning in the upper abdomen. Patients often call this heart burn. It may come before eating, during the meal, or soon after eating. Certain foods may make this burning worse, like hot spices, alcoholic drinks, some fruits. This burning often comes from gastritis, or from an ulcer in the stomach or the upper intestine.

3. Intermittent pain in the abdomen, or colic. This comes often in diseases of the intestines.

4. Diarrhea. Ask the patient what his stools look like, how often they come, and if he has pain when passing his stools.

5. Constipation. This means stools that are hard. They come out infrequently and with difficulty. Constipation can come from a disease of the intestines or the rectum. It also comes in many other diseases that affect how the patient eats.

6. Blood in the stools. This usually comes from a disease of the stomach, the liver, the intestines, the rectum, or the anus. Ask the patient what is the color of the stools.

   - Bright red blood comes from the anus or rectum.

   - Dark blood comes from the large intestine.

   - Black stools, like tar, come from much bleeding in the stomach or the small intestine. Bleeding in liver disease also may give black stools.

Symptoms of the liver and the gall bladder

1. Pain in the upper right quadrant of the abdomen. The pain is usually continuous and heavy. But it may be sharp like a knife. Sometimes the pain is worse during or after eating, especially if there is much fat in the food.

2. A yellow coloring of the skin, the white part of the eyes, and the mucus membranes. We call this jaundice. It is a sign of disease, but often the patient knows it is there and tells us about it. It comes from having too much bile in the circulation. It can come in diseases of the liver or of the gall bladder. It can also come in severe anemia.

3. A deep brown color of the urine. This comes with the jaundice. But the urine also becomes dark when a person is dehydrated. This is when a person has lost much liquid, or does not drink enough liquids. So learn to tell the difference between the brown urine of jaundice and the dark urine of dehydration.

4. Intermittent severe pain, or colic, in the right upper region of the abdomen. This is a symptom of gall bladder disease. Often there is vomiting with it.

5. Nausea, the desire to vomit.

6. Vomiting.

7. Loss of appetite which we call anorexia. The patient has no desire to eat.

REMEMBER:

Diseases of the stomach and diseases of the liver can cause the same symptoms.

Symptoms of the urinary system - urinary symptoms

1. Frequent urination, or frequency. The patient must urinate quickly and often.

2. An increase in the quantity of urine. We call this polyuria. This is different from frequency. In frequency, the patient must urinate often, but the quantity of urine each time is small. In polyuria, the patient urinates often and there is much urine each time. Polyuria comes in certain diseases of the kidney, in heart failure, and also in diabetes.

3. Pain on urination. We call this dysuria. This comes from a disease of the bladder, of the urethra, and sometimes of the uterus or the vagina.

4. Difficulty in passing urine. The patient must push hard in order to pass the urine. The urine comes out slowly, and the stream of urine is very small. This comes from an obstruction in the bladder or in the urethra. If the obstruction becomes complete, the patient will be unable to urinate at all. We call this urinary retention.

5. Pus in the urine. We call this pyuria. This comes from an infection in the bladder.

6. Pus coming from the opening of the urethra, or meatus. This comes from an infection of the urethra.

7. Blood in the urine, or hematuria. This is an indication of a very serious disease.

Symptoms of the female genital organs - gynecological symptoms

1. Liquid, usually thick, coming from the vagina. We call this leucorrhea.

2. Itching around the vagina. This can come from a fungus infection, from a parasite called trichomonas, or from lice.

3. Pain associated with the menstrual cycle. It may come before, during, or after the menstrual period. We call it dysmenorrhea.

4. An increase of bleeding during the menstrual period. We call this menorrhagia.

5. An absence of periods, or amenorrhea. This is normal during pregnancy and in older women after the menopause. But it can also come in younger women who have a serious general disease, like diabetes, malnutrition, tuberculosis, heart disease, liver disease, or others.

6. Bleeding from the vagina not coming with the menstrual periods. It can come between the periods, or in older women after the menopause. We call it metrorrhagia. It is a sign of serious disease in the genital organs.

7. Pain during sexual relations, or dyspareunia.

Symptoms of the male genital organs

1. Pain in the penis or in one or both testicles or spermatic cords.

2. Pain in the lower abdomen, the lower back, or around the anus. This can come from an infection of the prostate.

3. Swelling in the scrotum on one or both sides. This can come from a local disease, like a hydrocele, filariasis, or an infection. Or it can come from a disease that causes swelling elsewhere, like a disease of the heart, the liver, the kidneys, a severe anemia, or malnutrition.

4. Itching: from a fungus infection of the skin, or from parasites like scabies or lice.

Symptoms of the bones and joints - skeletal symptoms

1. Pain in a joint. Often movement makes the pain worse. It comes from an inflammation in the joint.

2. Swelling in a joint. This means there is liquid inside the joint. It comes from a disease of the joint. This is sometimes an infection in the joint.

3. Pain in one or several bones. This can come from an injury, an infection, a tumor, or in sickle cell anemia.

Symptoms of the muscles

1. Pain in the muscles.

2. Pain during movement of the muscles. This comes from an injury, or from an infection in the muscles.

3. Swelling in the muscles. This can come from an injury, or from an infection of the muscles which we call pyomyositis.

Symptoms of the nervous system - neurological symptoms

1. Headache.

2. Dizziness. Things look cloudy, or unsteady.

3. Vertigo. The patient thinks everything is turning around. He may have difficulty in standing up.

4. Convulsions. Find out what they are like, how often they come, and how long they last. See page 31.

5. Loss of consciousness, or coma.

6. Difficulty in talking.

7. Loss of feeling in a part of the body. We call this anesthesia.

8. Paralysis. The patient cannot move a part of his body, usually an arm or a leg, or one side of the face, or an eye.

9. Nervousness. The patient is worried and agitated. He may have bad dreams.

10. Insomnia. He cannot sleep well at night.

Symptoms of the eyes - ocular symptoms

1. Blurring or loss of vision. The patient cannot see clearly. Or he cannot see at all. This is a symptom of serious disease.

2. Pain in one or both eyes. Often bright light makes the pain worse. We call this photophobia, which means fear of light. This can come from an infection, or from a disease inside the eye. It can be serious.

3. Tears coming from the eyes. Tearing comes when the eyes are irritated.

4. Itching around the eye.

Table 2 - Symptom review by systems			
Organs	**Symptoms**	**Organs**	**Symptoms**
General	weakness weight loss fever aching all over		
Heart	cough sputum chest pain dyspnea orthopnea liver pain edema nocturia	**Lungs**	cough sputum chest pain dyspnea orthopnea wheezing
Stomach and Intestines	abdominal pain heart burn nausea vomiting colicky pain diarrhea blood in stools constipation	**Liver and Gall bladder**	pain in right upper quadrant loss of appetite nausea vomiting colicky pain jaundice dark urine black stools
Urinary system	frequency polyuria pain on urination dysuria pus in urine or from urethra hematuria	**Female Genital Organs**	leucorrhea vaginal itching dysmenorrhea menorrhagia amenorrhea metrorrhagia dyspareunia

Male	pain in genital
	  organs, in lower
	  abdomen, back or
	  around anus
	swelling in scrotum
	itching		

Organs	Symptoms	Organs	Symptoms
Bones and Joints	bone pain joint pain joint swelling	Muscles	muscle pain muscle swelling
Nervous system	headache dizziness vertigo convulsions confusion coma speech difficulty anesthesia paralysis nervousness	Eyes	blurred vision loss of vision pain in eye or eyes many tears itching around eyes

This list seems long. There are many questions to ask. But the symptom review by systems is not difficult. It usually takes only a little time. You can often go through the review quickly. Do it like this.

1. Ask the patient if he coughs, has trouble breathing, or has pain in his chest. If his answer is "no" to these questions, probably his heart and lungs are normal. On the other hand, perhaps he has one or more of these symptoms. If so, ask carefully about all of the others.

2. Ask the patient if he has a good appetite and if he eats well. Does he have nausea, or vomiting, or diarrhea? If he eats well, and has no digestive symptoms, his stomach, intestines, liver, and gall bladder are probably in good order.

3. Ask the patient if he has trouble urinating, or has blood or pus in the urine. If the answer is negative, the urinary system is probably normal.

4. If the patient is a woman, ask her if her periods are normal. If they are, she probably has no disease of her genital organs.

5. Ask the patient if he has pain in his back, neck, arms, or legs. If not, his bones, joints, and muscles are probably in good order.

6. Ask if there are headaches, dizziness, or any difficulty talking or walking. If not, the nervous system is probably normal.

7. Does the patient see well? Does he have pain in the eyes? If he sees well and there is no pain in the eyes, then his eyes are probably normal.

In this way, you can go through the symptom review by systems quickly with many patients. You can finish it in one or two minutes. Do it in order. This will help you to avoid forgetting the symptoms of any organ or system.

But a patient may have a serious or a complicated disease. He may have one or more symptoms of one or several organs. In this case, the symptom review will take more time. Go through each system carefully. Ask about every symptom.

This is why it is important for you to learn these symptoms well. You must be able to remember automatically the symptoms of each organ and system. Then the symptom review by systems will be easy. You will be able to do it carefully, and you will forget nothing.

It is important to know all the symptoms which the patient has had during his illness. In some cases, it is also important to know which symptoms are absent.

For example, a patient may have pain in the abdomen but no urinary symptoms. The disease giving the pain is therefore probably not in the urinary system.

Another patient may have swelling of the scrotum but no pain. Therefore he probably does not have an infection in the scrotum.

So pay attention to all the symptoms which the patient has had. Write them down. Pay attention also to the symptoms which are absent. Write down the important symptoms which are absent. This will help you make the right diagnosis.

REMEMBER:

The symptom review by systems is a very important part of taking the history.

Questions for study

1. Look at the list of symptoms of each organ or system of organs. How can you learn each list well? Can you make up a song, or write a poem, about each list that will help you learn it well?
2. In what kind of diseases can you do the symptom review quickly?
3. In what kind of diseases must you do the symptom review more slowly and carefully?
4. Why must you know if certain symptoms are absent?
5. Why is it important to write down all the symptoms that are present and certain important ones that are absent?

2.5.10 The family history

Contagious diseases

Certain diseases are contagious. They go from one person to another.
Hepatitis, tuberculosis, amebiasis and many other infections are examples
of this.

Ask the patient if anyone in his family or among his close friends has an
illness like his illness. Ask him if anyone has a contagious illness. Perhaps
the patient got his illness from someone else in the family.

It is also possible that the patient has given his illness to someone else
in his family or among his friends. If someone else in his family or among
his friends is ill, tell the patient to have this person come to the clinic. You
must examine this person also. He may need treatment.

Hereditary diseases

Some diseases exist in certain families and not in other families. They
are not contagious diseases. But they are frequent in members of the same
family. Some of these diseases go directly from the parents to the children.
They are hereditary diseases, like sickle cell anemia.

Familial diseases

Other diseases are not hereditary, but are more frequent in some families. We call them familial diseases. Epilepsy, diabetes, asthma, high blood
pressure are examples of familial diseases.

So find out about the health of all the other members of the patient's
family. If possible, find out the cause of death of the family members who
have died.

Questions for study

1. Why is it important to know about the health of the members of the patient's
    family?
2. What diseases can exist in several members of a patient's family? What
    are the reasons why this can happen?
3. What is the difference between a contagious disease and a familial
    disease?

2.5.11 The Past History

Find out about the patient's health during the past years, before this present illness. This is very important. Perhaps the patient has always been in good health. This means that the patient is a strong person. He has much resistance to disease.

Another patient may have had many illnesses. Then he has less resistance to disease. Perhaps this present illness has come from a disease that the patient had in the past years.

So ask each patient about his previous health. Ask about any illnesses in the past.

1. Have you had a serious illness in the past, such as tuberculosis, diabetes, jaundice, malnutrition, or a disease of the heart, the liver, the stomach, or another serious disease?

2. Have you ever been a patient in hospital before? If so, for what reason?

3. Have you ever had a surgical operation?

4. Have you ever had a serious accident, or an injury?

5. Have you ever had a reaction to any medicine you have taken? If a patient has had a reaction to a medicine, such as penicillin, we say that he is allergic to that medicine. He must never take that medicine again. Write this at the top of the patient's record: ALLERGIC TO _____!

The response to these questions will help you care for your patient. A patient with good health in the past will probably get well quickly. On the other hand, a patient who has had many illnesses will have more difficulty in getting well. This patient will need more care from you.

2.5.12 The living conditions of the patient

Living conditions affect health

Certain diseases come because of the way we live. Others come because of the conditions in which we live. Some diseases come because the patient does not follow good rules of hygiene. For example, malnutrition can come for many reasons: being poor, having too many children in the family, having little knowledge about food, and many other reasons.

1. Ask questions about the conditions of the patient's home.

   ● Where do you live? In a city? In a village? On a farm?

   ● What is your house like?

   ● How big is it?

- How many rooms does it have?
- How many persons live in it with you?

2. Ask about the patient's family.
   - Are you married?
   - How many children do you have?
   - Have some of your children died? If so, why did they die?
   - Does your family all live together? Or do some of your family live somewhere else?

3. If the patient has been married but is not married now, ask about this.
   - Has your wife, or husband, died? If so, when, and why?
   - Are you separated, or divorced?
   - Who helps you at home?

4. Ask the patient about his or her job.
   - Do you have a job?
   - What is your job?
   - How much money do you get in a month?

5. Ask the patient about his or her food.
   - What did you eat today? - What did you eat yesterday?
   - How many times a week do you eat meat, fish, or eggs?
   - How many times a week do you eat maize, rice, groundnuts, beans, soya, other cereals?
   - Do you raise animals or chickens?
   - Where do you keep these animals? In the house? In the kitchen? In another special place?
   - How often do you eat any of these animals or chickens?

6. Ask about the sanitary conditions.
   - Do you have a privy? If so, what is it like? If not, why do you not have one?
   - Do the other houses near you all have privies?
   - Where do you get your water for drinking?
   - Do you do anything to the water to make it safe to drink?

Beliefs affect health

Many people believe that diseases come from their enemies, or from the spirits of persons who have died. These beliefs can cause feelings such as fear, anger, hatred, and jealousy.

These feelings can make many physical symptoms. They can also diminish the resistance of the patient to diseases. They can diminish the ability of the patient to get well. Therefore, you need to know how the patient feels about his disease. Ask the patient these questions.

1. Where do you think your illness has come from?
2. What do your parents, your uncles, your grandparents, think about this illness?
3. Is there someone in the family who tried to make you ill?
4. Has someone put a curse on you? If so, why?
5. How do you feel about this?

REMEMBER:

A patient's beliefs and emotions can affect his health.

These questions are personal questions. They can make the patient feel uncomfortable. Perhaps he will not want to answer them. But they are important questions. They are about things that affect his health.

So ask these questions carefully and politely. Explain to the patient that these questions are about matters that affect his health. You must know about these matters to find out what his disease is and to help him get well.

The response to these questions will also help you to treat your patient. A very important part of the treatment is the instructions you give to the patient. To give good instructions, you need to know how the patient lives and how he feels. For example:

- To give him instructions about his food, you must know what he eats and what foods he will be able to get.
- To give him instructions about his family, you will need to know about his family.
- To give him instructions about hygiene, you must know about what his living conditions are like. You must know what he will be able to do about them.
- To help him with problems about his beliefs and feelings, you must find out about them first.

SUMMARY

There are eleven important things you must find out about the patient and his illness.

1. What are the important symptoms? What is each one like?
2. When and how did the illness start?
3. How has the illness developed?
4. Is there a possible cause for the illness?
5. How serious is the illness?
6. What treatment has the patient already had for this illness?
7. Has the patient had attacks of this illness in the past?
8. What are all of the other symptoms the patient has had?
9. What is the health of the other members of the family?
10. What was the patient's health in the past? What serious illnesses, operations, or accidents has he had?
11. What are the living conditions of the patient and his beliefs about this illness?

2.6 How can you learn to take a good history?

2.6.1 Learn good habits of history-taking

To do a job well, you must learn how to do it. You must know all you have to do in order to do the job well. It is good to understand why each thing has to be done. You must understand why it is important to do it well. Then practice each part of the job. Do it over and over again until it becomes easy.

When you practice doing the job, and doing each part of the job, it is important to develop good habits. These are the good habits you must learn.

1. Do each part of the job completely. Finish it before going to another part of the job. For example, finish taking the history of the present illness before taking the past history.
2. Do each part of the job in the right order.
3. Think carefully about what you are doing and why you are doing it. After doing the job, ask yourself if you have:
   - Done it carefully.
   - Done it in order.
   - Done it well.

If you have not done it well, do it over again.

2.6.2 Practice taking histories

Practice taking histories with your fellow students. You can pretend to have an illness. One of your fellow students can take the history. See if he can take a complete history. See if he can get a good idea of the disease you are pretending to have. But be careful to give the right symptoms for that disease.

Then your fellow student can pretend to be ill. You take the history from him. See if you can make the right diagnosis. Do this many times together.

When you take a history from a patient, do it carefully and slowly. Do not be in a hurry. Write down the information as you receive it. Think carefully about each part of the history. Finish it before going on to the next part.

At first this will be slow. It will take time. But continue practicing with your fellow students and with your patients. Soon you will be able to go faster. You will remember the right order and be able to follow it. You will be able to remember more information. You will write it down correctly.

Remember, however, that taking the history is only one part of your job. Making the diagnosis is also only one part of your job. Your real job is to help the patient get well. Therefore, you take a good history in order to make a good diagnosis. You make a good diagnosis in order to give good treatment. You give good treatment in order to help your patient get well.

SUMMARY

1. A good history helps to make a good diagnosis.
2. A good diagnosis shows you what treatment to give.
3. Good treatment will help your patient get well.

Questions for study

1. What do you need to know about the health of the patient in the past years?
2. What do you need to know about the living conditions of the patient? Why is this important?
3. Why is it important to know how the patient feels about his illness?
4. Why is history-taking the most important part of the examination of the patient?
5. What are the rules to follow to take a good history?

The history gives you much information about the illness of the patient. The history gives you the symptoms of the disease. It shows you how they began, how they developed, and what the patient has done about them.

Now you must find the signs of disease in your patient. You must examine the patient carefully. You must look for the changes which the disease has made in his body.

We said at the beginning of this chapter that a good history can often lead you to the right diagnosis. In this case, is it necessary to do a physical examination? If you already know the diagnosis, is there any need to examine the patient? Yes there is, for these important reasons.

1. Your diagnosis may not be right. The physical examination will show you signs leading to the right diagnosis.

2. You may find signs that indicate how serious the disease is.

3. You may find signs of another disease, a second disease.

4. The patient wants you to examine him.

In a real sense, taking the history and doing the physical examination are part of the treatment of the patient. They help gain the confidence of the patient. The patient will know that you have done a good job. He will feel that you have done all you can to help him. He will then be more willing to follow your instructions.

So always do a physical examination. It will help you do a complete job. It will help you make the right diagnosis and give good treatment.

Chapter 3
THE PHYSICAL EXAMINATION

3.1 The plan of the examination

3.2 The principles to follow to do a good physical examination

3.3 The physical signs to look for

3.1 The plan of the examination

Most diseases make changes in the body of the patient. You can find many of these changes, or signs, by doing a careful examination of the body. These signs will give you more information about the disease of the patient. So look for them carefully. We call the examination of the body the **physical examination** (PE). There are four main techniques to use in doing a complete physical examination.

3.1.1 Observe

Look at the patient carefully. We call this **observation**. See what signs you can find simply by looking at the patient. Often you can find important signs of disease just by looking at, or **observing**, the patient. ALWAYS observe each part of the body of the patient before feeling the patient with your hands.

3.1.2 Palpate

Examine the patient with your hands. With your hands feel carefully each part of the body. We call this **palpation**. Palpation will help you find signs of disease in the deeper tissues and in the internal organs. It will also show you where the patient is tender. **Tenderness** is where the patient has pain when you feel or touch with your hands.

3.1.3 Percuss

Tap gently on the patient with your fingers. This is **percussion**. Listen to the sound you make by percussion. Percussion can help you find signs of disease in the chest and in the abdomen.

3.1.4 Auscultate

Listen to the patient through the stethoscope. We call this **auscultation.** This will help you find other signs of disease in the chest and abdomen.

Learn how to use each of these four techniques well. Practice each one carefully. Observe others using these techniques and learn from them.

SUMMARY

1. **Observation**: Look carefully at the patient.
2. **Palpation**: Feel the body of the patient carefully with your hands and fingers.
3. **Percussion**: Tap gently on the chest and abdomen with your fingers.
4. **Auscultation**: Listen to the chest and abdomen through your stethoscope.

3.2 The principles to follow to do a good physical examination

In order to do a good physical examination, there are certain rules to follow.

3.2.1 Follow the same order

Do the physical examination in a planned order. Use the four techniques in order. Look first. Then palpate. Then percuss, and finally use your stethoscope.

Always start at the same place. The best place to start is to observe the overall condition of the patient. Then take the vital signs. These are very important and you must never forget to take them. Then examine the head and neck. Continue on down the rest of the body of the patient.

Follow this same order with each patient. Then you will not leave out anything important.

3.2.2 Be complete

Do a complete physical examination. If you do not examine a certain part of the body, you may miss an important sign of disease. For example, a patient has had diarrhea for some weeks. In such a case, always to a rectal exam. The patient may have a tumor in the rectum. If you do not do a rectal exam, you will not find the tumor.

3.2.3 Be gentle

Be gentle, especially with palpation. This will gain the confidence of the patient. It will help the patient relax. You will then be able to find more signs of disease.

3.2.4 Compare both sides of the body

Compare the two sides of the body, one side with the other. Normally the two sides of the body look alike. We say they are "symmetrical."

If you find something on one side which is absent on the other side, this may be an important sign of disease. For example, a swelling on one side of the chest but not on the other may indicate a tumor or an infection.

See if one side of the body is different from the other side. For example, the knee reflex on the right knee may be strong, but the reflex of the left knee may be weak or absent. This is not normal. This difference is a sign of a disease somewhere in the nervous system.

3.2.5 Observe carefully

Make careful observations. If you find an abnormal mass, or an organ that is too big, describe it. Make a careful note on the patient's record. Describe it exactly as you find it. Note how big it is, if it is smooth or irregular, if it is hard or soft, if it is tender (painful) or not, and if you can move it or not.

By following these rules, your examination will be complete and precise. You will get much information from it about the patient and about the disease. This will help you make the correct diagnosis.

SUMMARY

1. Follow the same order.
2. Be complete.
3. Be gentle.
4. Compare both sides of the body one with the other.
5. Observe carefully and write down carefully what you find.

Questions for study

1. What are some signs of diseases you can find by observation?
   - By palpation?
   - By percussion?
   - By auscultation?
2. In doing the PE, why is it important to follow a certain order?
3. How can being gentle help you find signs of disease?
4. Why is it important to look at both sides of the body?
5. What are some of the things to write in the patient's record about what you found in the PE?

3.3 The physical signs to look for

3.3.1 The overall condition

The whole patient

First of all, **look carefully at the patient**. Observe him while he is talking to you. This is very important. You can learn many things about the disease simply by looking carefully at the patient.

- Does he look ill?
- Does he seem to be in pain?
- Does he seem to be sad or worried about the illness?

If the patient sits quietly and is relaxed, probably he is not very ill. But if he is restless, sad, or worried, the disease may be serious.

Breathing

Look at the patient's breathing.

- Is the breathing quiet, without difficulty?
- Or is the breathing rapid, or with difficulty?

Nutrition

Look at the nutrition of the patient. Does he seem well nourished? Or are there signs of malnutrition?

- A loss of weight.
- Swelling of the feet or legs.
- Changes in the color of the skin or hair.

Hydration

Look for signs of dryness, or dehydration.

- Dry lips, often with cracks.
- Dry eyes, sunk into the eye sockets, and with no tears.
- Dry skin, with many folds and a loss of elasticity. Pinch the patient's skin gently, then let it go quickly. If the skin stays pinched for a few seconds, this is a sign of dehydration.

Consciousness

Observe how the patient talks.

● Does he talk quietly and clearly?

● Or does he seem confused?

A patient who cannot talk clearly about himself or about the illness may be very ill. We call this "delirium." This can come from a high fever. It can be a sign of a brain disease. Or it can come because the patient has drunk much wine or taken drugs.

The whole body

It is important to look carefully at the part of the body where the patient has pain. But it is also very important to look at the whole body. A serious disease can make changes in the whole body. If you do not look at the whole body, you will miss important signs of the disease.

Before starting the physical examination, ask the patient to take off some clothes. A man should take off his shirt. A woman may take off her blouse. In some cases, the patient must undress completely. But be polite about this. Show respect to the patient. Protect the patient's dignity.

Look for small cuts in the skin made by the patient or by a traditional healer. These cuts show where the patient feels pain. Note any special smell or odor. There may be a special odor of the patient's breath, or of certain secretions, or of a sore.

Looking at the patient carefully for signs of disease is like looking at the sky. A clear blue sky is a sign of good weather. Dark clouds are a sign of rain. So look carefully at the patient to find all the signs you can about the disease.

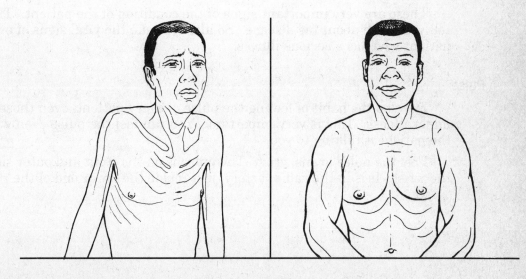

Look at the two pictures from the previous page carefully.

- Which patient looks very ill?
- What do you see that makes you think he is very ill?
- Which patient does not look very ill?
- Why do you think that this patient is not very ill?

Questions for study

1. What should you observe about the patient while you are taking the history?
2. What kinds of disease can you find by observing the patient's
   - Breathing?
   - Nutrition?
   - Hydration?
   - Consciousness?

3.3.2 The vital signs

There are five signs which we call the vital signs.

1. The pulse.
2. The breathing, or respirations.
3. The blood pressure.
4. The temperature.
5. The weight.

These are very important signs of the condition of the patient. They can tell you much about his disease. So **always** take the vital signs of every patient who has a serious illness.

Pulse

Develop the habit of feeling the pulse of every patient, even those with a minor illness. This is very important. You can feel the pulse even while the patient is talking to you.

Feel the pulse at his wrist. The pulse is on the front and outer side of the wrist. It is in the radial artery, just inside the lower end of the radius.

Or place your hand gently on the back of the patient's wrist. Put your fingers around the wrist. You will then be able to feel the radial pulse with the ends of your fingers on the front of his wrist.

There are three important things to note about the pulse.

1. How fast it is.

2. How strong it is.

3. The rhythm: is it regular or irregular?

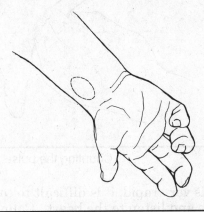

Where to count the pulse.

Count the pulse

You need a watch with a big second hand that goes around one time every minute. **The pulse is the number of heart beats in one minute**. We call this the **pulse rate**. There are two ways to count the pulse.

1. You can count it for one full minute (60 seconds). This will give you the pulse rate.

2. Or you can count it for 15 seconds (one quarter of a minute) and multiply this number by four. This will also give you the pulse rate.

How fast is the pulse? Normally the pulse is between 60 and 100 beats per minute in an adult. A pulse of more than 100 beats per minute in an adult at rest is a sign of serious disease. It can come from a high fever, anemia, shock, or heart disease. But sometimes the pulse is rapid only because the patient is very nervous or has just done much exercise.

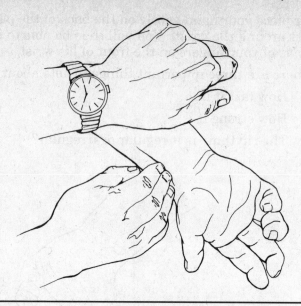

Counting the pulse.

If the pulse is very rapid, it is difficult to count it at the wrist. Then use your stethoscope and listen to the heart. Count the beats of the heart as you listen.

Feel how strong the pulse is

Is the pulse strong or weak? A pulse that is weak is often difficult to feel. A weak pulse is a sign of poor circulation of the blood. The pulse is weak or even absent in shock. It can be very weak in severe anemia or dehydration, in a disease of the heart, or in a serious infection. A pulse that is rapid and very weak we call a thin or "thready" pulse.

Note the rhythm of the pulse

Normally the pulse beats are regular. You can tap your foot at the same rhythm as the pulse of the patient. But if the pulse of the patient is irregular, it is impossible to tap your foot in the rhythm of his pulse.

An irregular pulse is often a sign of heart disease. Make a note of it. Read also on page 92 about the rhythm of the heart.

Respirations

Observe the breathing

Look at the patient as you count the respirations. Is the breathing difficult? Is it fast?

Rapid breathing

Rapid breathing is not always difficult breathing. Fever, anemia, shock, nervousness, or exercise can cause rapid breathing. But there is no difficulty. Rapid and very deep breathing comes in dehydration or in coma from diabetes or from serious kidney disease. Rapid breathing with the chest muscles but with no movement of the abdomen comes in peritonitis.

Difficult breathing

Difficult breathing, called **dyspnea**, comes in diseases of the heart or lungs. Difficulty in taking air into the lungs is a sign of an infection of the lungs, of the bronchi, or of the larynx. It is also a sign of heart failure. Difficulty in pushing air out of the lungs comes in asthma. See the strategies on dyspnea on pages 260 and 264.

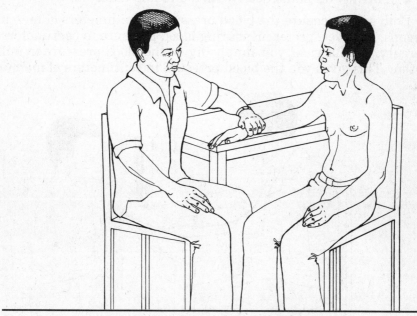

Counting the respirations.

Count the respirations

Count the number of respirations per minute. This is the **respiratory rate**. Normally an adult breathes from 12 to 20 times in one minute while sitting quietly.

If an adult breathes rapidly - more than 20 times per minute - there may be a serious disease. Rapid respirations can come from a high fever, anemia, shock, a serious infection, or a disease of the heart or lungs. It can also come because of nervousness and from exercise. Persons who live at high altitudes normally have faster breathing.

The best time to count the respirations is while you are feeling the pulse. First, count the pulse. Then before letting go of the wrist of the patient, look at the breathing and count the respirations. In this way the patient will not know you are counting the breathing. Count the respirations for one full minute. Or else count the respirations for 15 seconds and multiply by 4.

Blood pressure (BP)

There are two sorts of blood pressure machines, or manometers.

- A mercury manometer with a column of mercury in a glass tube.
- An aneroid manometer with a dial and a needle.

Both sorts measure the blood pressure in millimeters of mercury. Some persons, however, prefer measuring blood pressure in centimeters of mercury. In this case, you simply divide the blood pressure in millimeters by ten. This gives you the blood pressure in centimeters of mercury.

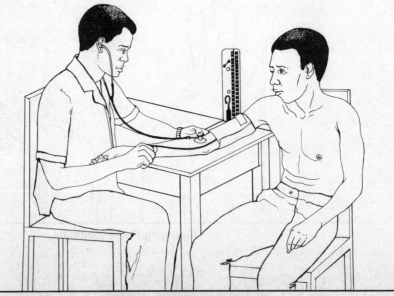

Taking the blood pressure.

Taking the blood pressure

When you take the blood pressure, the patient must sit down or lie down. Have him put one arm on a table or on the bed. Make sure his arm muscles are relaxed. Put the blood pressure cuff tightly around his upper arm. Feel for the pulse at the elbow. Then put your stethoscope over the place where you feel the pulse.

Pump air into the cuff until the column of mercury, or the needle, goes up above 200 mm (20 cm). Then let out the air slowly by opening the valve a little bit. As the air goes out slowly, listen for the pulse through the stethoscope.

When the mercury is above 200 mm, no blood will go through the artery (unless the blood pressure is very high). When blood does start to go through the artery, you will hear a dull thud sound like that of a hammer.

Systolic/diastolic blood pressures

Note the blood pressure - the column of mercury or the needle - at the moment you first hear the pulse. This is the top, or **systolic**, blood pressure. Let out more air slowly from the cuff. Note the pressure the moment you can no longer hear the pulse. This is the bottom, or **diastolic**, blood pressure. Be sure to let out all the air from the cuff before you take it off the arm of the patient.

Recording the blood pressure

Record the blood pressure by putting the systolic pressure over the diastolic pressure. In adults the normal BP is between 90/50 and 140/90 mm (9/5 and 14/9 cm).

High blood pressure

A high BP, above 140/90, sometimes comes from nervousness. But often it is a sign of disease. Perhaps you are not certain if the patient's high blood pressure is due to disease or simply to nervousness. In this case, take the patient's blood pressure every day for three days. Take it with him sitting up and again when he is lying down. If the pressure remains high, above 140/90, then he has high blood pressure.

Low blood pressure

A low BP, below 90/50, may be normal. Often, however, it is a sign of a serious circulatory weakness or of the beginning of shock. In this case, the pulse will be rapid and very weak or thready.

Temperature

Normal temperature

Fever, or an elevated temperature, is an important sign of disease. So always take the temperature of each patient. The normal temperature is between 36° and 37° C (96.8° and 98.6°F). There are three places in which you can take the temperature.

1. In the mouth: the **oral** temperature.
2. In the rectum: the **rectal** temperature.
3. In the armpit: the **axillary** temperature.

Shaking the thermometer

Always look at the thermometer first. Make sure that the mercury is at 37° C (98.6°F) or below. If it is above this, shake the thermometer until the mercury comes down to this point or below. Make sure also that the thermometer is very clean.

Taking the temperature

Oral temperature

Place the mercury bulb of the thermometer in the patient's mouth under the tongue. The patient must close the lips tightly but not the teeth. Leave the thermometer there for three minutes. Then take it out and look at the column of mercury. This will show you the degree of temperature of the patient. Record this on the patient's record. Clean the thermometer carefully in alcohol, in another antiseptic solution, or in water with soap before using it for another patient.

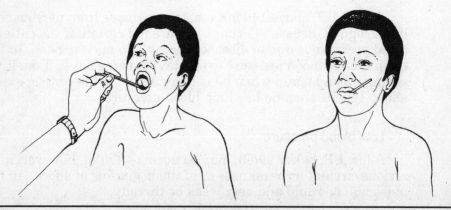

Taking the temperature by mouth.

Rectal temperature

To take the rectal temperature, place a small amount of vaseline on the bulb of the thermometer. The patient must be lying down, preferably on one side. Place the thermometer gently into the rectum. Leave it there for three minutes. Then take it out and look at the column of mercury. Write down the temperature on the patient's record. Clean the thermometer with an antiseptic solution before putting it away or using it again.

Axillary temperature

Place the bulb of the thermometer in the patient's armpit. Tell the patient to hold the arm tightly against the chest for three minutes. Then look at the column of mercury and read the temperature. Note it on the patient's record.

Note that it is the axillary temperature. This temperature is always a little below the true temperature, about one half degree Celsius, or one degree Fahrenheit.

To find the causes of a fever in a patient, see the strategy on fever on page 461.

Weight

If possible, weigh every patient who has a serious illness. This is important for two reasons.

Drug dosage by weight

The dose of many medicines changes according to the weight of the patient. A patient who weighs much gets a big dose. A patient who weighs little, like a baby or a child, will get a small dose. You must know the weight of the patient in order to know how much medicine to give. The size of the dose depends, therefore, on the weight of the patient in kilograms.

Weight change with treatment

Weight loss because of treatment

Some diseases cause swelling, or edema. The patient quickly gains weight because there is too much liquid in the body. When you start giving treatment, he begins to lose this liquid. Therefore, he loses weight, and this is good. If you weigh the him each day, you will see his weight go down. This means that your treatment is working well.

Weight gain because of treatment

Other diseases, like tuberculosis, malnutrition, or other chronic diseases, can make the patient lose weight. The patient is thin. But he will gain weight once you start giving good treatment. In this case, a gain in weight is a good sign. It means he is getting better on the treatment you are giving. To find the causes of loss of weight in a patient, see the strategy on loss of weight on page 468.

REMEMBER:

The vital signs are vital. They tell you much about the condition of the patient and about the disease.

Questions for study

1. What are all of the things to observe about the pulse of your patient?
2. What signs of disease can you find by taking the patient's pulse? What diseases can cause these signs?
3. What are all of the things to observe about the breathing of your patient?
4. What signs of disease can you find by looking at the patient's breathing?
5. Why is it important to take the blood pressure of your patient?
6. How do you take the blood pressure?
7. Why is it important to take the temperature of your patient?
8. Why is it important to weigh your patient before starting to give treatment?

3.3.3 The head

The head

Tumor

Look for swellings or tumors. A tumor which is fixed to the bone and which you cannot move is probably serious. A soft tumor which you can move is probably not serious. It may be a cyst or a fatty tumor (lipoma).

Injury

If there has been an accident, look for signs of injury - a wound, a swelling, or a dark color of the skin called **ecchymosis**. The dark color comes from bleeding into the skin. An ecchymosis around the eye can come from a fracture of the head bone, or skull.

Blood or clear water coming from the ear is a sign of a serious skull fracture. If the patient does not also have a cold, clear water coming from the nose after a head injury is also a sign of a serious skull fracture. The clear water coming from the ear or from the nose is spinal fluid.

Sores

Look for sores on the face and on the scalp (the skin with hair on top of the head). Look for signs of infection around these sores: swelling, tenderness, heat, big lymph nodes in the back of the head or in the neck. Look also for very small insects in the hair. These are lice.

Malnutrition

Look at the hair and the skin for signs of malnutrition. The hair becomes red or gray, short, and fragile. The skin shows spots with less color. There is often swelling around the eyes.

The eyes

Lids

Swelling of the lids of both eyes with no pain is a sign of a general disease. Look for other signs of a disease of the heart, the liver, the kidneys, or of malnutrition or anemia.

Swelling of the lids of one eye with no pain or fever can come from a filaria infection or from an allergic reaction. Swelling of the lids of one eye with pain and often fever is a sign of a serious infection around the eye.

Conjunctiva

Look inside the eyelids at the membrane, or conjunctiva.

Redness

Redness of the conjunctiva is a sign of infection. Look carefully to see where the redness is the most strong, or intense. In **conjunctivitis**, the redness is strongest inside the eyelids and in the angles between the lids and the eyeball.

The redness may be strongest, or most intense, right around the edge of the cornea. This is a sign of a serious infection inside the eye. Such a patient must go to hospital right away.

The redness may be only in the angles of the eye. We call this angular conjunctivitis. This comes because of hot sunshine, much wind, or much dust in the air. It is not serious and does not need treatment. Sometimes

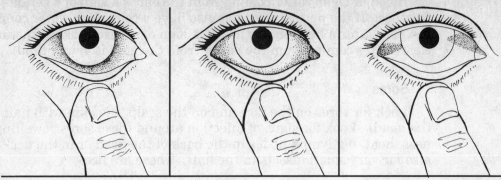

Conjunctivitis.   Serious infection in the eye.   Angular conjunctivitis.

the redness of the angular conjunctivitis grows out onto the cornea. We call this a pterygium. No treatment is necessary unless the pterygium grows to the center of the cornea.

Sometimes there is a bright red spot in one small part of the conjunctiva. This is a hemorrhage under the conjunctiva. It is not serious. It will go away in a few days and needs no treatment.

Red bumps of the conjunctiva, or thick bands between the eyelids and the eyeball, are signs of a serious disease called **trachoma**.

Foreign body

A small piece of matter on the conjunctiva such as sand, or a seed, or a piece of metal causes pain. Look carefully inside the upper and lower lids for such a foreign body in any patient with pain in the eye. If you find one, take it out with a small piece of clean cotton.

To look inside the upper eyelid, turn the lid inside out. Take a small stick. With your thumb and fingers of one hand, take hold of the upper eye lashes. Pull down gently. Now push against the middle of the upper eyelid with the stick. This will turn the lid inside out. You can now look at the inside of the lid for the foreign body.

Iris and light reflex

Look carefully inside the eye at the brown membrane, or **iris**. Look also at the **pupil**. This is the round black hole in the middle of the iris.

Use a small flashlight. Shine the light into the eye. Normally the light will make the pupil contract, or get smaller. The pupil will dilate, or get bigger, immediately after you take away the light. This is the **light reflex**.

If there is no light reflex, the pupil will not contract when you shine the light into the eye. This is a sign of a serious disease either in the eye or in the brain.

Eye muscles and movements

Test the movements of the eye. Hold a small object in front of the patient. Tell the patient to look steadily at it. Move the object slowly to the left and to the right, then up and down. Tell the patient to look at the object as you move it. But the patient must move only the eyes and not the head.

Normally the two eyes move together: both to the left, both to the right, both up and both down. But sometimes one eye moves and the other does not move in the same way. This is a sign of a serious disease. It means that one or more of the muscles of the eye is not working and is paralyzed.

Vision

In every patient who has trouble with one or both eyes, test the vision of each eye. If possible, use a standard eye chart. This has many letters of different sizes on it. Put the eye chart on the wall in a good light. Put it 6 meters (20 feet) from where the patient will sit. Be sure the chart is in a good light.

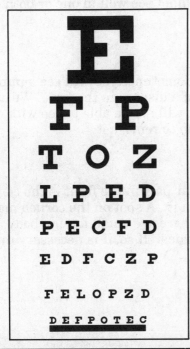

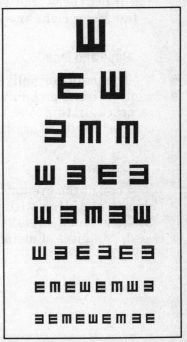

| Eye chart. | Eye chart for people who cannot read. |

If you do not have a standard eye chart, you can make one. Use a piece of white cardboard. Put black letters on it. The big letters go on top. The letters become smaller as you go down the chart.

Test the vision in each eye. Tell the patient to cover the right eye with his hand, or to hold a small piece of paper in front of it. Tell the patient to read the letters in each line of the eye chart with the left eye. Make a note of the smallest letters he can read without making an error.

Now tell him to cover the left eye and to read the letters with the right eye. Make a note of the smallest letters he can read with the right eye without making an error.

Perhaps he can see clearly with one eye, as well as you can see. But he cannot see clearly with the other eye. This means there is a disease in the poor eye. It may be that he cannot see clearly with either eye. Then there is a disease in both eyes.

A patient may not be able to read or name the letters. In this case, use the **E** chart. Ask him in which direction the **E** points. Or else stand 6 meters (20 feet) from the patient. Hold up one or two fingers of your hand. Ask the patient to tell you how many fingers you are holding up. Have the patient do this with each eye separately.

Use also a few objects such as a pen or a coin. See if the patient can identify them correctly with each eye separately. If not, there is a disease in one or both eyes. Patients who cannot see well in one or both eyes must go to the doctor right away.

Pupil and lens

The pupil normally is black. Sometimes you will see a pupil that is very white. This is probably because of a disease in the lens. We call this a cataract. In this case, the patient will not be able to see with that eye. A cataract needs a surgical operation to remove it.

Cornea

Look at the eye itself. The clear part in the front is the cornea. It is smooth and clear, with no spots on it. A spot on the cornea may be an ulcer. Look also very carefully to see if there is a small foreign body, like sand, or a seed, or a piece of metal on the cornea. If so, it is necessary to take this off.

Eyeball

The normal eyeball is white. A yellow color of the eyeball is called **jaundice**. This is a sign of liver disease or of certain anemias. Redness right around the edge of the cornea is a sign of serious infection inside the eyeball. Often there is much pain. The patient must go immediately to hospital.

The ears

Look in the ear canal. Use a strong light. A special light, called an **otoscope,** is very good for this. Pull up on the top of the outside of the ear. In this way you can see better inside the ear canal.

A thick brown lump in the canal is ear wax. You can often get this out by a gentle irrigation of the ear canal with warm water. If not, put some warm baby oil into the canal in the evening. This will help the wax come out by itself.

Try to look at the ear drum, the gray membrane at the far end of the canal. A red ear drum is a sign of infection in the ear. There is usually much pain. There is also pain when you pull on the outside of the ear or press on the bone behind or under the ear. Thick yellow liquid, or pus, coming from the ear canal is also a sign of infection in the ear.

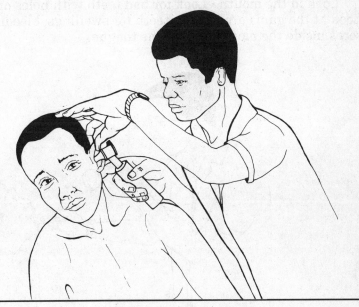

Examining the ear canal.

The nose

Look up the nose. A clear or thick liquid coming from the nose is a sign of a cold. Blood coming from the nose, called **epistaxis**, often is not serious. But it may be a sign of disease. Examine the nose to look for an ulcer, a swelling, or a tumor.

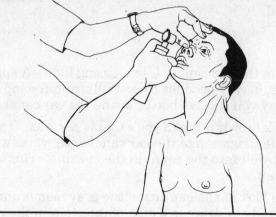

Examining the nose.

The mouth

Look in the mouth. Look for bad teeth with holes or cavities in them. Look at the gums around the teeth for swellings, bleeding, or pus. Look for sores inside the mouth and on the tongue.

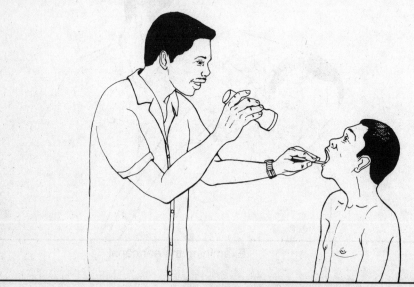

Examining the mouth.

The pharynx

Look in the back of the mouth. We call this the **pharynx**, or throat. Use a strong light and a flat instrument to push down gently on the back of the tongue. Tell the patient to say "AH." A red pharynx is a sign of a cold.

At each side of the pharynx is a small lump of tissue called the **tonsil**. Swelling of the tonsils with redness, and especially with white spots on them, is a sign of a serious infection called **tonsillitis**.

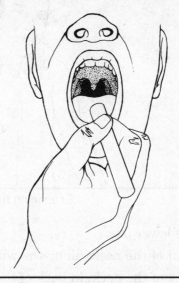

Examining the pharynx.

3.3.4 The neck

Observation

Look carefully at the neck from the front. The neck normally is symmetrical. This means that the two sides look the same. See if the two sides are the same. If they are not the same, a disease is probably present.

Palpation

Now palpate the neck. To do this, stand in back of the patient. Feel gently both sides of the neck with your fingers. Feel for swellings, tumors, and lymph nodes. Feel also for painful spots. Feel carefully in all of these places.

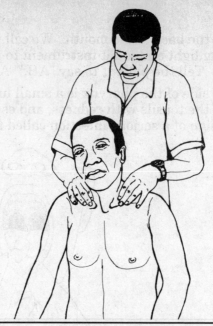

Examining the neck.

1. Under the lower jaw.

2. In the front of the neck, along the windpipe, or trachea.

3. At the back of the neck, in back of the thick **sterno-mastoid** muscle. This muscle goes from the end of the clavicle to the bone in back of the ear.

4. In the hollow place above the clavicles. We call this the **supra-clavicular fossa**.

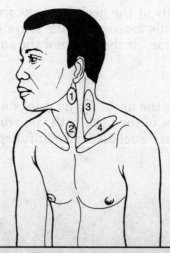

Regions of the neck.

Thyroid gland

The thyroid gland is in the low front part of the neck. It is in two parts, one on each side of the trachea. It moves up and down with the trachea when the patient swallows. The normal thyroid is very small. It is impossible to feel it.

If the gland is big, you can feel it easily. Stand behind the patient. Place the tips of your fingers gently on each side of the trachea below the larynx. Tell the patient to swallow. If the thyroid is big, you will feel a mass move up and down with the trachea. A big thyroid gland is most probably a goiter.

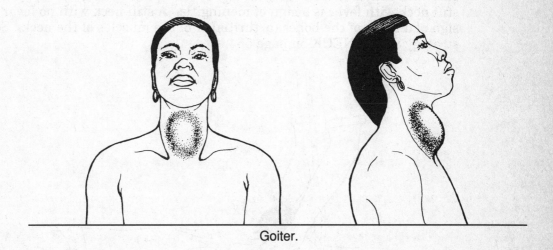

Goiter.

Lymph nodes

1. Big nodes with much pain and often with fever come from an acute infection.

2. Big nodes under the chin and under the ears come probably from infections of the mouth, the teeth, the pharynx, the tonsils, or the ears.

3. Big nodes in the back of the neck or in the supra-clavicular fossa with a little pain come probably from tuberculosis or from an infection in the ear or of the skin of the head.

4. A series of small nodes in the back of the neck with no pain may come from:

   - Trypanosomiasis (African sleeping sickness).

   - Filariasis.

   - A general infection like syphilis or hepatitis.

5. Big hard nodes with no pain can come from a tumor.

6. One node in the supra-clavicular fossa is a sign of disease in the abdomen. It may be tuberculosis. It may be a malignant tumor.

7. A small opening in the skin of the neck from which pus comes is called a **sinus**. It is a sign of tuberculosis or of another chronic infection of the lymph nodes.

See the strategy on BIG LYMPH NODES on page 550.

Stiff neck

See if the patient can bend the neck up and down and to each side. A stiff neck which bends with difficulty or with pain is a sign of disease. A stiff neck with fever is a sign of meningitis. A stiff neck with no fever is a sign of disease of the bones (arthritis) or of the muscles of the neck. See the strategy STIFF NECK on page 564.

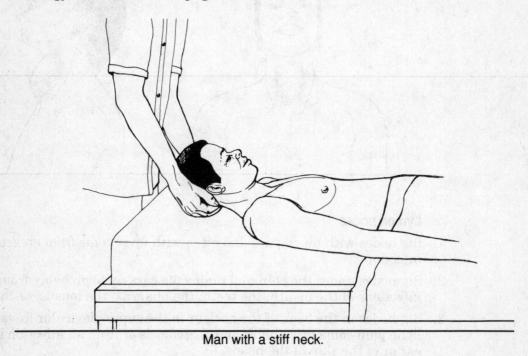

Man with a stiff neck.

3.3.5 The breasts

Observation

With the woman sitting down, look carefully at her breasts. Look for these signs.

1. Symmetry. Do the two breasts look alike?
2. Swelling of one breast.
3. A lump or a mass in one breast.
4. A change in the skin: edema, which makes the skin look like an orange peel.
5. An ulcer or a sinus.
6. Secretions or blood coming from the nipple.

Ask the woman to lie down. Now look again at the two breasts for the same things.

Palpation

Feel carefully both breasts, first with the woman sitting up, then with her lying down. Feel for these things.

Tenderness

This usually means infection. In a breast infection, there is usually a big hard tender area. There is often a fever. There may be fluctuation. This is a sign of pus inside the breast. During pregnancy, and also right after the mother gives birth, both breasts may be tender. This is normal.

Lumps

A lump in the breast can be:

- A cyst.
- A benign tumor.
- A malignant tumor.

It is important to send a woman with a lump in the breast to hospital immediately. But if the lump is smooth and round, it may be a cyst. If so, it is full of liquid. Try to aspirate this liquid with a sterile syringe and needle. This is how to do it.

- Clean the skin carefully with an antiseptic solution.
- Hold the lump firmly between the fingers of your left hand.

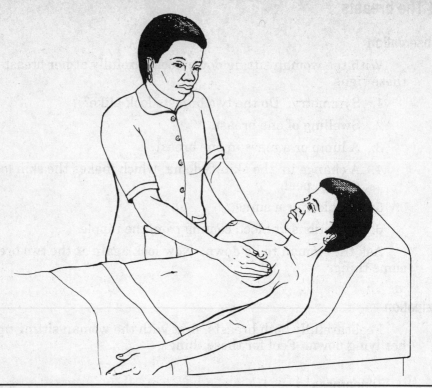

Examining the breast.

- Push the needle into the lump.
- Draw back on the barrel of the syringe.
- Take out all of the liquid.

If there is no liquid, send the woman to hospital.

Lymph nodes

Feel for lymph nodes in the armpit and at the base of the neck. Big lymph nodes can come from:

- An infection, or mastitis.
- A malignant tumor.

Questions for study

1. What signs of disease must you look for on the head?
2. Make a list of all the signs of disease you can find in the eyes.
3. Why is it important to test the vision of anyone with an eye disease?
4. What signs of disease can you find:
   - In the ears?
   - In the nose?
   - In the mouth?
5. What signs of disease can you find in the neck?
6. When you find one or more lymph nodes in the neck, what should you note about them?
7. What are the common diseases that cause big lymph nodes in the neck?
8. How must you examine a woman's breasts?
9. What diseases should you look for in a woman's breasts?
10. What signs does each breast disease give?

3.3.6 The chest and the lungs

Observation

Look at the chest carefully. Does the chest look the same on both sides? In other words, is the chest symmetrical? If not, find out why. Look for lumps, sores, or wounds.

Observe the breathing of the patient. You have already counted the respiration rate when you took the vital signs. Look at the rhythm of the breathing.

1. Is it regular or irregular?

2. Do both sides of the chest move the same amount?

3. Or does one side move more than the other side?

Palpation

To palpate the chest, stand or sit behind the patient. Feel for these things:

Breathing

Put your hands on the chest, one on each side. Tell the patient to breathe deeply. Look at how your hands move when he breathes deeply. Does one hand move more than the other? If so, there is a disease in the chest. It is probably in the lung on the side of the chest that moves only a little.

Lumps or masses

Feel for lumps or masses in the skin, in the subcutaneous tissue, in the muscles, and in the bones. For each lump or mass, note:

- How big it is.
- If there is tenderness.
- If it is hard or soft.
- It you can move it or not.

Pain or tenderness

Feel for tender spots. A tender spot can mean an infection or a tender mass. Look for other signs of infection, like heat or swelling.

If there has been an injury and the patient has pain in the chest, look for a fracture of one or more ribs. There are two ways to look for a rib fracture.

1. With one finger, feel gently along each rib. A spot on a rib which is very tender is a sign of a fracture.

2. With both your hands, push gently on the chest, front and back. Then push from each side. Much pain in one spot when you push this way is a sign of a fracture of one or more ribs.

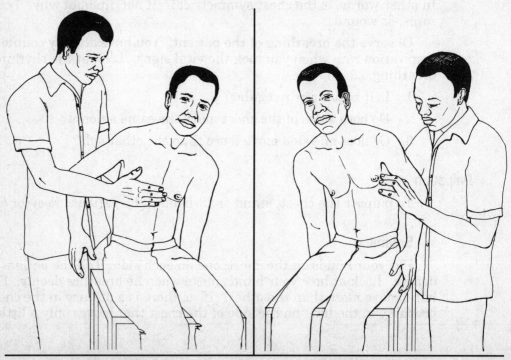

| Feeling each rib. | Pressing on the chest. |

If there are signs of a rib fracture, listen carefully to the breath sounds. See page 86.

Pain in the ribs can also come from arthritis. In this case, there are tender spots. But there is no history of an injury and no signs of infection.

Vibrations

Feel for vibrations when the patient talks. Tell the patient to say, "ninety nine." Normally you can feel faint vibrations of the voice with your fingers on the chest. These vibrations come through the lungs when the patient talks. Compare the force of the vibrations on the two sides of the chest.

The vibrations are weak or absent if there is liquid in the lungs or in the pleural space around the lungs. They are also absent if there is air in the pleural space. We call air in the pleural space **pneumothorax**.

Percussion

Percussion of the chest is very helpful in finding signs of disease in the chest and lungs.

Technique of percussion

Put the middle finger of your left hand flat and firmly on the chest of the patient. Tap gently on the middle of this finger with the tip of the middle finger of your right hand. Be sure to curve the right middle finger.

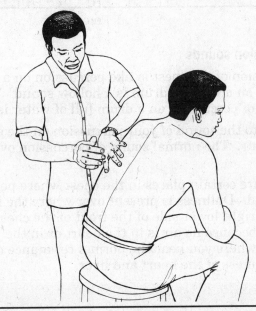

Percussion.

When tapping, or percussing, move the whole right hand at the wrist. Move the whole hand and not just the middle finger. Keep your right arm steady. It must not move. Percuss only with the right hand and middle finger. Or percuss with the left hand and middle finger if you are left-handed.

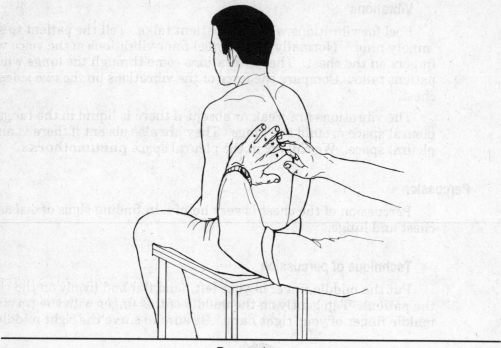

Percussion.

Percussion sounds

Percussion of the chest is like percussion on a drum. The sound of percussion on an empty drum is a hollow sound. We call it **resonance**. The sound of percussion on a drum full of water is flat or **dull**.

Listen to the sound of your percussion on the chest. Normally the lungs are full of air. The normal sound of percussion over the lungs is therefore resonant.

There are certain places in the chest where percussion normally makes a dull sound. Dullness is present over where the heart is. There is dullness also in the right lower side of the front of the chest. This is where the liver is. This is because no air is in the heart or in the liver. The next drawing shows you where you hear the normal resonance of the lungs and the normal dullness of the heart and liver.

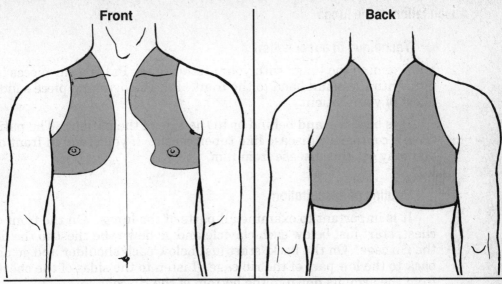

Front   **Back**

Normal resonance of the chest.

Percussion signs of disease

Some diseases cause liquid to come into the lungs or into the chest. This can be the liquid of edema, of infection, of pus, or of blood. The sound is then not resonant. It is dull. It is like percussing on a drum full of water.

When you hear a dull sound where normally the sound is resonant, you know there is liquid inside. The liquid may be in the lungs. This occurs in:

- Pneumonia.
- Tuberculosis, usually at the top of the lungs.
- Heart failure, usually at the bottom, or base, of the lungs.

The liquid can be in the space around the lungs, the pleural space. This liquid can come from:

- The liquid of edema from heart failure.
- The liquid of infection.
- Pus as a result of a severe infection. We call this an **empyema**.
- Blood, from an injury such as a rib fracture or a wound.

REMEMBER:

Resonance means air.

Dullness means liquid or solid tissue.

Auscultation of the lungs

Technique of auscultation

Examine the lungs with your stethoscope. Put the ear pieces in your ears with the small bend to the front. Put the listening piece solidly on the chest of your patient.

It is best to stand behind or to the side of the patient. The patient may have a contagious disease like tuberculosis. If you stand in front of him, you may get this disease from him.

Routine of auscultation

It is important to examine all parts of the lungs. On the front of the chest, start just below each clavicle and go down the chest to the bottom of the rib cage. On the back, start just below each shoulder and go down the back to the low part of the rib cage. Listen to the sides of the chest also, from the armpits down to the bottom of the rib cage.

Move the stethoscope from one side of the chest to the other. Compare the sound on one side with the sound on the other side. Tell the patient to open his mouth and to breathe a little more deeply than normal.

Breath sounds

Through the stethoscope you can hear air coming into the lungs. This is **inspiration**. You can also hear air going out of the lungs. This is **expiration**.

The sound you hear is like that of the wind blowing softly through the trees. The sound of air coming in takes a little more time. The sound of air going out of the lungs takes a little less time. Inspiration is therefore a little more long than expiration.

Normal breath sounds

Listen to the lungs of persons who are well. This will teach you the normal sounds of respiration. There are two sounds to hear: **breath sounds** and **bronchial sounds**.

The **breath sounds** are soft. This is the sound of air coming into the air spaces or alveoli and then going out again.

Bronchial sounds are loud and high. They are like air going through a pipe. You hear them normally over the trachea. You also hear them at the top part of the front of the chest.

Listen to the two sides of the chest, front and back. Do the two sides sound the same? If not, there is probably a disease present in the chest.

Abnormal breath sounds

Consolidation

During some kinds of infection, part of a lung can become solid. This is because this part of the lung is full of liquid. We call this **consolidation**. Where there is consolidation, you will hear only bronchial breath sounds. The vibrations will be more strong. When you percuss over this area, you will hear a dull sound and not a resonant sound. These are the signs of a serious infection of the lungs. We call it **lobar pneumonia**.

Pleural fluid

If liquid comes into the chest around the lung, then the breath sounds become weak and difficult to hear. The vibrations will also be weak or absent. You will hear a dull sound on percussion and not a resonant sound. This is often at the bottom of the lung. It may be only on one side of the chest.

Air in the chest

Sometimes air comes into the pleural space around the lungs. This can happen after a rib fracture. Or it can happen in certain lung diseases. We call this a **pneumothorax**.

The breath sounds and the vibrations are very weak or absent. But the percussion sound is now very resonant. Look for these changes in every patient with a rib fracture. If you find them, send the patient immediately to hospital.

Voice sounds

Tell the patient to say "ninety nine." Listen to this through your stethoscope. Listen in different parts of the chest. The voice sounds are transmitted through the normal lungs. They change in certain diseases.

1. The voice sounds increase in pneumonia with consolidation.
2. The voice sounds decrease or are absent:
   - If there is much liquid in the pleural space.
   - In pneumonia with no consolidation.
   - If there is much air in the pleural space - pneumothorax.

Rhonchi

These are loud sounds, high or low. They come from liquid in the bronchial tubes. You hear them during inspiration or during expiration, or sometimes in both inspiration and expiration.

They are signs of disease in the bronchi, or air tubes. Rhonchi during inspiration are signs of bronchitis. High rhonchi during expiration are signs of asthma. We call this **wheezing**.

Crackles

Crackles, sometimes called rales, are soft sounds like softly boiling water. They come when there is some liquid in the small air spaces or alveoli. You hear them during inspiration and not often during expiration. Pinch your hair between your fingers near one of your ears. Rub your fingers together. This makes a sound much like the sound of crackles.

These are some of the diseases that can cause crackles.

1. A lung infection like **pneumonia** can cause crackles in any part of the lungs.
2. **Tuberculosis**. The crackles are usually in the top part of the lungs.
3. **Heart failure**. The crackles are often at the bottom part, or base, of the lungs.

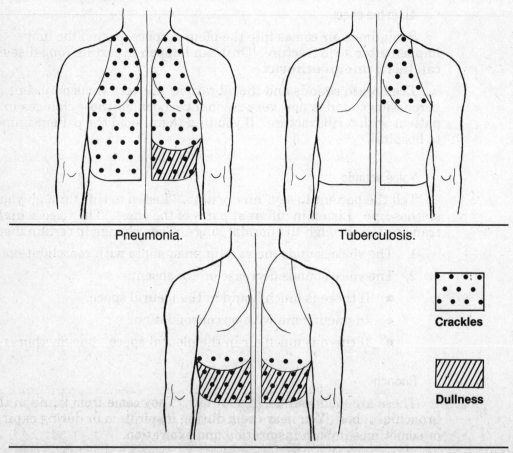

Pneumonia.

Tuberculosis.

Heart Failure.

Crackles

Dullness

REMEMBER:

Rhonchi mean liquid in the bronchial tubes. Crackles mean liquid in the air spaces or alveoli.

SUMMARY

1. Pneumonia without consolidation makes dullness, crackles, weak or absent breath sounds, and weak or absent voice vibrations and sounds.

2. Consolidation makes dullness, bronchial sounds, and increased voice vibrations and sounds.

3. Pleural fluid makes dullness, weak or absent breath sounds, and weak or absent voice vibrations and sounds.

4. Pneumothorax makes much resonance, absent breath sounds, and absent voice vibrations.

5. Tuberculosis makes crackles, usually at the top of the lungs.

6. Asthma makes high rhonchi, or wheezes, during expiration.

3.3.7 The heart

The heart is in the front of the chest. It is just behind the breast bone or sternum and a little to the left side.

Observation

Look carefully at the front of the chest. Look for the **apical pulse**. This is a spot on the chest where you can often see the heart beat. At this spot the point, or apex, of the heart hits the inside of the rib cage every time the heart beats.

In thin persons you can see this apical pulse. A small area of the skin "beats" when the heart beats and hits the inside of the chest. However, in persons with thick muscles or with much fat you cannot see the apical pulse.

Palpation

Now feel for the apical pulse with your hand. Find out exactly where it is. Normally it is just under the left nipple. It is in the fourth or the fifth rib space.

In some diseases the heart becomes big. Then the apical pulse will move and be in a different place. It will be more to the left, often on the side of the chest.

If the heart is big, the apical pulse can also become much stronger. It may cover a big area of the chest wall. So a big apical pulse to the left of the left nipple is a sign of heart disease.

A serious disease of the heart valves can cause vibrations of the chest wall, usually at the apical pulse. You can feel these vibrations with your fingers or hand. We call these vibrations a **thrill**.

Percussion

Normal cardiac dullness

The heart is made of thick muscle. It is full of blood. When you percuss over the heart, you hear a dull sound. Therefore, there is a dull sound on the front of the chest just to the left of the sternum. We call this **cardiac dullness**. This figure shows you the normal area of cardiac dullness.

To percuss the heart, percuss in each rib space on the left side of the front of the chest. Start at the side and move toward the sternum in each space. With your pen make a mark on the skin in each rib space where the resonance changes to dullness. When you finish, these marks will show you how big the heart is.

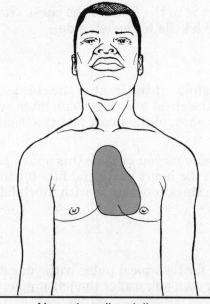

Normal cardiac dullness.

Big heart

In certain diseases of the heart, the heart becomes very big. The area of cardiac dullness also becomes big. Sometimes the cardiac dullness can go over to the side of the chest. This means that the heart is very big.

Auscultation

Normal heart sounds

The heart pumps blood to all of the body. With the stethoscope you can hear the sounds of the heart pumping blood. The heart makes two loud sounds, or thumps, each time it pumps. The sounds are like this:

lub - dub   lub - dub   lub - dub   lub - dub   lub - dub.

Each lub - dub is one heart beat. The two sounds come from the closing of the different valves in the heart.

You can learn many things about the heart by listening to it with your stethoscope.

1. How fast the heart goes: the **heart rate**.

2. The heart rhythm: if the heart beats are regular or irregular.

3. If there are abnormal heart sounds which we call **murmurs**.

To listen to the heart, stand or sit on the right side of the patient. Or else stand in back. There are four places on the front of the chest to listen to the heart. This figure shows you these four places.

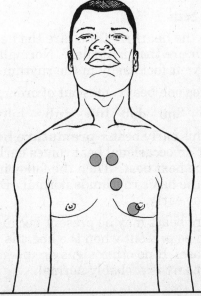

Four places to listen to the heart.

Normal heart rhythms

Heart rate

Count the heart beats. This is the heart rate. Is it fast or slow? A heart rate, or pulse, of more than 100 beats per minute in an adult at rest is a sign of disease.

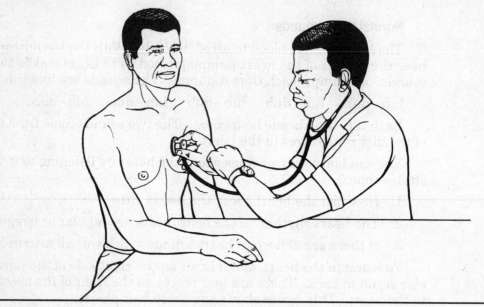

Counting the heart rate.

Premature beats

Listen to the heart rhythm. Are the heart beats regular, like the ticks of a clock? Or are they irregular? Normally the heart rhythm is regular. You can tap your foot easily in the rhythm of the heart rate.

Sometimes one beat comes out of order, too early, like this:

lub - dub   lub - dub   **lub - dub**   lub - dub   lub - dub

We call this early beat a **premature beat**. The basic heart rhythm is regular. But an occasional beat comes early. This is followed by a longer interval to the next beat. Then the following beats come in the regular rhythm. So the basic rhythm is normal. But in this rhythm an occasional beat comes too early.

Premature beats may be present because of a disease of the heart. But they can also be present when the heart is normal. So look for other signs of heart disease. If no other signs are present and the basic heart rhythm is regular, the heart is probably normal.

Irregular rhythm with breathing

In young persons the heart rhythm is sometimes irregular. This irregular rhythm changes with the breathing. The beats are fast during inspiration. They become slow during expiration. This rhythm is normal. It is not a sign of heart disease. Do not tell the young person that the heart rhythm is irregular.

Signs of heart disease

Completely irregular rhythm

A very irregular rhythm is a sign of serious heart disease. It is often fast and difficult to count. When the rhythm is very irregular, you will be unable to tap your foot with the heart rhythm.

When the heart rhythm is very irregular, many heart beats do not get to the radial artery. So when you take the pulse, you cannot count all of the beats. You can count the heart beats well only by listening to the heart with your stethoscope. In this case, the pulse rate at the wrist and the heart rate are different. The heart rate is fast but the pulse rate is slow. This is because many weak beats do not get to the wrist where you feel the pulse.

Heart murmurs

Heart murmurs are strange sounds that come between the lub - dubs. They are like the sound you make when you blow air across the opening of a bottle. The murmur comes with every beat. It may be a high sound or a low sound.

A heart murmur is a sign of disease. Most often it is a sign of a disease of one of the heart valves. The valve may be too large so that it cannot close well. The valve may be too small, and the blood has trouble going through the valve. Or the valve may have much scar tissue on it. In any case, the blood going through the diseased valve makes a noise, or murmur.

The valve disease makes the heart work harder to pump blood. This can cause heart failure after some months or years. Heart murmurs can also occur in other diseases like a disease of the heart muscle, or in severe anemia.

Heart failure

Certain diseases make the heart work harder. High blood pressure, a disease of the heart valves, severe anemia and severe infections make the heart work very hard. After some time the heart can no longer do all the work it must do. So the heart begins to "fail." We call this **heart failure**.

Heart failure causes certain changes in the circulation and in the body. These changes make signs which you can find in your examination. Look for these signs in every case of high blood pressure, heart valve disease, severe anemia and severe infection. These are the signs:

1. **Rapid pulse or rapid heart rate**, more than 100 beats per minute in an adult at rest.

2. **Rapid respirations**, often with difficult breathing.

3. **Crackles** in the lungs, especially at the base of the lungs. These crackles come from liquid or edema in the alveoli of the lungs.

4. **Dullness** on percussion at the bottom of the lungs. This is because there is edema liquid in the base of the lungs or in the pleural space around the lungs.

5. **Swelling**, or edema of the ankles, the legs, and sometimes of the abdomen and the face. When you push on this swollen tissue with your finger, your finger makes a hollow pit or depression. This pit goes away in a few seconds or minutes. We call this pitting edema. But push gently, for it may be painful.

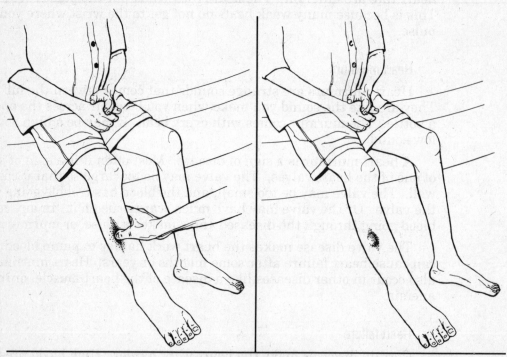

Swelling of the legs.

6. **Swelling of the abdomen** caused by edema liquid inside the abdomen. We call this **ascites**. Turn to page 110 to find out how to look for ascites.

7. **Big tender liver**. The liver becomes big and tender because there is swelling or edema in the liver.

8. **Big spleen**, also because of edema.

9. **Swollen veins in the neck**. Swollen neck veins can occur because of heart failure. But they can also be normal. So you must find out if swollen veins in a patient are normal or a sign of heart failure.

Ask the patient to sit up. Look carefully at the swollen veins in the neck. Put your finger on a vein at the top of the neck under the chin. Press on it to close it and hold your finger on it.

With a finger of your other hand, press on this vein from just below your other finger down to the clavicle. This will make the vein become empty of blood and therefore flat. Now take off your bottom finger.

If the vein fills with blood from the clavicle up toward the neck, this is a sign of heart failure. But if the vein remains empty and flat, then the swelling of the vein is normal. It is not a sign of heart disease.

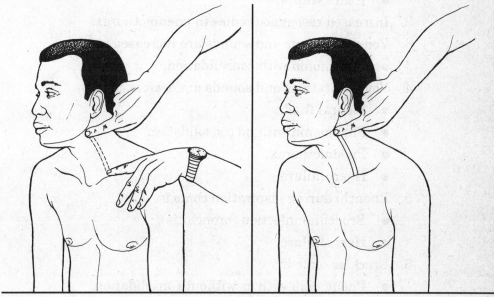

Swollen veins in the neck.

A patient with heart failure may have three or four of the above signs but not the others. A patient with pneumonia may have crackles but not dullness or changes in the voice vibrations or sounds. A patient with a small infection of tuberculosis may have normal lung sounds.

Also, different diseases can give the same signs. Tuberculosis can sometimes look like pneumonia. Heart failure can sometimes look like asthma.

So you must be very careful in making a diagnosis of a disease of the lungs, the heart, or the pleural space.

1. Always take a good history. Take note of every symptom.
2. Do a careful and complete physical exam.
3. Do the necessary laboratory exams.
4. Follow the strategies of each important symptom and sign.

In this way you will find out all you can about the disease of your patient. You will be able to make the right diagnosis.

SUMMARY

1. Dullness comes in:
   - Pleural fluid from edema, infection, pus, or blood.
   - Pneumonia with consolidation.
   - Heart failure.
2. Increased resonance comes in pneumothorax.
3. Voice vibrations and sounds are increased in:
   - Pneumonia with consolidation.
4. Voice vibrations and sounds are decreased in:
   - Pleural fluid.
   - Pneumonia with no consolidation.
   - Pneumothorax.
   - Heart failure.
5. Rhonchi during inspiration come in:
   - Bronchial infection (bronchitis).
   - Heart failure.
6. Crackles come in:
   - Pneumonia with or without consolidation.
   - Tuberculosis, usually near the top of the lungs.
   - Heart failure, especially at the base of the lungs.
7. Heart murmurs come in:
   - Diseases of the heart valves or muscle.
   - Severe anemia.

Questions for study

1. What signs of disease can you find by observation of the chest?
2. What signs of disease can you find by palpation of the chest?
3. What signs of disease can you find by percussion of the chest?
4. What signs indicate fluid in the pleural space?
5. What signs indicate infection in the lungs?
6. What do crackles mean?
7. What signs can you find in the chest in heart failure?
8. What do you hear in the lungs in asthma?
9. What are all the signs of disease to look for when you examine the heart?
10. Heart failure can give nine different signs. What is the reason why heart failure can cause each one of these signs?

3.3.8 The abdomen

We divide the abdomen into four different regions by drawing two straight lines. One line is vertical, or up and down. It goes down the middle of the abdomen from the bottom of the sternum through the umbilicus to the pubic bone. The other line is horizontal. It goes across the abdomen at the level of the umbilicus.

Each part of the abdomen is called a quadrant. This means a "quarter" or one fourth. There are four quadrants.

1. **The right upper quadrant**.

2. **The left upper quadrant**.

3. **The right lower quadrant**.

4. **The left lower quadrant**.

We also sometimes talk about other regions.

1. The **epigastric region**, which is in the middle just below the bottom of the sternum.

2. The **umbilical region**, which is the area around the umbilicus or navel.

There are many important organs in the abdomen. These are the stomach, the small and large intestines, the liver, the spleen and the pelvic organs.

You must know the anatomy of the abdomen very well. You must know where each of these organs is. You must know where a patient feels pain coming from a disease of each different organ. This figure shows you the place where the patient feels pain coming from each one of the important organs in the abdomen.

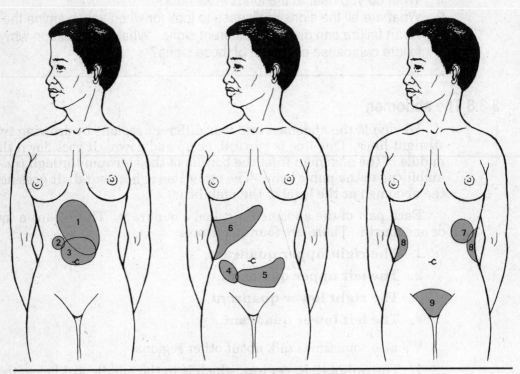

Areas of pain in the abdomen.

Observation

The patient must lie flat on his back on the examining table or on the bed. His arms must be at his sides and not up by his head. Tell the patient to bend his legs at the knees. This will help the muscles of the abdomen to relax.

Make sure that a good light falls on the abdomen. This is essential. It will permit you to look very carefully for signs of disease. Look especially for these signs:

A big abdomen

There are four possible reasons for the abdomen to become very big or "distended."

1. Much **fat**. The patient is "obese." There will be much fat in other places as well - chest, arms, legs.

2. **Liquid** in the abdomen. This can come in diseases of the heart, the liver, the kidneys, or in malnutrition, anemia, or peritonitis.

3. Much **gas** in the intestines.

4. In a woman, a **pregnancy**.

A thin abdomen

This can be normal. Or it can come from malnutrition or a serious disease like tuberculosis, cancer or diabetes.

A big organ, a mass, or a tumor

This may be one of these things.

1. **A big liver**.
2. **A big spleen**.
3. **A full bladder**.
4. **A pregnancy**.
5. **A tumor**.

Waves of peristalsis in the intestines

There are regular waves of contraction which move down the intestines. We call these **peristaltic waves**. These waves of contraction are very important for the digestion of our food. They push the food down through the intestines. A wave of peristalsis comes every few minutes. Normally, you cannot see these waves. Sometimes, however, in a very thin patient, you can see the normal waves of peristalsis.

If there is a block, or obstruction, in the intestines, the intestines become very full of liquid and gas. The waves of peristalsis become very strong. Now you can see these waves very clearly. They move from one side of the abdomen to the other. They give the patient much pain as they move.

Movements of respiration

Normally the front wall of the abdomen moves out when the patient breathes in. This is because the diaphragm moves down during inspiration. The diaphragm is the big thin muscle between the lungs and the abdomen. As it moves down, it pushes the organs in the abdomen down. This pushes the front wall of the abdomen out. When the patient breathes out, the wall of the abdomen then goes back in.

In an infection of the inside of the abdomen, called **peritonitis**, the patient has much pain in the abdomen. Every movement causes pain. The wall of the abdomen now will not move during respiration. The patient will breathe only with the chest muscles. So in a patient with much pain in the abdomen, look very carefully at the abdomen. See if the abdomen moves out and in with breathing. If the abdomen is rigid and does not move with breathing, the patient probably has peritonitis.

Palpation

How to palpate the abdomen

Now you are ready to feel the abdomen. Tell the patient to lie on his back and bend his legs at the knees and to keep his arms at his sides. This will help make the muscles of the abdomen soft. The patient must try to relax the abdominal muscles and keep them soft while you feel the abdomen. Then you can palpate the abdomen easily.

If possible, examine the abdomen of the patient from the right side. Your arm must be on the same level as his abdomen. If the table or the bed is low, sit down, or else kneel on the floor. This will permit you to examine the abdomen gently.

Ask the patient where he feels pain. Start palpating on the side of the abdomen where there is no pain. Then move slowly to the part where there is pain. This will gain the confidence of the patient. It will help the patient to stay relaxed.

Push very gently on all parts of the abdomen. Push with the flat part of your hands. Do not push only with the tips of your fingers. Do not push strongly at first. If you push strongly at first, the patient will feel pain. The abdominal muscles will then contract and become rigid. You will be unable to find signs of disease. So always be VERY GENTLE.

Talk to the patient while you are examining the abdomen. This will help him to relax because he will be thinking about other things. You will then be able to feel more signs of disease.

First, feel gently all parts of the abdomen. Note if the muscles are soft and relaxed or if they are contracted and rigid. Rigid contracted muscles in the abdomen are a sign of inflammation in that part of the abdomen. Note exactly where the muscles are rigid and contracted.

After you have felt everywhere gently, you can then push harder. You will be able to feel more deeply. You can feel the parts of the abdomen that are deep inside.

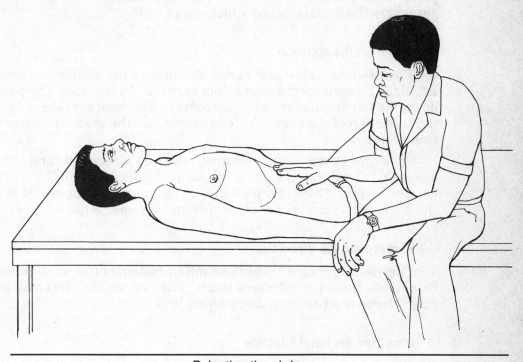

Palpating the abdomen.

SUMMARY

1. Be gentle.
2. Tell the patient to relax the abdominal muscles and make them soft.
3. Tell the patient to bend his legs and keep his arms at his sides.
4. Palpate with your whole hand and not just with your fingers.
5. Make sure your arm is on the same level as the patient's abdomen.
6. Feel first where there is no pain.
7. Feel gently every part of the abdomen first to note where there is pain.
8. Only then, push more strongly to feel the deeper parts of the abdomen.

Signs to look for in the abdomen by palpation

Tenderness

Pain in the abdomen on palpation is a sign of disease. Pain on palpation we call **tenderness**. Most often it is a sign of inflammation or of infection.

Each organ in the abdomen causes pain and tenderness in a certain place. Find out exactly where the patient is tender. This will help you find out where the disease is and which organ is ill.

Pain from the stomach

This is in the upper part of the abdomen in the middle and often to the left side. Sometimes the stomach is very big. In this case, the pain may go down the left side as far as the iliac crest. Tenderness is the only sign of inflammation of the stomach. You cannot feel the stomach unless there is a tumor in it.

Sometimes there is an inflammation or an ulcer at the end of the stomach, the pyloric end. Or it can be at the beginning of the small intestine, the duodenum. This gives pain in the right upper quadrant. It is just below the liver. This pain is in a small spot and the spot is quite tender.

Pain around the umbilicus

This usually means there is an inflammation of the small intestine. Sometimes there is tenderness there. But you can feel the small intestine only if there is a tumor or much liquid in it.

Pain from the large intestine

This pain is sometimes in the lower abdomen, across the low part. A disease of the appendix or at the beginning of the large intestine, the "cecum," causes pain and tenderness in the right lower quadrant. This is a little above the right inguinal ligament. A disease in the left part of the large intestine causes pain in the left lower quadrant.

Pain in the right upper quadrant

This comes most often from the liver. It can also come from the **gall bladder**. Feel carefully for the liver. Is it tender? Hit gently the lower right side of the chest. If the liver is inflamed, this will cause pain.

Pain in the left upper quadrant

Often this comes from the **spleen**. Feel carefully for the spleen. Hit gently the lower left side of the chest to see if the spleen is tender.

However, pain in the right upper quadrant or in the left upper quadrant can also come from a disease in the **lungs**. So look carefully for signs of lung disease.

Pain in the flank and back

Pain here comes often from the **kidneys**. Push gently on the flank. Hit the flank gently as well. Look for other signs of kidney disease by doing a careful examination of the urine.

Pain in the lower part of the abdomen in a woman

This pain can come from a disease in the **pelvic organs**: the uterus, the tubes, the ovaries. It can also come from a disease of the **bladder**. Feel for tenderness and also for a mass.

Infection or bleeding inside the abdomen can also cause pain in the lower abdomen. Look for signs of infection and of anemia. Be sure to examine the urine.

Pain in the lower part of the abdomen in a man

This pain can come from an inflammation of the **prostate gland** or from the **bladder**. Always do a rectal exam and a good examination of the urine.

Pain in the lower part of the abdomen in both men and women

Arthritis of the lower back can cause pain in the lower abdomen in a man or a woman. We call this "radiated" pain because it "radiates" from the back. The pain is worse when the patient bends forward or lifts a heavy load. But there is no tenderness in the abdomen. So examine the back carefully in any patient with pain in the lower abdomen.

For any patient with pain in the abdomen, follow the strategies on pain in the abdomen on pages 364 and 370.

Severe pain and tenderness in the abdomen

These are signs of serious disease. They can come from a serious infection, or from bleeding inside the abdomen. The muscles of the abdomen are hard and rigid. The patient has much tenderness when you palpate the abdomen.

Rebound tenderness

There is one very important sign to look for in a painful abdomen. Press gently on the abdomen with your hand. Then take your hand off the abdomen very quickly. If the patient cries with pain when you take off your hand quickly, the patient has **rebound tenderness**.

This is a sign of a severe inflammation of the lining of the abdomen. We call it "peritonitis." It can come from a serious infection inside the abdomen or from bleeding inside the abdomen.

In this case look for signs of infection: fever and a high white blood cell count. Look also for signs of anemia: low blood pressure, rapid thready pulse, pale color of the mucus membranes, and a low hemoglobin. Do also a rectal exam to feel for tenderness.

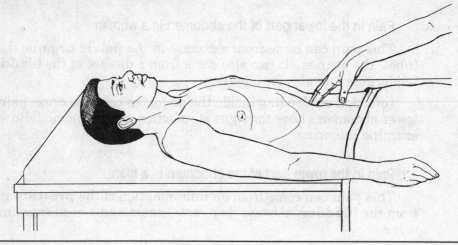

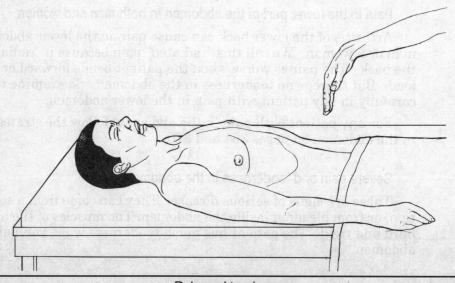

Rebound tenderness.

Liver and gall bladder

The normal liver

The liver is in the right upper quadrant. It is behind the lower ribs. Normally you cannot feel it. The liver moves down when the patient takes a big breath. This is because the diaphragm moves down when the patient breathes in. The diaphragm pushes the liver and the spleen down with it.

Before feeling for the liver, percuss on the right lower chest for liver dullness. Continue percussing down into the right upper quadrant. See how far down the liver dullness goes. This will give you an idea of how big the liver is. Put a mark on the skin at the lower edge of liver dullness.

To feel the liver, put your hand flat on the right upper quadrant below the edge of liver dullness. Feel for the lower edge of the liver with the tips of your fingers. The lower edge of the normal liver goes in the same direction as the lower edge of the rib cage.

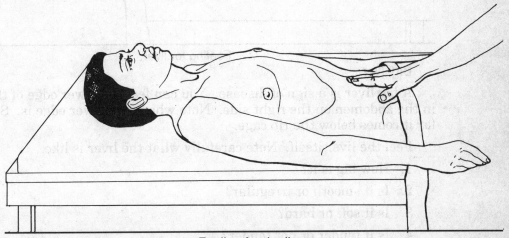

Feeling for the liver.

Tell the patient to take a deep breath. You can usually feel the edge of the liver move down. You can feel this with your finger tips. Note what the edge of the liver is like.

1. Is it smooth or irregular?
2. Is the edge sharp or round?
3. Is it tender or not?

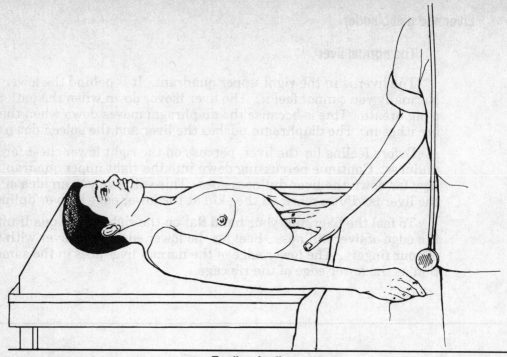

Feeling for liver.

Big liver

A big liver is a sign of disease. You can feel the lower edge of the liver in the abdomen on the right side. Note where the lower edge is. See how far it comes below the rib cage.

Feel the liver itself. Note carefully what the liver is like.

1. How big is it?

2. Is it smooth or irregular?

3. Is it soft or hard?

4. Is it tender or not tender?

A hard irregular liver comes in cirrhosis. If the liver is big and tender, the patient may have hepatitis, a virus disease of the liver. Look for signs of hepatitis: fever and jaundice. Or the cause could be heart failure. So look for signs of heart failure. See page 94.

A big lump in the liver is probably a liver tumor. But it could be an abscess. So look for signs of infection: fever, much tenderness, and a high white blood cell count.

Write down a good description of the liver on the patient's record. If the liver is big, follow the strategy BIG LIVER on page 512. If the patient has jaundice, follow the strategy JAUNDICE on page 526.

Gall bladder

The gall bladder is a small sack filled with liquid, the bile. It is under the middle of the liver. Normally you cannot feel it. But sometimes the gall bladder becomes big and inflamed. Then you can feel it. It is a small, round, tender mass just below the middle of the edge of the liver. It moves down when the liver moves down.

SUMMARY

If the liver is big, take note of these things.

1. How big is it?

2. Is it smooth or irregular?

3. Is it soft or hard?

4. Is it tender or not?

5. Is there is a big lump in it? If so, is it tender?

6. Are there signs of infection?

7. Is there jaundice, or signs of heart failure?

The spleen

The spleen is in the left upper quadrant. It is behind the lower left ribs. When the spleen is normal you cannot feel it.

Feel for it as you feel for the liver. Place your hand flat on the left side of the abdomen. Your fingers should be pointed toward the patient's head. Tell the patient to take a deep breath. Feel for the tip of the spleen. It will move down when the patient takes in a deep breath.

If it is very big, you can feel it as a round mass under the left ribs. It moves down when the patient takes a big breath.

A big spleen comes often from frequent attacks of malaria. It can also come in sickle cell anemia, in heart failure, in some other infections, or in certain tumors. If you can feel the spleen, write down how big it is.

The next drawing shows you how to tell how big it is.

> \+ when you can just feel the end of the spleen during a deep breath.

> ++ when you feel the end of the spleen even with no deep breath.

> +++ when the end of the spleen is at the level of the umbilicus.

> ++++ when the end of the spleen is below the level of the umbilicus.

> +++++ when the end of the spleen is below the level of the iliac crest.

In a patient with a big spleen, follow the strategy BIG SPLEEN on page 536.

REMEMBER:

The liver and the spleen move down when the patient breathes in.

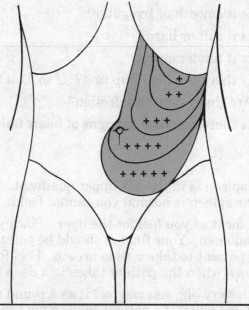

Big spleen.

Stomach and intestines

Normally it is impossible to feel the stomach and the intestines. However, in thin persons there is often a small lump in the left lower quadrant a little above the inguinal ligament. This lump is not tender and it moves a little when you push on it. It is the sigmoid part of the large intestine. It is normal and is not a sign of disease.

Masses (lumps)

A big mass or lump in the abdomen is probably a sign of a serious disease. Find out where it is, how big it is, if it moves when the patient breathes or when you push on it, and if it is tender or not.

In the right upper quadrant

A big mass which moves down when the patient breathes in is the liver.

In the left upper quadrant

A mass which moves down when the patient breathes in is the spleen.

In the upper part of the abdomen

A mass which does not move down when the patient breathes in is probably a tumor of the stomach, the intestines, or even the pancreas.

In the flank

A mass which does not move when the patient breathes is probably in the kidney.

In the lower part of the abdomen in a woman

A big mass may be a pregnancy or a tumor of the uterus or of an ovary.

In the lower abdomen

A big mass may be a full bladder. Tell the patient to urinate. If the mass goes away, it was a full bladder.

Many small masses in the abdomen

They may be big lymph nodes. Follow the strategy BIG LYMPH NODES on page 550.

Fecal matter or tumor

Sometimes you can feel a lump or lumps of fecal matter in the abdomen, especially in the left lower quadrant. Fecal matter in the abdomen is normal. It usually does not require treatment.

Perhaps you cannot be sure if this is fecal matter or a sign of disease. In this case, give the patient an enema. Examine him after he has passed stools. If the lump or lumps have changed or gone, you know they were simply fecal matter. But if the lump or lumps are the same, it is a sign of disease - a tumor, or lymph nodes. Send the patient to hospital.

REMEMBER:

For any mass in the abdomen, find out:

- Where it is.
- How big it is.
- If it moves when the patient breathes or when you push on it.
- If it is tender or not.

Percussion

Gas

Air or gas makes a resonant sound on percussion. Normally there is some air in the stomach and intestines. So there is normally resonance in some parts of the abdomen.

Some diseases cause much air to come into the intestines, like obstruction of the intestines or peritonitis. There is also much air in the intestines in the condition we call ileus. We will talk about ileus under auscultation. In these diseases, or in ileus, there will be resonance in all or almost all of the abdomen. The abdomen will also be big, or swollen.

Liquid

Liquid comes into the abdomen in many diseases. We call liquid inside the abdomen ascites. Ascites comes in diseases of the heart, the liver, the kidneys, in malnutrition, in anemia, and in peritonitis. The abdomen becomes big or swollen. Percussion will show you if there is ascites in the abdomen.

Percuss the abdomen like you percuss the chest. With the patient lying down on the back, percuss across the abdomen. Note where there is resonance and where there is dullness.

If there is much ascites, or liquid, there will be some resonance around the umbilicus. But there will be dullness on the sides and in the flanks. This is because the gas in the intestines makes the intestines float, or stay on top of the liquid. The intestines with gas will therefore be just inside the umbilicus.

Make a mark on the skin of the patient's abdomen where the percussion sound changes from resonance to dullness. Now turn the patient on one side. Percuss again. Make a mark where the sound changes from resonance to dullness.

If there is much ascites, the place where the sound changes will move as the patient turns. This is because the liquid always moves to the low part. The intestines stay on the top. We call this **shifting dullness**.

Look at the marks you have made on the skin, the mark when the patient is on his back, and the mark with him on one side. If the two marks are close together, there is little or no ascites. But if the marks are a few centimeters apart, he has ascites. If he has ascites, follow the strategy ASCITES on page 516.

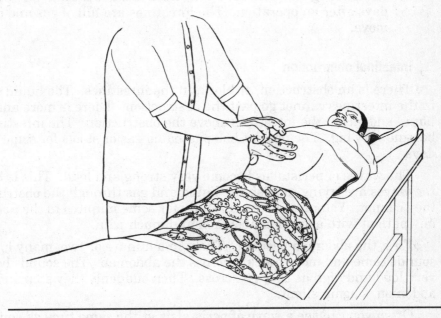

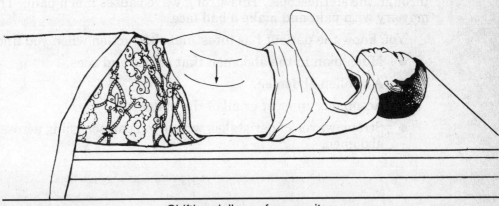

Shifting dullness from ascites.

Auscultation

Listen to the abdomen through your stethoscope. Listen to the sounds of the waves of peristalsis. They make a quiet sound, like water running in a small river. They come and go every few seconds. They come and go all the time, day and night. But they change in certain diseases.

Ileus

In this case there are no waves of peristalsis. The abdomen is silent because the intestines do not move. Ileus comes in:

1. **Peritonitis**, a very serious infection inside the abdomen.
2. **After a big abdominal operation**. This is normal for two or three days after an operation. The intestines are full of gas and do not move.

Intestinal obstruction

There is an obstruction, or block, in the intestines. The liquid and gas in the intestines cannot go past the obstruction. There is more and more liquid and gas in the intestines above the obstruction. The intestines become very big. The patient has passed no gas or stools for some hours or days.

The waves of peristalsis become very strong and loud. This is because the waves are trying to push the liquid and gas through the obstruction, but they cannot. You must listen carefully for some minutes to the abdomen of any patient with a swollen abdomen and much pain.

First the abdomen is silent. Then, in a minute or two, many loud sounds come and move quickly across the abdomen. The sounds become very loud and high as they go across. Then suddenly they stop and the abdomen is again silent.

Often you can see a wave of peristalsis at the same time as you hear it through the stethoscope. This strong wave causes much pain. The patient may cry with pain and make a bad face.

You know the patient has intestinal obstruction when you find:

- Much pain in the abdomen that comes and goes.
- A swollen abdomen.
- Resonance in most or all of the abdomen.
- Strong waves of peristalsis which you can see going across the abdomen.

- Loud sounds of peristalsis which come when you see the waves and when the patient feels much pain.
- The patient has passed no stools or gas for some hours or days.

This is a very serious disease. The patient needs an operation immediately. Send the patient quickly to hospital.

3.3.9 Hernia

Simple hernia

A hernia is a small sack of peritoneum which comes out through the muscles of the abdomen. It makes a soft swelling under the skin. This swelling comes when the patient stands, pushes hard, or coughs. This is because an organ inside the abdomen goes into the sack. The organ may be a loop of intestine.

The swelling goes away when the patient lies down or when you or the patient push on it gently. This means that the organ in the sack has gone back into the abdomen. We say that the hernia is now **reduced**.

A simple hernia is a swelling under the skin around the abdomen that comes and goes. It can be reduced easily. Normally a hernia causes little pain and is not tender. A hernia is a surgical disease. The patient needs an operation. The patient must go to hospital.

Kinds of hernia

There are four places where a hernia can come.

In the inguinal region

This is the most common place for a hernia. The swelling is a little above the middle of the inguinal ligament. It may be very small. Or it may go down into the scrotum of a man or into the vulva of a woman. We call this an **inguinal hernia**.

In the middle line of the abdomen

The middle vertical line of the abdomen is somewhat weak. A hernia can come somewhere in this line. It may come in the epigastric region and form an **epigastric hernia**. Or it may come at the umbilicus and form an **umbilical hernia**.

In an old surgical incision

We call this an **incisional hernia**.

In the flank, in the back

It is just under the back of the rib cage and to the side of the big back muscles. We call this a **lumbar hernia**.

Examining for hernia

Have the patient stand in front of you. Look at the place where the swelling comes. Tell the patient to take a big breath and push down hard. Or have him cough. See if a swelling comes when he does this. If it does, push gently on it to see if it will go away or reduce. If it does, it is a hernia.

Now put your fingers on the place where the swelling comes. Tell the patient to push or cough. Feel for a swelling coming under your finger tips. If a swelling comes, push gently on it to see if it will reduce. If it does, it is a hernia.

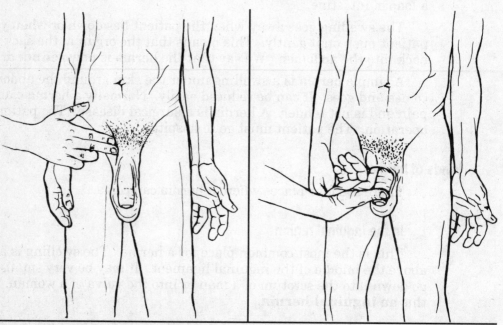

Feeling for hernia at inguinal ring.   Feeling for hernia inside scrotum.

A small inguinal hernia may be hard to find. In this case, in a man, put your index finger on the side of the scrotum. Push it gently up into the inguinal canal. Tell the patient to push or cough. Even if the hernia is very small, you can find it this way.

Strangulated hernia

A hernia may suddenly become **strangulated**. This means that the hernia is swollen but the swelling cannot go away. It is "stuck." It cannot be reduced.

The hernia is very painful and tender. The abdomen becomes swollen and often the patient has much vomiting. The patient develops signs of intestinal obstruction. The swelling is quite hard. It will not go away when you push gently on it. But NEVER push hard on it. This is an emergency. Send the patient quickly to hospital for an operation.

SUMMARY

1. A hernia is soft, not hard.
2. The hernia swelling comes when the patient stands, pushes, or coughs.
3. The hernia goes away, or reduces, when you or the patient pushes on it.
4. A simple hernia causes little or no pain and no tenderness.
5. A hernia that has much pain and tenderness and will not reduce is strangulated. Send such a patient immediately to hospital.
6. Do not push on a strangulated hernia.

Questions for study

1. What kinds of disease can you find by looking at the abdomen?
2. If the abdomen is very big, what signs must you look for to find out why the abdomen is very big?
3. If the abdomen is tender, what other signs must you look for?
4. What organs give pain in the upper abdomen?
5. What organs give pain in the lower abdomen?
6. To palpate the abdomen, in what position must you put the patient?
7. What rules must you follow to palpate the abdomen well?
8. If the liver is big, what things must you describe about it? What other signs of disease must you look for?
9. What are the signs of a severe infection in the abdomen?
10. If there is a mass in the abdomen, what must you find out about it?
11. How can you tell if a patient has ascites?
12. What are the signs of peritonitis?
13. What are the signs of intestinal obstruction?
14. Where are the places to look for a hernia?
15. How can you tell a hernia from another kind of swelling under the skin, like a fatty tumor?

3.3.10 Lymph nodes

There are lymph nodes in many parts of the body. Normally they are very small and impossible to feel. Big lymph nodes are a sign of an infection or a tumor. When there is an infection or tumor, the lymph nodes in that part of the body become big.

Size and pain of nodes

1. In an **acute infection**, the nodes are big and tender. There may also be a fever.

2. In **tuberculosis** and in **chronic skin infections**, the nodes are big. They are often in a group and are "stuck" together. They give little pain and sometimes no pain. Often they have been present for some weeks or months.

3. In a **tumor**, the nodes are big, hard, and not painful. Often they are "stuck" together in a group.

4. In **filariasis**, the nodes may be big. They are often in a group and may or may not be painful or tender.

5. In **African sleeping sickness (trypanosomiasis)**, the nodes are in a line or series going down the back of the neck. They are quite small and are not painful.

Location of lymph nodes

Look for big lymph nodes in all of these places:

1. In the back of the head. These come from diseases of the skin of the head.

2. In the neck. See page 77.

3. Under the armpits. These come from diseases on the arms or hands, on the chest, or in the breast.

4. In the inguinal region. These come from diseases of the feet, the legs, the buttocks, or the genital organs.

5. In the femoral region. These come from diseases of the feet or legs.

6. In the iliac region. These lymph nodes are inside the abdomen. They are a little above the inguinal ligament and are fixed to it. You cannot move them. They are just to the outside of the iliac artery. You can feel the pulse in this artery at the middle of the inguinal ligament. Big iliac nodes are a sign of disease in the abdomen or in the pelvic organs. Often they come from tuberculosis.

7. Inside the abdomen. You can feel these nodes as you palpate the abdomen. Often there are many of them. You can move them a little when you push on them.

In a patient with big lymph nodes, follow the strategy BIG LYMPH NODES on page 550.

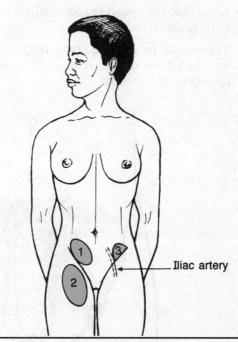

Iliac artery

Lymph nodes in lower abdomen.

3.3.11 The male organs

Observation

Penis

Look on the penis for sores, ulcers, or tumors. Be sure to look carefully under the foreskin on the end of the penis.

1. Small sores that itch may be scabies or pubic lice.

2. A sore that is very painful is an acute infection.

3. A round, raised sore or ulcer that is not painful may be the first, or primary, sore of syphilis. We call this a **chancre**.

4. A sore on the penis of an older man that grows big may be a tumor, or cancer. It will not go away after treatment by antibiotics. Send a man with such a sore to hospital.

Scrotum

Look at the scrotum.

1. Small sores that itch are probably scabies or pubic lice.
2. Look also for small insects called lice. They also make small sores with much itching.
3. There may be a large spot on the scrotum that itches. Often this spot is between the scrotum and the leg. It is probably a fungus infection of the skin.

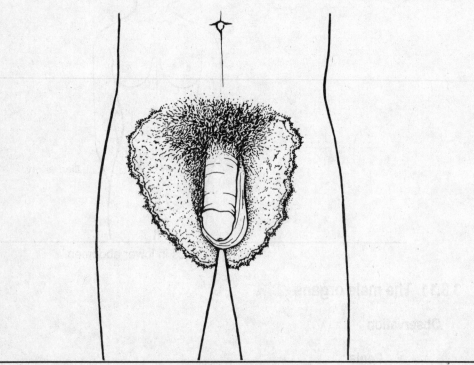

Fungus infection in genital area.

Palpation

Penis

Look in the opening of the penis for liquid. A liquid like milk is a sign of gonorrhea. Put a rubber or plastic glove on your hand. Hold the penis at the top, or base. Squeeze gently on the penis from the place where it is joined to the body down to the end. If there is liquid or pus in the urine canal, it will come out as you do this.

Put a drop of the liquid on a microscope slide. Look at it under the microscope to look for white blood cells. If possible, do a gram stain and look for the bacteria of gonorrhea. These are small round red bacteria in pairs. They are INSIDE the white blood cells. If the bacteria are not inside the white blood cells, they are not the bacteria of gonorrhea.

But be careful! Always put on a glove before examining the penis and the scrotum. This will protect you from getting a disease like syphilis or AIDS.

Scrotum

1. Feel gently the testicle and the cord that comes down to it from the inguinal region. This is the "spermatic cord." Sometimes the veins of the spermatic cord are very thick. They feel like worms, but cause no pain. This is a **varicocele**. It does not need treatment.

2. A **hydrocele** is a big swelling around the testicle with no pain. It is full of liquid. It will not go away when the patient lies down or when you push on it. You cannot feel the testicle because the testicle is inside the hydrocele. If you hold a strong light from a torch against the back of the hydrocele, you can often see some light coming through the hydrocele.

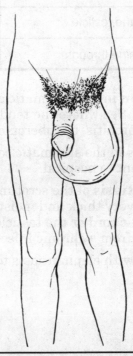

A big inguinal hernia.

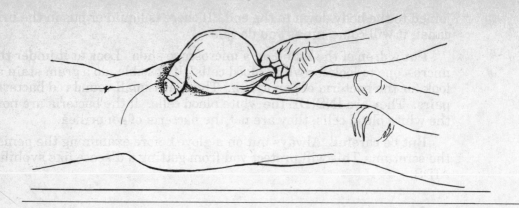

Testicle outside of hernia sack.

3. An **inguinal hernia** often comes down into the scrotum. It makes a big mass in the scrotum. But it is different from a hydrocele. This is how you can tell a hernia from a hydrocele:

Hernia	Hydrocele
Can be reduced	Will not reduce
Does not include the testicle	Includes the testicle
Will not let light shine through	Will let light shine through

4. An **infection** in the spermatic cord or testicle causes pain and tenderness. See where the tenderness is. The patient may have gonorrhea, orchitis, or tuberculosis.

5. A hard mass in the spermatic cord or testicle may be a tumor. Send such a patient to hospital.

6. In **elephantiasis** of the scrotum, the scrotum becomes very big. The skin is very thick and moist, with many folds. You cannot feel the spermatic cord or the testicle inside. Elephantiasis comes from filariasis or from a chronic infection of the inguinal lymph nodes.

Send a patient with elephantiasis to the doctor.

3.3.12 The rectal exam

Reasons for doing a rectal exam

1. Blood in the fecal matter.
2. Constipation for a long time.
3. Pain in the rectum.
4. Pain in the lower part of the back.
5. Pain in the lower part of the abdomen.
6. Diarrhea for a long time.
7. Difficulty on urination or a block in the urine.
8. Blood in the urine.
9. Hemorrhoids.

Position of the patient

There are three positions in which you can put the patient. Put the patient in the position that makes it easy for the patient and also easy for you to do the examination.

1. On his side on the table or bed, with his knees bent.
2. On his back on the table or bed, with his legs bent at the knees and spread apart.
3. Standing on the floor and bending forward over the table or bed. His legs must be straight, but spread apart.

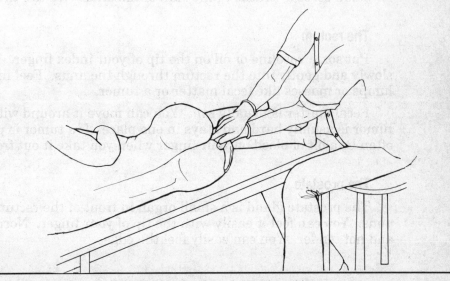

Rectal examination. Lateral position.

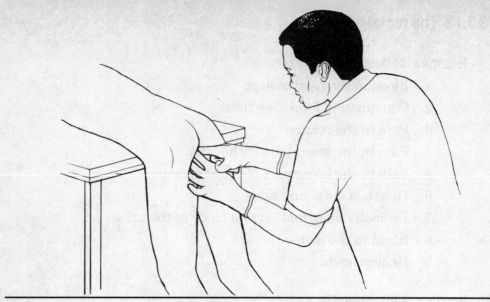

Rectal examination. Upright position.

Technique of the examination

The anus and buttocks

Put a glove on your hand. Push the buttocks apart. Look at the skin of the buttocks for sores, swellings, or small openings from which pus comes.

Look carefully at the opening or "anus." Look for small swellings called **hemorrhoids**. These are small swellings at the edge of the anus. Look also for small sores or cracks in the skin of the anus. We call these **fissures**.

The rectum

Put some vaseline or oil on the tip of your index finger. Push your finger slowly and gently into the rectum through the anus. Feel inside for any lumps or masses like fecal matter or a tumor.

Fecal matter is usually soft. You can move it around with your finger. A tumor is usually hard and stays in one place. If a tumor is present, there will often be a bit of blood on your finger when you take it out from the rectum.

The prostate

The prostate gland is a small organ in front of the rectum just inside the anus. You can feel it easily with the tip of your finger. Normally it is smooth and not tender. You can easily feel the edges.

See if the prostate is tender. Tenderness is a sign of infection in the prostate. See if it is big. A big prostate can cause difficulty on urination and even a blockage of the urine. A man with a big prostate gland must go to the doctor right away.

Practice doing rectal exams

Doing a good rectal exam requires practice and experience. Do a rectal exam on many of your patients. Do also a rectal exam on some of your fellow students. This will show you what a normal prostate is like.

Also, let a fellow student do a rectal exam on you. You will then learn how a rectal exam feels. This will help you know better how a patient feels during the rectal exam. Always wash your hands carefully after doing a rectal exam.

Questions for study

1. What diseases can cause big lymph nodes?
2. How can you tell which disease is probably causing the big lymph nodes?
3. What diseases can come on the penis?
4. What diseases can come in the scrotum? Make a list of the signs of each of these diseases.
5. How can you tell if a mass in the scrotum is a hernia or a hydrocele?
6. What are all of the reasons for doing a rectal exam?
7. For each reason, what are the signs to look for? What are the diseases to look for?

3.3.13 The female organs

Diseases of the female organs are often difficult to diagnose. A woman who has a disease of these organs should go to the doctor. But you can diagnose some diseases of the female organs by their signs and symptoms.

Liquid coming from the vagina

Many women have liquid coming from the vagina. We call this **leucorrhea**.

1. Liquid coming during pregnancy is usually normal.
2. The liquid may be urine. In this case there is an opening, or **fistula**, between the bladder and the vagina. This fistula has probably come because of a long and difficult delivery.

3. Liquid which is thick, white, and causes itching may come from a **fungus infection**. Or it may come from an infection caused by a parasite that we call **trichomonas**.

4. Liquid which is white like milk probably comes from **gonorrhea**.

Put a drop of the liquid on a microscope slide. Look at it under the microscope. Look for trichomonas or for fungus. Trichomonas are small single-cell parasites that move quite rapidly in the liquid.

If possible, do a gram stain of the liquid. Look for the bacteria of gonorrhea. They are small round red bacteria in pairs. They are INSIDE white blood cells or epithelial cells.

Swelling coming from the vagina

There are muscles around the vagina which hold the bladder and the uterus in their places. After many deliveries these muscles may become weak. They can no longer hold the bladder or the uterus in place. So a woman who has many children may have a swelling which comes out of the vagina. This swelling comes when she stands up or coughs. The swelling can be a:

1. **Cystocele** when the front wall of the vagina comes down and out of the vagina. Often a woman with a cystocele has trouble holding her urine in the bladder. A little comes out when she stands, pushes, or coughs.

2. **Rectocele** when the back wall of the vagina comes down and out of the vagina.

3. **Prolapse** of the uterus when the uterus itself comes down and out of the vagina.

Sometimes a woman has two, or all three, of these swellings together. The treatment for each one is a surgical operation. The woman must go to hospital.

Tumors

A tumor can develop in the uterus or in one of the ovaries. Often you can feel this tumor by palpation of the lower abdomen. This requires a surgical operation. Send the woman to hospital.

Change of monthly periods

Many women have irregular monthly periods. Some have pain with their periods. Others may have bleeding between their monthly periods. Send these women to the doctor.

Older women normally stop having monthly periods. We call this the **menopause**. But an older woman who has stopped having periods may again have bleeding from the vagina. This is very serious. She may have a tumor of the uterus. Send her immediately to the doctor.

REMEMBER:

A woman with bleeding after the menopause probably has a very serious tumor. Send her immediately to the doctor.

A woman who has no periods

A woman who has no periods has **amenorrhea**. A woman normally has amenorrhea during pregnancy. She may have amenorrhea while she is breast-feeding her baby. Monthly periods can also stop because of a serious disease.

A young woman with amenorrhea who is not pregnant and not breast-feeding may have a serious disease. Look for signs of a chronic disease, or for signs of malnutrition. If you cannot find out why she has amenorrhea, send her to the doctor.

Much pain and tenderness

A woman who has much pain and tenderness in the lower abdomen, with rebound pain, has a very serious disease.

1. If she has signs of infection, like fever and a high white blood cell count, she probably has **peritonitis**.

2. If she has anemia and no fever, she probably has a pregnancy out-side the uterus. We call this an **ectopic pregnancy**. This ectopic pregnancy causes bleeding inside the abdomen. The woman may be in shock. Send her immediately to hospital for an operation.

3.3.14 Pregnancy

Signs of pregnancy

Pregnant mothers will often come to you for an examination and for help. You must be able to tell if a woman is pregnant or not. These are the most important signs of pregnancy.

1. The woman has amenorrhea for one or more months. Try to find out the day when her last normal period began. This will help you know how many months the pregnancy is. It will also help you know about what date she will deliver her baby.

2. The breasts grow and become full and sometimes a little painful.

3. Often there is vomiting, or the desire to vomit, especially in the early morning.

4. A round smooth swelling in the lower abdomen comes after two months. It grows a little each month. This swelling is the pregnancy. The size of the pregnancy will show you how many months the pregnancy is.

5. After five months you can feel the baby move inside the pregnancy. You can also hear the heart beat of the baby inside the uterus with a special stethoscope.

Measure the size of the pregnancy with a tape measure. Put the zero line of the tape measure on the top edge of the middle of the pubic bone. Palpate the pregnancy with your other hand. Find the very top of the pregnancy. With the tape measure, see how many centimeters this is above the pubic bone. Table 3 shows you the age of the pregnancy in months for the number of centimeters between the top of the pubic bone and the top of the pregnancy.

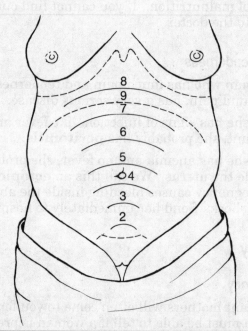

Size of pregnancy in months.

Table 3 - Age of pregnancy in months	
Number of centimeters above pubis	**Age of pregnancy in months**
9 cm	3 months
16 cm	4 months
20 cm	5 months
24 cm	6 months
28 cm	7 months
32 cm	8 months
31 - 34 cm	9 months

Abnormal pregnancies

There are some serious diseases that come during pregnancy. These are some of the important diseases and the signs they make.

Threatened abortion

This comes during the first five months of the pregnancy. The woman has strong pain in the lower abdomen. This is a sign that the uterus may try to push the baby out.

Probable abortion

Bleeding from the vagina during the first five months of the pregnancy is a sign that the uterus is beginning to push the baby out.

Placenta previa

This comes during the last three months of the pregnancy. We call this the **last**, or **third trimester**. There is much bleeding. This is very serious. It is a sign that the placenta covers the opening of the uterus. The placenta is bleeding. The woman must go to hospital immediately. If not, she may die from bleeding.

Toxemia of pregnancy

This comes also during the last trimester. There are three important signs of this disease.

- Swelling of the ankles, legs, face, or hands.
- Protein in the urine.
- High blood pressure, above 130/90 mm.

In every pregnant woman with swelling during the last trimester, look for the other two signs. Look every week. If you find two or all three of these signs, the woman has toxemia of pregnancy. Send her to hospital.

Pregnant mothers at risk

Some pregnant mothers are very likely to have a difficult delivery. We call these women **mothers at risk**. Look for them in the prenatal clinic. These signs indicate that the pregnant mother is **at risk**.

1. A mother with a height of less than 150 cm.
2. A mother who has had a cesarian section in the past in order to deliver a previous baby.
3. A mother who has had a difficult delivery in the past.
4. A mother who has given birth to one or more dead babies. We call these **stillbirths**.
5. A mother who has had more than six deliveries.
6. A mother who has delivered one or more premature babies in the past.
7. A mother who has had severe bleeding or a retained placenta after a delivery in the past.
8. A mother who limps or has a deformity or paralysis of one or both legs.
9. A mother who has bleeding during this pregnancy, or signs of toxemia.
10. A mother who has another serious disease.

Anemia of pregnancy

Anemia comes often during pregnancy. Look for signs of anemia in every pregnant mother.

1. Pale color of the mucus membranes.
2. Swelling of the legs or the face.
3. A hemoglobin of 8 grams or less.

Send such a woman to hospital. She may need a transfusion.

Questions for study

1. How can you find the cause for leucorrhea?
2. For what symptoms or signs of the female organs should you send a woman to the doctor?
3. Which of these are very urgent?
4. How can you tell if a woman is pregnant?
5. How can you tell the age of the pregnancy? Name two methods.
6. What dangerous symptoms and signs can occur during pregnancy?
7. How can you diagnose an abortion?
8. How can you diagnose toxemia of pregnancy?
9. What must you do to find out the pregnant mothers at **risk**? Make a list of the ten **risk factors**. Put this list on the wall where you have the prenatal clinic.
10. How can you recognize anemia during pregnancy?

3.3.15 The back

Many patients have pain in the back. Often the pain is in the lower back. We call this the "lumbar region." This pain can come from a disease of:

- The bones of the spinal column.
- The muscles and ligaments of the back.
- The nerves of the back.
- Diseases of other organs like the kidneys, the female organs, or the prostate gland.

Examine carefully every patient with low back pain. Follow the strategies on pain in the lower back of a man and also of a woman - pages 364 and 370.

Observation

Curves of the back

Tell the patient to take off all his clothes. You must be able to look at the whole back, the buttocks, and the legs. Look carefully at the back while the patient is standing. Normally the back is symmetrical. The two sides look alike.

Look for strange bumps or curves. A curve of the spine to one side is a sign of disease. A bump, or a backward curve of the bones of the spine is also a sign of disease. It can come from:

- An old fracture of the bones of the spine.
- Tuberculosis of the bones of the spine. We call this **Pott's disease**.

If there is a backward curve, ask the patient if he has had a serious accident in the past with an injury to the back. If not, look for signs of a chronic infection: fever, loss of weight, pain and tenderness in the bump in the spine. Ask also if the patient has had tuberculosis in the past. Ask if someone else in the family has tuberculosis, or has had it in the recent past. If there are signs of a chronic infection, the bump probably comes from tuberculosis. Send the patient to hospital.

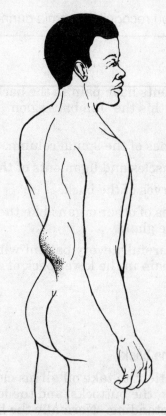

Tuberculosis of the spine.

Lumps and masses

Look for lumps and masses. A soft lump under the skin in the flank may be a lumbar hernia. Push gently on it. If it disappears, it is a hernia. If it does not disappear, it is probably a fatty tumor, or **lipoma**.

Movements of the back

Tell the patient to bend forward. Ask if this causes pain. Look at the curve of the back. This drawing shows the normal curve of the back.

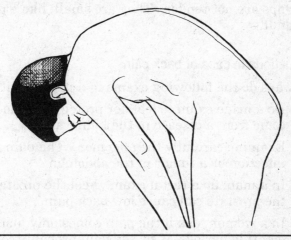

Normal back.

If there is a disease of the bones of the spine, the patient will not be able to bend well. The spine may look like this.

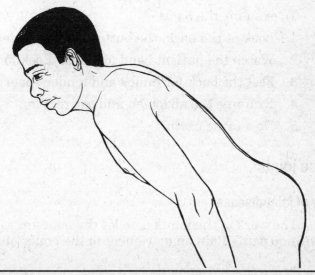

Pain in the low back.

Palpation

Feel the back carefully. Look for tender spots in the bones and in the muscles. A tender spot in the muscles is a sign of disease in the muscles, the ligaments, or the nerves of the back.

Push firmly on the flank just below the last rib and just outside the big back muscle. Tenderness here may be a sign of a disease of the kidney.

In an area where there is much onchocerciasis, feel along the bones of the back, the shoulders, the pelvis, and the hips. Look for very small hard lumps under the skin. These are cysts where the Onchocerca filaria live. The lumps are not tender. They are small, like a grain of rice or a groundnut.

Other examinations in case of back pain

Always do the following exams in a patient with back pain.

1. Do a urine exam to look for protein and blood cells. The pain may come from a disease in the kidneys.

2. Examine carefully the abdomen. The pain may come from an infection or a tumor in the abdomen.

3. In a man, do a rectal exam. Feel the prostate gland. An infection of the prostate can cause low back pain.

4. In a woman, ask if the pain comes only just before or during the monthly periods. If so, the pain probably comes from a disease in the female organs.

SUMMARY

To examine the back,

1. Look at the back, the buttocks, and the legs carefully.
2. Watch the patient bend forward. Look for abnormal curves.
3. Feel the back for lumps and tender spots.
4. Examine the abdomen and the rectum.
5. Do a urine exam.

3.3.16 The joints

History of joint disease

The work of the joints is to let the bones move. A normal joint moves with no pain. Pain on movement of the bones of a joint is a sign of inflammation in the joint. We call this **arthritis**. The pain is in the joint. Ask the patient how this pain came.

1. Was there an accident?
2. Were there signs of infection, like fever and much tenderness?
3. Did the pain come right after the patient did much heavy work?

People who are fat often have arthritis in the back, the hips, or the knees. This is because of the extra weight. The joints have extra work to carry the extra weight.

Examination of the movements of each joint

Examine the movements of each joint. First, tell the patient to move each joint. See if there is a full range of movement. Ask the patient if these movements cause pain. Then you move each joint. Move the joints gently. The patient must relax the muscles. Ask if this causes pain.

Here is a list of the movements of each joint together with the normal range of movement of each joint.

The neck

The normal movements are:

1. Flexion: touch the chin to the top of the chest.
2. Extension: look straight up.
3. Turning or rotation: touch the chin to the top of each shoulder.

The shoulder

Normally a person can move his arm:

1. Straight up.
2. Straight out.
3. Straight to the front.
4. A little way to the back.

The elbow

The normal movements are:

1. Flexion: the hand can touch the shoulder.
2. Extension: the arm is straight.

The wrist

The normal movements are:

1. Flexion to a 90 degree, or right, angle.
2. Extension: back up to 45 degrees.
3. Turning the hand completely up and completely down.

The fingers

The normal movements are:

1. Flexion: the finger is very curved.
2. Extension: the finger is straight.
3. Bringing the tip of the thumb to the tip of each of the other fingers.

The hip

Tell the patient to lie flat on his back. Normally the patient can do these movements:

1. Extension: hold the leg straight out and a little back.
2. Flexion of the hip: touch the knee to the chin, with the neck bent forward.
3. Rotation: turn the leg in and out.

The knee

The normal movements are:

1. Flexion: the knee bent, bringing the heel close to the buttock.
2. Extension: the leg straight out.

The ankle

The normal movements are:

1. Flexion: the foot is straight up to more than a right angle with the leg. We call this **dorsi-flexion**.
2. Extension: the foot is down. We call this **plantar-flexion**.
3. Rotation: the foot can turn a little in and out.

Signs of injury

If the patient has had an accident, look for signs of an injury to a joint.

Sprain

This means a tear in the ligaments around the joint. These are the ligaments that hold the joint together.

1. Tenderness on one side of the joint or all around the joint.
2. Pain on movement of the joint.
3. Swelling of the joint.
4. A dark blue color under the skin around the joint. We call this an **ecchymosis**. It comes from bleeding under the skin.
5. No signs of a dislocation or of a fracture.

Dislocation

This is when the end of one bone comes out of the joint socket.

1. Severe pain in the joint.
2. Loss of power. The patient cannot move the injured part.
3. Change in the shape of the injured part.
4. Change in the length of the injured arm or leg.
5. No swelling. There may be a hollow place over the joint.
6. No "crepitation." See signs of fracture on page 137.

Send to hospital immediately any patient who may have a dislocation.

Arthritis

If there is arthritis in a joint, there will be:

- Pain on movement of the joint.
- Inability to do one or all of the joint movements.
- Sometimes swelling of the joint.

The two common types of **arthritis** are **arthritis of age** which we call **osteoarthritis**, and **rheumatoid arthritis** which usually comes in young persons. In rheumatoid arthritis, there are often:

- Attacks of pain and tenderness which come and go.
- A low fever.
- Swelling of the first joint of each finger, the joint near the hand.

In osteoarthritis, there is:

- Pain on movement of the joint but little or no tenderness.
- No fever.
- Swelling with no pain of the second, or last, joint of each finger.

For a patient with joint pain, follow the strategy PAIN IN A JOINT on page 396.

Examination of joint fluid

Sometimes liquid can come into a joint, especially into the knee. The knee swells and is painful. When you push on the small knee bone, which we call the **patella**, you can feel the liquid inside. It is important to know what makes the liquid come into the knee. To find the cause, take out the liquid and look at it.

Tell the patient to lie down with the leg straight. Clean the knee very carefully with soap and water and then with an antiseptic solution. Use a sterile syringe and needle. Put the needle into the joint just below the side of the patella. Draw out the liquid. Look at a drop of the liquid under the microscope. Look for:

1. Clear liquid with no cells: osteoarthritis.
2. Many red blood cells in the liquid: an injury.
3. Many polynuclear white blood cells: an acute infection.
4. Many mononuclear white blood cells. This can be tuberculosis. Send this patient to hospital.

3.3.17 The bones and muscles

Bones

Pain in the bones is a sign of serious disease. Feel along the bone for tender places, lumps, or swellings. Look for signs of infection, like fever and a high white blood cell count. Look also for sickle cell anemia.

A disease in a bone usually causes no pain when the patient moves the bone. Pain on movement is a sign of disease in a joint or the muscles, but not in bone.

If the patient has had an accident, look for signs of a fracture.

1. Severe tenderness at the point of the injury.
2. Swelling at the place of the injury and pain.
3. Movement in the bone where there should be no movement.
4. Loss of power. The patient cannot move the injured part.
5. Change in the shape of the injured part. It may be turned or bent.
6. Change in the length of the arm, finger, or leg.
7. A feeling of "scraping" of the bone ends at the place of the injury when you move the injured part. We call this **crepitations**. Always move an injured part very gently.
8. Sometimes an ecchymosis at the point of the injury.

Look for a small hole in the skin covering the bone. See if there is pus coming from this hole. We call a hole like this a sinus. This is a sign of a serious bone infection, or **osteomyelitis**.

Muscles

The patient may have pain in the muscles. Ask the patient when and how this pain came.

1. Was there an accident?
2. Was there a fever?
3. Did the pain come just after the patient did much hard work or physical activity?

Feel the muscles. Look for tenderness and swelling in the muscles. See if there is pain in the muscles when the patient moves the limb or the painful area. See if there is pain in the muscles when you move the limb or the painful area.

A hard tender group of muscles with signs of infection indicate a muscle infection. We call this **pyomyositis**. There will be much pain on moving this group of muscles. Send the patient to hospital. It is necessary to make an incision to let out the pus from this group of muscles.

If the patient has had an accident, look for signs of a contusion.

1. Tenderness in a group of muscles.
2. Pain on movement of those muscles.
3. Swelling in these muscles.

In a patient with pain in the bones or muscles of one or more limbs, follow the strategies PAIN IN ONE LEG on page 400 and PAIN IN MORE THAN ONE LIMB on page 406.

Questions for study

1. What are all of the diseases that can cause pain in the lower back? Make a list of them.
2. What are the signs of disease that you can find in examining the back?
3. Ask a fellow student to let you examine his or her joints. Note carefully the movements of each joint. Note exactly how far each movement of flexion, extension, and rotation can go.
4. Make a list of the diseases that can cause an inflammation, or arthritis, of a joint. What must you do to find the cause of the arthritis?
5. A patient has pain in his leg. How can you tell if the pain is in the bones or the muscles or in a joint?
6. What are the signs of an injury to a joint?
   - To a bone?
   - To the muscles?
7. How can you tell a fracture from a sprain?
8. How can you tell a fracture from a dislocation?

3.3.18 The nerves

Examining the nerves

Nerves do three things.

1. They feel.
2. They make muscles move.
3. They make reflexes which help protect us from injury.

Some diseases of the nerves take away feeling. We call this **anesthesia**. Other diseases make the muscle movements weak or impossible. We call this **paralysis**. Other diseases of the nerves take away the reflexes and sometimes cause reflexes that are abnormal. To examine the nerves we must look at all three of these things that nerves do.

Examining for anesthesia

There are three important sorts of anesthesia.

1. **Anesthesia to pain**. The patient cannot feel pain.
2. **Anesthesia to temperature**. The patient cannot tell hot and cold in the area where the nerve goes.
3. **Anesthesia to touch**. The patient cannot feel even a gentle touch.

Anesthesia to pain

A nerve may be cut or killed by disease. The patient will then feel nothing in the part of the body where the nerve goes.

Use a sharp pin or needle. Tell the patient that you will touch gently different parts of his body. The patient must tell you where you are touching the skin of the body.

Tell the patient to keep his eyes closed. The patient must not look at you during the exam. If the patient sees you touching the skin, the patient may say that he feels it. But in reality the patient may not feel it at all. The patient simply sees you touching the skin but thinks that he should be feeling it.

There is no anesthesia to pain if the patient can tell you exactly

- Each time you touch the skin.
- Just where you touch the skin each time.

Anesthesia to temperature

Leprosy is a disease of the nerves. It causes anesthesia to pain, to temperature, and to touch. These sorts of anesthesia come in the spots of less color that leprosy makes on the skin. They may also come on the hands and feet. Test for anesthesia to temperature and to touch in the spots on the skin or on the fingers and toes.

For the temperature test, take two ordinary test tubes from the laboratory. Fill one with cool water. Fill the other with hot water, but not hot enough to burn the patient.

Tell the patient you will touch many places on the skin with each tube, one at a time. He must tell you which tube is touching the skin, the hot tube or the cool tube.

Tell the patient to close his eyes. He must not look at you during the test. Then touch the skin on different places, sometimes on normal skin and sometimes on a skin spot. This is how you can tell if he has anesthesia to temperature or not.

1. The patient is unable to tell which tube is touching the spots. But he can tell each time which tube is touching the normal skin. The patient has anesthesia to temperature in the spots and probably has leprosy. Send the patient to the doctor.

2. The patient can tell which tube is touching the skin on both the normal skin and on the spots on the skin. The patient does not have leprosy.

3. The patient cannot tell which tube is touching the skin on both the normal skin and on the spots on the skin. In this case, the patient does not understand what you are doing. Repeat the instructions clearly and do the exam again.

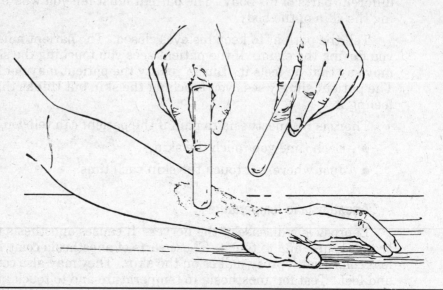

Testing for anesthesia to temperature.

Anesthesia to touch

Use a small piece of cotton wad. Tell the patient you will touch the skin gently in different places. Ask him to tell you when and where you are touching the skin. He must close his eyes and not look at you during the test.

Touch sometimes the normal skin. Touch the skin spots at other times. This is how you can tell if he has leprosy or not.

1. He knows when and where you touch the normal skin. But he cannot tell you when you touch a skin spot. He has anesthesia to touch and probably has leprosy. Send him to the doctor.

2. He can tell you each time when and where you are touching both the normal skin and the skin spots. There is no anesthesia and he probably does not have leprosy.

3. He cannot tell when or where you are touching the normal skin or skin spots. This means that he does not understand what you are doing. Repeat the instructions and try again.

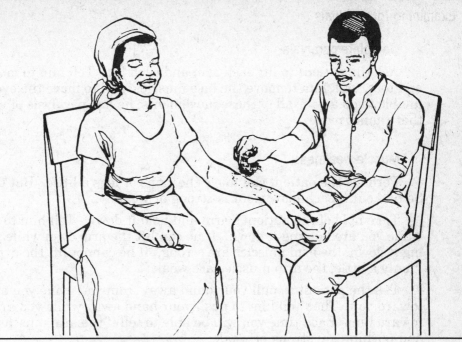

Testing for anesthesia to touch.

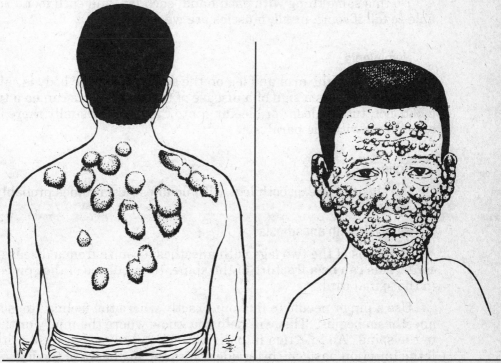

Tuberculoid leprosy.   Lepromatous leprosy.

Examining for paralysis

Complete paralysis

Ask the patient to lift each arm and each leg. Tell him to move the fingers and toes. Ask him to move the face muscles, and to move the eyes. If he is unable to do any or all of these movements, he has paralysis of the muscles that cannot move.

Muscle weakness

Perhaps the patient can move the arms or legs a little. But they are weak. So find out if each movement is strong or weak.

Take hold of the patient's arm and hold it down. Tell him to lift the arm while you are holding it down. If he can lift the arm even while you are holding it down, the arm muscles are strong. If he cannot lift the arm, or can lift it only a little, the arm muscles are weak.

Tell the patient to pull your hand away from you while you are pulling it toward you. Then tell him to push your hand away while you are pushing it toward him. Each time you will be able to tell if the arm muscles for pulling and pushing are strong or weak.

Do this same thing with each hand, each leg, and each foot. You will be able to tell if some, or all, muscles are weak.

Hemiplegia

Paralysis of the arm and leg on the same side of the body is called **hemiplegia.** It is a sign of a disease of the brain. This can be a tumor, a blood clot, tuberculosis, or bleeding into the brain. Usually there is no anesthesia with the paralysis.

Polio

Paralysis of one or both legs with no anesthesia comes probably from polio.

Paralysis with anesthesia

Paralysis of the two legs with anesthesia comes from a disease of the spinal cord. This can be a fracture of the spine, tuberculosis of the spine, or a tumor in the spinal cord.

Use a pin or needle to find out exactly where the feeling stops and the anesthesia begins. This will help you know where the injury or the disease is in the spine. An injection into the buttock can cause paralysis with anesthesia if the injection has gone by accident into the big nerve of the leg.

For a patient who has paralysis of one or both legs, see the strategy PARALYSIS OF ONE OR BOTH LEGS on page 568.

DIFFERENT CAUSES OF PARALYSIS

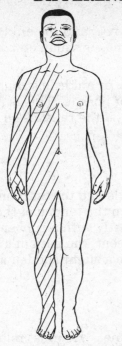

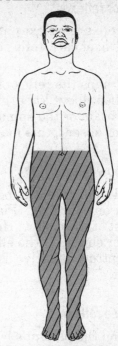

1. Brain disease with hemiplegia.   2. Spine disease with paralysis and anesthesia.

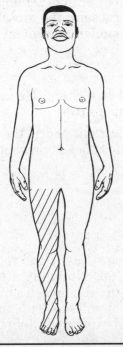

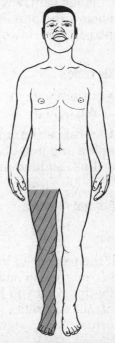

3. Polio with paralysis of one leg and no anesthesia.   4. Injury of leg nerve.

 Paralysis   **Anesthesia**

Examining for reflexes

There are reflexes at the elbow, the knee, and the ankle. The force, or strength, of each reflex should be the same, or equal, on both sides of the body.

Perhaps the reflex of one elbow, knee, or ankle is strong. But the one on the other elbow, knee, or ankle is weak or absent. This is a sign of disease in the brain or the spinal cord. However, if the reflexes on both sides are weak or absent, this may be normal.

Elbow reflex

Tell the patient to bend the arm a little and to rest it on the table, the bed, or on your arm. Place your thumb on the tendon of the biceps muscle in front of the elbow. Hit your thumb gently with a rubber hammer or another object. If the elbow reflex is present, the patient's biceps muscle will contract slightly. The arm will make a slight sudden movement of flexion.

Knee reflex

Bend the patient's leg a little at the knee. He must relax the leg completely. Find the tendon just below the patella.

Hit the leg gently with a rubber hammer or another object on the tendon below the patella. If the reflex is present, the muscles of the thigh will contract. The lower leg will make a sudden movement forward.

Ankle reflex

The patient can sit, lie down, or kneel on a chair. He must let the leg relax. Take hold of the foot and bend it up a little.

With a rubber hammer or another object, hit gently the tendon in back of the ankle and just above the heel. If the reflex is present, the foot will make a slight sudden movement down.

Abnormal reflexes

Clonus

Tell the patient to lie down with the leg straight and relaxed. Bend his foot up strongly and suddenly and hold it up. Normally there is no reaction. But sometimes, as you hold the foot bent up, the muscles in the lower leg will contract and relax in rhythm. The foot will move up and down. We call this **clonus**. It is a sign of disease in the brain or the spinal cord.

Babinski reflex

Tell the patient to lie down with the leg straight and relaxed. Take a blunt metal object. Draw it across the bottom of the foot. Start at the heel. Move up the outside of the bottom of the foot to the base of the toes. Then move across the base of the toes to the base of the big toe. Push quite hard.

Normally the toes will move down. But sometimes the big toe will move up in extension. We call this upward movement of the big toe the **Babinski reflex**. It is a sign of a disease in the brain or in the spinal cord.

REMEMBER:

Unequal reflexes are not normal.

Questions for study

1. How do you test for the different kinds of anesthesia?
2. What equipment do you need for each test?
3. Practice each test on your fellow students and let them practice on you.
4. What are the nerve signs of leprosy?
5. How do you test reflexes to find diseases of the nerves?
6. What diseases can cause anesthesia?
7. What diseases can cause paralysis?

3.3.19 The skin

The skin signs of disease

There are many diseases that make changes or "lesions" in the skin. Some diseases of the body cause changes, or eruptions, in the skin. Measles, chicken pox, malnutrition, and syphilis are examples of this. The skin changes come from the disease in the body.

Other diseases are only in the skin itself. The skin lesions come from the skin disease. The body is normal. Learn to tell quickly the most important diseases that cause changes in the skin. Look for these skin signs of disease.

1. **Macules**. These are very small flat spots on the skin. They are not thick.
2. **Papules**. These are very small raised bumps in the skin.
3. **Vesicles**. These are small bumps on the skin filled with liquid.
4. **Pustules**. These are small bumps on the skin filled with pus.

5. **Nodules**. These are big hard bumps in the skin.

6. **Plaques**. These are big flat spots on the skin. They may be several centimeters wide. They may be thick and raised, or flat. They come from an infection with bacteria or fungus. They may also come from leprosy.

7. **Ulcer**. This is a hole in or through the skin. At the base there is pus, or blood, or red tissue.

Ask the patient about any symptoms of pain, itching, or loss of feeling. Ask how long these skin signs have been present. Ask if there has been fever, or any other disease of the body. For a patient with itching, follow the strategy ITCHING on page 448.

Observation

Look at the skin lesions very carefully. Note:

1. On what part of the body the skin lesions are.

2. The color of the skin lesions. Are they very dark? Or do they have less color than the skin around them?

3. Signs of inflammation around the skin lesions, like tenderness and heat.

4. Lymph nodes in the area. Are they big and tender?

5. If the skin lesions are dry or moist. A moist skin lesion comes probably from an infection.

6. The edges of the skin lesions. Are the edges sharp and clear? Or are they unclear so that you cannot be sure where the skin begins to change?

7. If there are fine scales of skin on the lesions.

SUMMARY

For any skin signs of disease, note:

1. Where they are.

2. What they look like.

3. What symptoms they give.

4. How long they have been present.

5. If there are signs of a general disease.

Skin diseases

Ulcers

There are six important sorts of ulcers, or sores, of the skin. They often come on the lower leg.

Tropical ulcer

It is deep, painful, and often has a strong bad smell. There may be big tender lymph nodes in the inguinal region.

Infected ulcer

This comes from a small sore or wound that has become infected. There is pain and swelling around the ulcer. But there is not a bad smell.

Simple ulcer

An ulcer can come because of poor circulation of the blood. It is not deep. It has no signs of infection, pain, or smell. We call it a **simple ulcer**.

Bed sore

This is a flat ulcer that comes in patients who are paralyzed, or who must be in bed for a long time. The bed sores come because of poor circulation. They come where the skin is pressed against the bed for long periods of time.

Malignant tumor

If an ulcer has been present for many years, it may become a **malignant tumor**. The ulcer becomes very big. The edges grow very thick and irregular.

Mycobacterium ulcer

This is a skin ulcer that comes from a bacteria of the tuberculosis family. It is not common but it is very serious. It is often easy to tell this ulcer. The edges are smooth and **undermined**. You can pass an instrument under the skin around the edge of the ulcer. There is little or no pain and no bad odor in the ulcer.

SKIN ULCERS

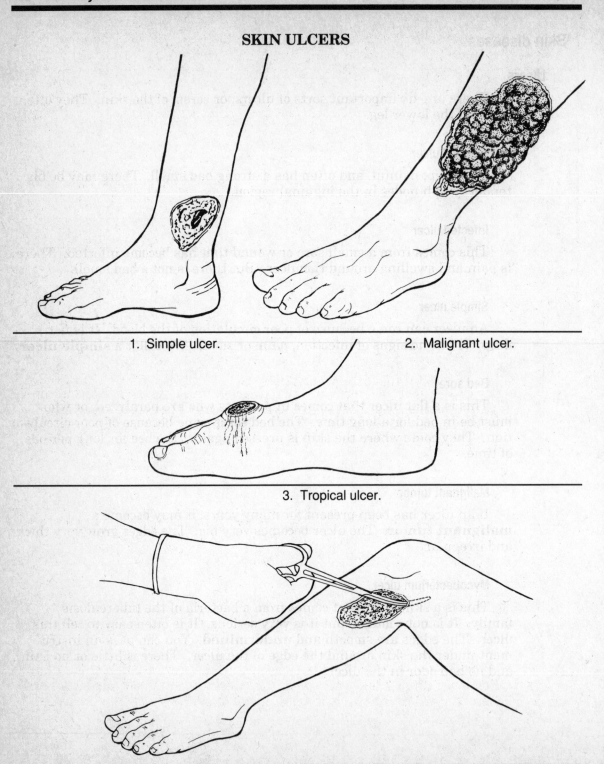

1. Simple ulcer.

2. Malignant ulcer.

3. Tropical ulcer.

4. Mycobacterium ulcer.

Table 4 - Skin ulcers

Ulcer Type	Pain	Pus	Odor	Big Lymph Nodes	Edges
Tropical	yes	yes	yes	yes	raised
Infected	yes	yes	no	yes	raised
Simple	no	no	no	no	flat
Bed sores	no	often	no	no	flat
Tumor	no	sometimes	sometimes	sometimes	very thick
Mycobacterium	no	no	no	no	undermined

Scabies

Scabies comes from little insects that make small bumps in the skin. They cause much itching. The bumps are on the body, the arms, and the legs. They usually are not on the face and head. They come especially in the folds of skin around the joints, like the elbows, the armpits, the inguinal region, and the knees.

Fungus infections of the skin

A fungus infection makes a flat plaque, or many plaques on the skin. The plaques have sharp edges and may be slightly raised. There are fine scales on the plaques. There is much itching. There is no anesthesia and no big lymph nodes. A fungus infection is often in the folds of skin or on the buttocks.

General diseases with skin signs

Malnutrition

Look at the color of the skin. Malnutrition makes the skin change color. Often malnutrition takes away some of the normal color of the skin, sometimes everywhere, but other times only in spots.

The skin becomes very smooth, especially on the legs. There are many fine lines, or cracks, in the skin. The skin looks like the skin of a lizard.

Urticaria

These are big irregular bumps in the skin with much itching. Each bump stays for only a few minutes or hours. But more come, often for several days. They come from an allergic disease.

Drug eruption

This is a very serious condition. There are macules and papules on much or all of the body. There is much itching everywhere. The skin begins to come off in thin sheets. The cause is a medicine which the patient is taking. The patient must stop taking this medicine IMMEDIATELY. Send the patient immediately to hospital.

Questions for study

1. Make a list of the signs of skin disease. After each sign, write down the names of the diseases you know that can cause this sign.
2. What must you note about each skin sign?
3. To find the cause of a skin ulcer, what must you look for?

Chapter 4
EXAMINING INFANTS AND CHILDREN

4.1 How are children different from adults?

4.2 How do you take the history of the illness of a child?

4.3 How do you do the physical examination of a child?

4.1 How are children different from adults?

Children are very special persons. Someday they will be adults. But you must remember that children are not small adults. They are different.

Making a diagnosis in children can be difficult. Often it is more difficult than in adults. Why is this so? There are several reasons for this.

4.1.1 Children are different

First of all, the body of a child is different in some ways from the body of an adult. A child does not feel things the same way as an adult feels things. A child's mind is different. A child thinks and talks like a child and not like an adult. It is important for you to know these differences.

4.1.2 Diseases in children are different

Diseases do different things in children than in adults. The symptoms are different because children feel things differently than do adults. Small infants are unable to tell you how they feel. So we cannot always know their symptoms and how they feel.

The signs of disease may be different in children. In some diseases in children there may be no specific signs at all.

Diseases can develop very quickly in children. In children death can come very quickly. Death usually comes more slowly in adults. So it is very important for you to make the right diagnosis in children. It is important to do this quickly.

For example, malaria in a small child is very severe. It can kill the child quickly. Usually malaria is not severe in an adult. Tuberculosis is also more acute and more severe in children. Often in children there are no specific signs of tuberculosis, such as tubercle bacilli in the sputum or crackles in the lungs. Tuberculosis is more chronic, or slow, in adults.

So give special attention to sick children. Examine them right away. Try to make the right diagnosis quickly. Start giving the treatment they need right away. You will save many lives by doing this.

4.1.3 The history often must come from another person

An infant cannot talk. A small child cannot talk well. Even a big child cannot always talk clearly.

Therefore, you must often take the history of the illness of a child from another person. Most often, you will take the history from the mother of the child. Sometimes you will take it from the father, from a grandparent, or from another person close to the child.

Always take the history from the person, or persons, who know the child well and who know about the illness. Older children can often tell you about some things. In this case, talk to the child and to the mother. In this chapter, we will presume that the mother is the person giving you the history.

To take the history of the illness of a child, follow the same rules as those for taking the history of the illness of an adult.

1. Be complete.

2. Find out all you can about each important symptom.

3. Follow the right order.

4.1.4 The order for taking the history is different in children

The order for taking the history of the illness in children is different. It is not the same as the order for the history of the illness in adults. There are special questions to ask the mother of the child. We do not ask these questions of an adult patient.

1. Ask about the mother's health when she was pregnant with this child.

2. Ask about the birth of the child.

3. Ask about his food and nutrition.

These questions are important. They will help you to understand better the health and the development of each child. They will also help you in caring for the child during the illness.

SUMMARY

Making the right diagnosis in children is very important. Making the diagnosis in children is different than in adults. Often it is more difficult in children.

1. Children are not small adults. They are different.

2. Diseases can act differently in children.

3. Diseases often develop more quickly in children.

4. Small children cannot give you a history. You must get the history from another person.

5. There are different questions to ask.

Questions for study

1. In what ways are children different from adults?
2. In what ways are diseases in children different from diseases in adults?
3. What difference does this make in how you make the diagnosis?

4.2 How do you take the history of the illness of a child?

Now let us look at the questions to ask in taking the history from the mother of the child.

4.2.1 What is the illness like?

First, ask the mother why she has brought the child to you.

- What is wrong with your child? or
- Why did you bring your child to the health center?

Let the mother talk about the illness. Listen carefully to what she says. She may also talk about what she has done to treat the child, or what others have done. Listen to this also. This is very important. It will give you much information about the disease and about the condition of the child.

After the mother stops talking, ask questions about certain things. First of all, ask about the most important symptoms. Find out all you can about each symptom.

4.2.2 What are the important symptoms like?

Fever

1. Does the child have fever?
2. When did the fever start?
3. How much fever has there been?
4. When does the fever come?
   - All of the time?
   - Only at night?
   - Only during the day?

Pain

1. Does the child seem to have pain? An infant cannot tell you that he has pain. But the pain will make him cry. Pain often makes the muscles become hard. Sometimes the infant will touch the place where he has pain. If there is pain in the ear, he will often pull on the ear. Ask about this.

2. Where does the mother think the pain is?
   - In the abdomen?
   - In the chest?
   - In the neck or head?
   - In the arms or legs?

3. Does the infant cry when she touches him?

4. On what part of the body does her touch make him cry?

5. Does he cry when she moves him, or when she moves a part of his body?

6. When does the pain come?
   - After eating?
   - With a cough?
   - With diarrhea?
   - With passing urine?

7. Does the pain keep the child from sleeping?

8. What does the mother do when the pain comes?

9. Can she seem to stop the pain by doing something to the child?

10. Do certain things seem to make the pain worse?

Cough

1. Does the child cough?

2. When does the cough come?
   - All the time?
   - Only at night?

3. Does the child seem to have pain with the cough?

4. Is the cough short, with 3 or 4 coughs and then a breath?

5. Or is the cough long, with many coughs before the child can take a breath? Whooping cough can give a very long cough. In whooping cough, often the lips become blue at the end of a long cough. The child may vomit at the end of the cough. Often there is very thick mucus in the child's mouth. The child has great difficulty in taking a breath at the end of this long cough. In a child of one year of age or more, this breath makes a loud sound which we call a "whoop."

See the strategy COUGH IN A CHILD on page 253.

Children do not often cough out sputum. They swallow it. It goes down into the stomach. But sometimes, in a serious pneumonia, there will be much sputum with pus. The child will then cough out this sputum. Most often, however, even with tuberculosis, children will not bring up sputum.

Vomiting

1. Does the child vomit?
2. When does he vomit?
   - All of the time?
   - Only with eating?
3. What does he vomit?
   - Milk or food only?
   - Much liquid from the stomach?
   - Blood?
   - Brown liquid that smells like fecal matter?

Many small infants vomit a little after taking breast milk. This is not serious. But it is very serious if a new infant of one to three weeks old vomits all of his milk every time. There may be an obstruction in the stomach. Send this child to hospital right away. See the strategies on vomiting in children on pages 294 and 298.

Diarrhea

1. Does the child have diarrhea?
2. What are the stools like?
3. Is there blood or pus in the stools?
4. Or is there only water and liquid fecal matter?
5. How many days has the child had diarrhea?

6. How many times has he had diarrhea today? How many times yesterday?

7. Does he have pain with the diarrhea?

8. Does he vomit with the diarrhea?

Many diseases with a high fever, like malaria, measles, pneumonia and others, cause diarrhea because of the fever. The stools are liquid, with no blood or pus.

But a disease of the intestines can cause diarrhea with blood, or pus, or both. We call this "dysentery." Often there is much pain with this diarrhea. There may be vomiting and fever. This can be very serious. See the strategy ACUTE DIARRHEA IN A CHILD on page 318.

Convulsions

1. Has the child had a convulsion?

2. If so, when?

3. Was it with a high fever? Or was there no fever?

4. How many convulsions did he have?

5. Does he often have convulsions?

6. If so, do they come only when he has a fever?

See the strategy CONVULSIONS IN A CHILD on page 422.

Trouble breathing

1. Does the child breathe fast? Fast breathing comes with a high fever or with an anemia. The breathing is fast but not difficult.

2. Does the child seem to have trouble breathing? This is when the child must work hard to breathe. Trouble breathing comes in diseases of the lungs or of the heart. Often there is a cough with it.

3. What is the trouble breathing like? Is it trouble getting air into the lungs? Or is it trouble pushing the air out of the lungs? In the second case, there is often a loud sound when the child breathes out. We call this a "wheeze."

See the strategy TROUBLE BREATHING IN A CHILD on page 264.

Questions for study

1. What must you find out about the child's fever?
   - About pain?
   - About cough?
   - About vomiting?
   - About diarrhea?
   - About convulsions?
   - About trouble breathing?
2. Write down in your notebook all that you must find out about each of these symptoms. Learn all of this by heart.

4.2.3 What are the other questions to ask?

Ask the same questions about the present illness that you ask of adult patients. Read again about these questions on pages 27 to 32. Briefly, these are the questions to ask.

1. When did the illness start?
2. How did the illness start?
   - Did it start quickly?
   - Or did it start slowly?
3. How has the illness developed?
4. Did anything happen to cause the illness?
   - Did the child fall?
   - Did the child drink bad water?
   - Did the child take a new sort of food?
   - Did the child eat or drink something bad, like paraffin (kerosene), or pills, or something poisonous?
5. How serious is the illness?
   - Does the child eat and drink well?
   - Does he sleep well?
   - Has the child lost weight?
   - Does the child cry much of the time?
   - Does the child play normally, or not?

6. What treatment has the child received?

- Did the mother give this treatment, or someone else?

- Did the mother take the child to another health center for treatment? If so, what treatment was given? What was the result?

- Did the mother take the child to a traditional healer? If so, what did the healer do? What was the result? Find out about this, for it is very important.

7. Has the child had any medicines?

- Did the mother give a laxative, like salts, or oil?

- If so, why? When? What was the result?

- Did the mother give an enema? If so, what was in the water? When did she give it? How much water did she give? What came out after she gave the enema?

8. Has the child been ill like this before? Even small children can have chronic diseases, like asthma, heart disease, malnutrition, or others.

9. Does anyone else in the family have an illness like that of the child?

4.2.4 Are there other symptoms?

The symptom review in a child is difficult. It is often impossible to know all that the child feels. But the mother can tell you about some things. So ask her if the child seems to have any of the important symptoms of the different organs.

1. General symptoms: weakness, fever, loss of weight.

2. Heart: trouble breathing, cough, swelling of the feet, the legs, or the eyes, a blue color of the lips. An infant with heart disease will often cough or become blue when taking breast milk or a bottle. Ask about this.

3. Lungs: cough, trouble breathing, wheezing. Ask the mother if the low part of the child's chest goes in and out every time the child breathes in and out.

4. Stomach and intestines: pain in the abdomen, loss of appetite, vomiting, diarrhea, constipation, blood in the stools.

5. Liver: jaundice, very dark urine, vomiting. Remember that jaundice can also come from some kinds of anemia.

6. Urinary system: pain on passing urine.

- Does the child cry every time he passes urine?

- Is there blood or pus in the urine?

7. Muscles, bones, joints: swelling, pain on movement, weakness.
8. Nervous system: convulsions, loss of consciousness, stiff neck, pain in the head, paralysis, bad dreams.

Questions for study

1. Why is it important to ask all of these questions?
2. Why is it important to know what treatment the child has received?
3. How can the symptom review in children help you make the right diagnosis?

4.2.5 How has the child grown and developed?

It is important to know about the early life of the child. It is important to know about the mother's pregnancy and the birth of the child. An illness of the mother during the pregnancy can affect the child even now. Difficulty during the birth can also affect the child. So ask questions about these things.

Pregnancy

1. Did the mother have trouble when she was pregnant with this child?
2. Did she have any serious illness or injuries during the pregnancy?
3. Did she have swelling or convulsions?
4. Did she have a high fever? or jaundice? or bleeding?
5. Did she have any other symptoms or signs?

Birth

1. Was the infant born in hospital or at home?
2. Was there any trouble with the birth? If so, what trouble?
3. How long was the labor before the birth?
4. What part of the infant came out first, the head or the feet?
5. Did the doctor or the nurse do any operation to help with the birth, like using a vacuum extractor or forceps, or doing a cesarian section?
6. Did the infant take a breath and cry quickly? If not, how many minutes was it before he started to breathe?
7. Did the infant have trouble breathing, or trouble taking breast milk during the first few days of life?

8. Did the infant have any infection right after the birth?

9. How much did the infant weigh at birth? The mother may know this. If so, this is important information. Infants with a low birth weight, below 2.5 kg, often have many illnesses. They need special care and good food.

The first month of life

1. Did the infant have any fever or infection during the first month of life?

2. Were there any other illnesses? If so, what?

3. Did the infant breathe well and take breast milk well?

4. Was there much vomiting?

5. Did the infant have jaundice?

Growth of the infant

There are certain things an infant can do at certain times. We call these things the "markers" of growth. They are like the signs by the side of the road that show how many kilometers, or miles, there are to the next city. These are the important markers of growth.

1. At 3 months of age, a normal infant can hold his head up.

2. At 6 months of age, a normal infant can sit up without help.

3. At 6 months of age, the teeth start to come in.

4. At 9 months of age, a normal infant can walk on his hands and feet. We call this "crawling."

5. At 11 months of age, a normal infant can stand up. But he must hold on to something.

6. At 13 months of age, a normal child starts to walk.

7. At 12 to 15 months of age, a normal child starts to talk.

There are normal differences in the growth of children. Some infants can hold up their head at 2 months of age. Others can hold it up only at 4 months of age. This difference is normal. But infants who are unable to hold up their head at 6 months of age are not normal.

Teeth may start to come in at 3 months. Or they may start to come in only at 9 months. This is normal. But it is not normal for teeth to wait until after 12 months of age to start coming in.

* Table 5 - Age of appearing of different teeth	
First, or infant teeth	
Age in months	**Teeth to appear**
5 to 8 months	lower central incisor teeth
6 to 10 months	upper central incisor teeth
7 to 10 months	lower lateral incisor teeth
8 to 12 months	upper lateral incisor teeth
11 to 18 months	lower and upper first molar teeth
16 to 20 months	lower and upper first molar teeth
Second, or permanent teeth	
Age in years	**Teeth to appear**
6 to 7 years	lower central incisor teeth
7 to 8 years	upper central incisor teeth
7 to 8 years	lower lateral incisor teeth
8 to 9 years	upper lateral incisor teeth
9 to 11 years	lower cuspid teeth
11 to 12 years	upper cuspid teeth
10 to 12 years	lower first premolar teeth
10 to 11 years	upper first premolar teeth
10 to 12 years	upper second premolar teeth
11 to 13 years	lower second premolar teeth
6 to 7 years	lower and upper first molar teeth
12 to 14 years	lower and upper second molar teeth
17 to 30 years	lower and upper third molar teeth
* After LANGE	

You want to know if the growth of the infant or child is normal. To do this, you must first know the child's age. But often the mother will not remember the day of the birth of the child. She may not know even how many months or years old the child is.

Often, however, she will have an idea if the child can do the things that are normal for that age. She can do this because she sees other children born at the same time as her child. She will see what these other children can do and what her child can do. If her child cannot do the things that other children born at the same time can do, she will probably recognize this. She will know that the development of her child is slow.

There are ways you can use to find out about how old a child is. Ask the mother about what time of the year the child was born. Was it before or after a certain big day, like New Year's Day, or some other important day that everyone knows? Was it before or after the time to plant, or the time to harvest? Was it before or after the return of the rains, or the beginning of the dry season? Was it at the beginning or at the end of the cold season? or of the hot season? By asking these questions you can find out about when a child was born.

Questions for study

1. What must you know about the mother's pregnancy?
2. What must you find out about the birth of the child?
3. What must you find out about the first month of the child's life?
4. Why is it important to find out about these things?
5. Why is it important to know the growth markers of the child?
6. What are these markers? Learn them by heart.
7. Practice looking at many infants to see if their growth is normal or not.
   - Look at an infant of 5 months. Can he hold up his head?
   - Look at an infant of 7 months. Can he sit up? Does he have any teeth? What teeth does he have?
   - This practice will help you examine sick infants. You will learn quickly if their growth is normal or not.

Nutrition

The nutrition of children is very important. Good food helps them grow well. It makes them healthy. Poor food, or not enough food, keeps them from growing well. Their health will be poor. They will have many illnesses.

Ask the mother many questions about the food the child eats. Many mothers are afraid to talk about this. They may think you are being critical of them. So ask the questions carefully and politely.

Breast milk

Normally children take breast milk, or "nurse", until the age of 18 months or 2 years. This is good, because breast milk has good protein. If children stop nursing before this time, they may not get enough protein. Then they will not grow well. So ask about this.

1. Is the child still nursing?
2. If not, at what age did the child stop nursing?
3. If the child stopped nursing before the age of 18 months, what was the reason? Was the mother ill? Or was it because the mother had another pregnancy?

Solid foods

Often it is difficult to get a good history about food. A mother may not know what is important about food. She may forget how she fed her child in the past.

You can help her remember by asking specific questions. This takes time and patience. But it is very important. It will tell you much about the health of the child.

1. When did the child start eating solid foods?
2. What foods did he start eating?
3. What foods does he now eat every day?
4. What did the child eat today? How much did he eat?
5. What did he eat yesterday? How much did he eat?
6. What did he eat the day before yesterday? How much?

Foods with protein

Foods with protein are very important for children. They help them to grow well. Children must eat two or more different foods with protein every day. This will help them grow well. They must eat enough of each protein food.

If children do not eat like this, you know that their nutrition is poor. They will be weak. They will have many infections and other diseases. So ask each mother if her child eats these foods. Ask her how much the child eats of each one and how often.

1. When was the last time the child ate fish?
2. How much did he eat at that time?
3. How often does he eat fish?
   - One time a week?
   - One time a month?
   - Not at all?

Ask these same questions about eggs and meat. Ask about maize, beans, groundnuts and rice. Ask about soya, millet, green leafy vegetables, and any other foods in your area that have protein.*

4.2.6 What was the health of the child before this illness?

Other diseases

Ask the mother if the child has had measles, whooping cough, polio or chicken pox. A child can get each of these diseases only one time.

For example, the child may have had measles. In this case, you know that the present illness is not measles. Be sure the mother knows the child really had measles. She may tell you that it was measles. But in fact it was not measles, but another disease.

Ask about other diseases, like asthma, heart trouble, and jaundice. Ask about anemia. A child who often has anemia may have sickle cell anemia. Or the anemia may come from hookworm, or from malnutrition, or from many attacks of malaria.

Ask about other infections, like ear infections, tonsil infections, pneumonia, infections of the lymph nodes, diarrhea. A child who has had many infections is not strong. This child will need much good treatment, good food, and good care. The mother will need good education about how to help the child become healthy.

---

*There is a very good book about nutrition by Dr. Maurice King. The name of the book is Nutrition in Developing Countries. You can learn much about food and nutrition from this book. You can also learn how to take a good nutrition history.

Health care

If the child is less than 5 years old, ask the mother if she takes the child to the "preschool" or "under-five" clinic. If so, ask to see the chart from the clinic. If she does not have the chart, tell her to come with it as soon as possible. See if the child goes to the clinic every month. Look at the weight curve. Is it good? See if the child receives anti-malaria medicine each month.

If the mother does not bring the child to the preschool clinic, find out why. Tell her that it is very important for the child's health. She must bring the child every month. Explain to her the reasons for bringing the child to the clinic each month.

Ask the mother about vaccinations. Has the child had vaccinations against measles, polio, tetanus, whooping cough, diphtheria, and tuberculosis? Which vaccinations has he had, and when? If the child needs one or more of these vaccinations, make arrangements for the child to get it, or them, when he gets well.

Use this time of history-taking to give advice to the mother about the health care of the child. This can help the child to stay healthy in the future.

Questions for study

1. What must you find out about the nutrition of the child?
2. Why is this important?
3. Make a list of all the foods in your area that have protein.
4. What other diseases should you ask the mother about? Make a list of them. Learn this list by heart.
5. If the child does not go to the preschool clinic, what should you do? Why?
6. If the child needs one or more vaccinations, when should you give it, or them?

4.2.7 What is the family situation of the child?

Ask questions about the family of the child. Ask them in the same way that you ask about the family of an adult patient.

The marriage

1. Is the mother married?
2. Does she live with the father of the child?
3. Does the father work? If so, what does he do?

4. Do they have money to get good foods?

5. Does the father help take care of the child?

6. Is the father married to another woman? If so, how many wives does he have?

The family

1. Are there other children in the family?

2. Are the other children well? Are they often ill? Have any other children in the family died? If so, of what diseases?

3. Is this child the first, second, third, or fourth child?

4. Does the mother have another child born after this one? If so, look carefully at the child for signs of malnutrition.

5. If the mother is not married, who is the father of the child?

6. Does the mother work? Does she have money of her own?

7. Who helps the mother in the garden and in the house? Children of mothers who are not married often do not eat well. They are weak and malnourished. They often have many diseases.

If the mother has many children, this child or infant may not get enough food. If this is the case, talk to the mother about food. If possible, talk also to the father. Talk to them about what they can do to keep from having more children. See page 658 for the instructions to give about good nutrition.

Living conditions of the family

1. In what kind of a house does the family live? How many rooms are there? How many people live in the house?

2. Is there a sanitary installation (privy)?

3. Where does the family get its drinking water? Is this water safe for drinking?

4. Are there animals who live in or near the house? If so, what animals?

5. Are there many flies or mosquitoes in or near the house?

SUMMARY

The history seems long and difficult. In simple diseases, it is not necessary to ask every one of these questions. In more serious diseases, it is good to ask all of them. So learn how to do this well.

A good history is the most important part of the examination of children. Even in simple diseases, ask about the family and the living conditions of the child.

This is a very good time for health education. There may be things in the family or in the home of the child which are bad for health. Talk to the mother and father about them. Tell them to follow the rules of good health. This will help the child stay healthy when he gets well.

Questions for study

1. How does the health of the family affect the child?
2. What should you know about the family?
3. How does the living situation of the family affect the health of the child?
4. What should you know about the living conditions of the family?

4.3 How do you do the physical examination of a child?

The physical examination of children is different from the physical examination of adults. The body of the child is small. The organs of the child are small.

Sometimes the signs of a disease are different in children than in adults. Sometimes a disease in a child goes not give a certain sign. For example,

1. Pneumonia may not give crackles in the lungs of an infant. The only signs will be fever and changes in the breathing of the infant.

2. Tuberculosis may give a high fever in a child. But in adults, it usually gives only a low fever.

3. Meningitis may not give a stiff neck in small infants. But often it will cause a swelling in the fontanel, the soft part in the top of the head. This fontanel is not present in older children or in adults.

Small children are often afraid of the physical examination. They cry quickly. But crying can keep you from finding important signs of the disease.

Try to keep the child from crying. Talk to him gently. If the child can talk to you, talk about things other than the disease. Give him something to look at or to play with. Give him your hand. Show him that you are his friend.

It is important to look at the whole body of the child. Ask the mother to undress him. This may make him afraid. Ask her to take off his clothes slowly. If he is older, take off only some of the clothes at first, like the shirt or the dress. Take off the other clothes later.

Some children do not like to lie on a table. They are afraid that you are going to hurt them. In this case, let the child stay in the mother's arms. Look at him there. You can even do some of the physical examination with the child in the mother's arms. If it is an infant, he may start to cry. If he does, tell the mother to let him nurse. Or tell her to put him on her shoulder.

Sometimes it is necessary to do something painful to a child, like an injection, or a painful examination. If the child is older, tell him what you are going to do. This will gain his confidence. Then do the painful thing quickly. If you do not explain this first to the child, he will be upset. This will make the rest of the examination difficult.

The order for the physical examination in children is different than the order in adults. First you do the things which will not give fear or pain to the child. You do the painful things only at the end. In this way it is more easy to do a good examination. It is more easy to find the signs of disease.

There are three important steps in the examination of children. Do these steps in order.

1. Look at the child carefully. Look at every part of his body for signs of disease.

2. Examine him with your hands. Feel for signs of disease.

3. Examine him with instruments.

Questions for study

1. Why is the examination of children different from the examination of adults?
2. In what ways in the examination of children different from that of adults?
3. What must you do to examine children well?

4.3.1 Look carefully at the child - OBSERVATION

This is the most important part of the physical examination. You can often find many signs of disease simply by observing. Look at these things.

The general condition

Signs of serious disease.

First, see if the child is very ill or not. This is how you can tell.

1. See how the child acts. If he is awake and happy, he is probably not very ill. If he sits quietly and breathes quietly, the disease is probably a simple one.

2. Is the child awake or asleep? If the child is asleep, is it just sleep? Or is the child in a coma? If he is in a coma, this is very serious. You cannot wake him. Coma can come from a very high fever, cerebral malaria, a serious infection, serious dehydration, or the loss of much blood.

3. Does the child cry all the time? If so, this may be because he is very ill. It may be because he has pain. It may also be because he is afraid of you. Or perhaps it is because he is hungry.

   If an infant cries, tell the mother to let him nurse. If he stops crying, then his crying is not because of pain. Perhaps the infant is crying because of tight clothes, or because of a pin sticking into him. Look for this. The crying will stop when the mother takes off his clothes, or takes away the pin.

4. Does the child seem weak? Does he stay in the mother's arms without moving? Perhaps he does not talk or cry at all. He may even not look at what you are doing. This is a sign of serious illness, like malaria, meningitis, a high fever, or serious malnutrition.

Signs of chronic disease

1. Loss of weight.
2. Weakness.
3. A pale color of the lips or the inside of the eyelids.
4. Swellings or lumps anywhere.

Signs of dehydration

Dehydration comes in diarrhea, vomiting, high fever, or after a severe burn. It can be very serious and cause death. Look for these signs of dehydration.

1. Weakness. Dehydrated children lie very still. They do not make movements, even when you touch them. They do not cry.

2. Rapid deep breathing.

3. The pulse is fast and feeble. Sometimes you cannot feel the pulse at all. This means the child is in shock.

4. The eyes are dry. There are no tears. Often the eyes seem small and are sunk back in the eye sockets.

5. The skin is dry. It is loose, with many folds. Take the skin between your fingers. Press your fingers together to make a fold in the skin. Then let it go. In severe dehydration, the fold will stay for some seconds, perhaps even a minute.

6. In an infant, the fontanel is very deep, or shrunken. Look at page 188 to see what the fontanel is.

7. The muscles are feeble. When you lift an arm or a leg, the child cannot keep the arm or the leg up. It will fall back quickly.

8. There is little urine. Perhaps the child has not passed urine for many hours, or even for a whole day.

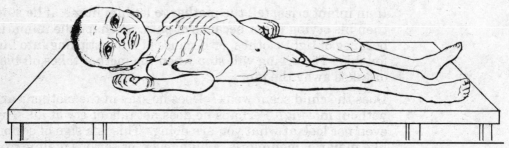

Child with dehydration.

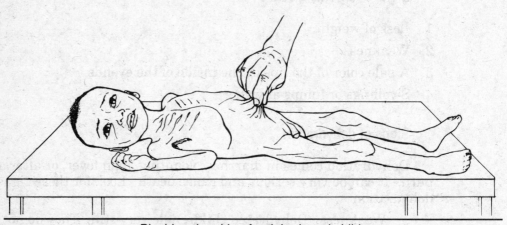

Pinching the skin of a dehydrated child.

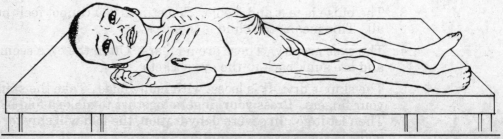

The skin stays folded for a few seconds.

Signs of malnutrition.

Malnutrition causes many changes in the body.

The hair.

The hair normally is black, smooth, and thick. In malnutrition, the hair becomes short and thin. It often becomes red or white. Much of it may fall out.

The skin.

The skin normally is smooth and soft. You can see light reflected from the skin. The color is the same all over the body except on the bottoms of the hands and feet. There it is much lighter.

In malnutrition, the color becomes different in different parts of the body. Some skin may be dark. Other skin may be light. There may be small dark spots on the skin. The skin looks thin and tight. There may be many thin lines on the skin, especially on the skin of the legs.

Often there are sores on the skin, and these sores may be big. Pieces of skin can come off, especially on the arms and legs. The skin under these pieces is very red and thin. In the folds under the arms and between the legs, the skin becomes red and thin.

Swelling

This is another sign of malnutrition. The lower legs swell, and sometimes the forearms,the hands, and even the face swell. The face can become almost round. Often there is swelling of the eyelids.

The abdomen

It becomes big and sticks out in front. We call this a "pot belly." This is because the muscles of the abdomen are weak. There may be liquid, or ascites, in the abdomen. The liver and the spleen may be big, causing the abdomen to be big.

Sadness

Children with malnutrition are not happy. They move little, and sit with their head down. They are sad, and do not smile. They will not talk to you when you talk to them. They may cry much. They do not eat well. They do not play with other children.

Loss of weight

The child loses weight even when there is swelling. The upper part of the arms and legs becomes thin. The ribs can be seen very easily.

Diarrhea

Often the child has diarrhea. The stools are like water, with very little brown fecal matter. There is no blood or pus in the stools.

SUMMARY

These, then, are the signs of malnutrition.
1. Short, thin hair which may be red or white.
2. Changes in the color of the skin, with thin skin and often many sores.
3. Swelling, often with a round face.
4. A big abdomen - "pot belly."
5. A sad look.
6. Loss of weight.
7. Diarrhea, like water.

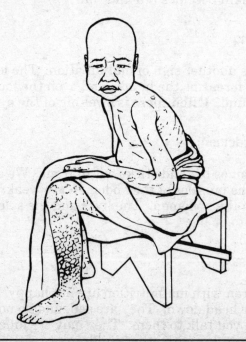

Signs of malnutrition.

Questions for study

1. How can you tell if a child has a serious illness?
2. How can you tell if a child has a chronic illness?
3. How can you tell if a child is dehydrated?
4. How can you tell if a child is malnourished?

The skin

Look carefully at the skin for signs of disease. Turn back to page 145 to see the different kinds of changes that can come on the skin. Look for these special conditions on the skin of the child.

Fungus infections.

Very small white spots on the skin of the chest and back come from a fungus infection called "tinea versicolor." This is not serious. Another fungus infection is called "ringworm." This causes big, round, light spots on the skin. There are fine scales at the edge. Often there is much itching.

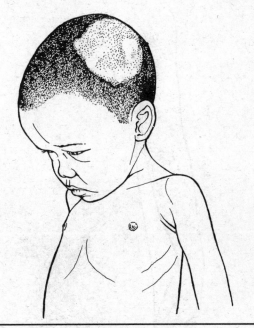

Fungus infection on head.

Measles

This causes an eruption of very small bumps all over the body. It starts on the face and behind the ears. Then it goes all over the body. On light colored skin the eruption, or "rash," looks red. On dark skin, you cannot see the red color. There is much fever and often a cough. The infant or child is very ill. The rash stays for 7 days, then goes away. Then fine scales of skin come off where the rash had been.

Scabies

This is a skin infection caused by small insect parasites that get into the skin. There are many small bumps, very irregular. The bumps are especially on the hands, at the elbows, under the arms, in the inguinal regions, and between the legs. There is much itching, with signs of scratching. Children with scabies often do not get good care at home. So look for signs of malnutrition.

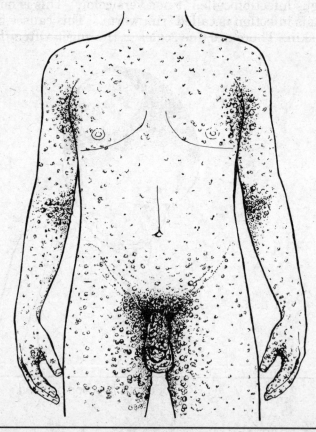

Scabies.

Lice

Small bumps on the face and head that look like scabies come from other insects, called lice.

Chicken pox

This causes an eruption of small bumps on the skin, with some fever. The bumps get big, then liquid comes into them. After 3 or 4 days, the liquid becomes pus. Then the bumps open and a crust comes on them. This soon falls off, and the disease is finished.

The bumps start first on the body. They then come on the arms and legs. At any one time, there are different sorts of bumps. Some are new. Some have liquid, others have pus. Some have crusts on them. The eruption goes away in 5 to 7 days. Usually the disease is not serious.

Infections of the skin

Infections can start in the bumps of scabies, lice, chicken pox, sores, or bites of insects. They can become open sores with pain and swelling around them. There can be big painful lymph nodes near by. Or the infection can stay under the skin. Then it causes a big round red spot with yellow scales on it. This is called "impetigo." It causes fever, and can make the child very ill.

The head

The head

Look for lumps, swellings, sores, and infections. Is the shape of the head normal? A very large head, a very small head, or an irregularly shaped head is a sign of serious disease. Send this child to hospital.

The eyes

1. Look for swelling of the eyelids. This may be a sign of anemia, of malnutrition, of a disease of the heart, the liver, or the kidneys. The swelling may be only of one eye. If there is no pain, this may be an allergic reaction. Or it can come from filaria. If there is much pain with the swelling, there is probably an infection in or around the eye. This is very serious.

2. A red color of the eye is a sign of conjunctivitis. But if there is much pain, there may be a serious infection inside the eye. Send this child to hospital.

3. A yellow color of the eyes, or jaundice, is a sign of either liver disease or of certain anemias.

4. Look at the cornea. This is the clear front part of the eye. Are there spots on it? A white spot with no signs of infection is from an old disease. No treatment will help. A spot or spots on the cornea with pain and redness is a sign of a serious infection. Send the child to hospital.

5. Look at the pupil. Normally the pupil is very black. If the pupil is white, or yellow, this is serious. There may be a tumor in the eye. Send the child immediately to hospital. See the strategy on pain in the eye on page 454.

The ears

Thick liquid coming from the ear is a sign of an ear infection. Often with this there is a sore on the skin outside the ear. The pus from inside causes this sore.

The nose

Look at the nose. Liquid from the nose, clear or thick, is a sign of a cold. Look at the sides of the nose. Do the sides move back and forth every time the child breathes? This is a sign of difficult breathing.

The lips

Sores on the lips come in chronic diseases with fever. They also come in malnutrition.

The teeth

Thick pus at the base of the teeth shows there is infection around the teeth. This comes in children who do not get good care. Often they have malnutrition. This pus can cause a serious infection in the mouth.

The neck

Look for lumps. If there is a lump, see in what part of the neck it is in - the front and middle, the side, the back, or right above the clavicles. Is the lump, or lumps, a lymph node or a tumor? See if there are small holes from which pus comes. This is a sign of tuberculosis of the lymph nodes.

The chest

Look carefully at the breathing of the child. This is the most important thing to do to find diseases of the lungs or heart.

1. Count the breathing. Is it fast, or slow? In a newborn infant, the respiration rate is between 30 and 60 times a minute. In a child of one year it is between 20 and 30 times a minute. In older children, it is slower.

2. Is the breathing difficult? Look at the lower ribs. Normally the lower ribs move out when the child breathes in. In difficult breathing, the lower ribs move in when the child breathes in. The spaces between the ribs also move in. We call this "retraction," and it is a sign of difficult breathing.

3. Look also at the nose. In difficult breathing, the sides of the nose move back and forth with breathing.

So there are three signs of difficult breathing.

1. Fast breathing.

2. Retraction of the lower ribs and the spaces between the ribs.

3. Movement, or "beating," of the sides of the nose during breathing.

You can find all of these signs simply by looking at the child. So in a child with symptoms of lung disease, look at him carefully. Look for these signs. This is the most important thing to do to make the diagnosis of lung disease. There may be no other signs, such as crackles or dullness in the chest.

The abdomen

Look carefully at the abdomen. Is it very big? If so, try to find out what is making it big.

1. Is there a big organ, like the liver or spleen?

2. Is there a big mass, or tumor?

3. Can you see waves of peristalsis? This is a sign of an obstruction in the intestines.

Malnutrition can cause the abdomen to become big. This is because the muscles are weak. Much liquid in the abdomen can also make it big. Malnutrition can also cause the abdomen to become thin. This comes when the child has very little to eat. A thin abdomen comes also in dehydration, and in many chronic diseases.

The back

Look at the spinal column. See if it is straight, or curved. Look for a strange bend, or bump, in it. This can be a sign of tuberculosis of the spine. A curved spine can come after an infection with polio. Look also for any lumps.

The genital organs

1   The urine opening - Is it in the right place?

2. The vagina - Is it open? If not, send the girl to hospital.

3. In a boy, look at the scrotum. Do the two sides look the same? If one side is bigger than the other, there is probably either a hernia or a hydrocele.

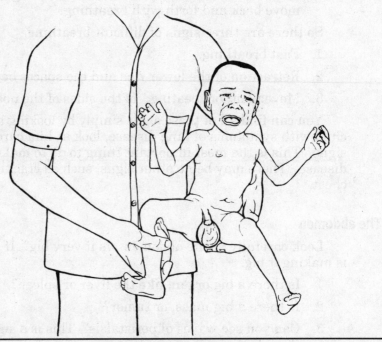

Boy with congenital hernia.

The arms and legs

1. Look for lumps or swellings. A big lump can be a big lymph node, an infection, an injury, or a tumor.

2. Look for swelling, or edema. Swelling of the hands and feet only is a sign of sickle cell anemia.

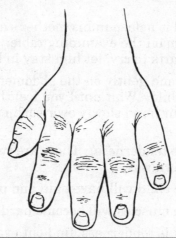

Swelling of fingers and hand in sickle cell disease.

Questions for study

1. What signs do you look for on the skin of children?
2. What signs do you look for in the eyes of children?
3. What signs do you look for in the ears, in the nose, and in the mouth of children?
4. What signs do you look for in the chest of children?
5. What will you see in a child who has pneumonia?
6. What can cause the abdomen of a child to become big?
7. What can cause the abdomen of a child to become very thin?
8. What signs do you look for in the back of a child?
9. What signs do you look for in the genital organs of a child?
10. What signs do you look for in the arms and legs of a child?

4.3.2 Feel for signs of disease - PALPATION

Now you are ready to examine the child with your hands. The order to follow in palpation is different in children than in adults. With young children, it is good to start with the abdomen.

When you examine children, move slowly. Children are afraid of fast movements. Children are also afraid you will hurt them. So always be gentle. Talk quietly to the child and to the mother during the examination. This will help the child relax.

The abdomen

If the child is asleep in his mother's arms, let him stay there. If he is awake, put him on the examining table. But he may be afraid to lie on the table. If he starts to cry, let him stay in his mother's arms.

Put your hand gently on the abdomen and let it stay in one place. Talk gently to the child. Wait until you feel the muscles of the abdomen relax. Then move your hand slowly over each part of the abdomen. At first, feel very gently.

1. Is there tenderness? There are two things that will show you if there is tenderness.

   ● The child will have pain and perhaps will cry.

   ● The muscles will become hard.

   If there is tenderness, find out exactly where it is.

2. Is there much pain when you take away your hand quickly? We call this "rebound" pain. It is a sign of peritonitis.

3. Feel for the liver. See page 105 for the way to examine the liver in adults. Normally, you can feel the lower edge of the liver below the last rib on the right. The edge is smooth and sharp. There is no tenderness. In an older child, often you cannot feel the edge of the liver at all. See if the liver is big. If it is big, look for these things.

   ● How big is it?

   ● What is it like? smooth, or irregular?

   ● Is it tender?

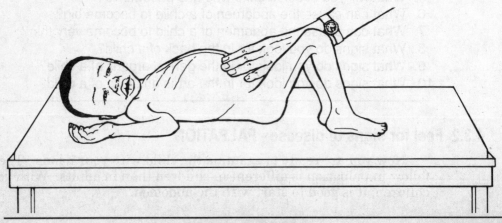

Feeling for the liver.

The big liver of heart failure is smooth and tender. The big liver of hepatitis is also smooth and tender. But there is usually fever and jaundice. The big liver of cirrhosis is irregular, often hard, with little or no tenderness.

4. Feel for the spleen. Normally it is not possible to feel the spleen. If you can feel it, this means the spleen is big because of disease. There are three ways to feel for the spleen.

- With the child lying flat on his back on the table or bed.
- With the child sitting up.
- With the child in his mother's arms over her shoulder.

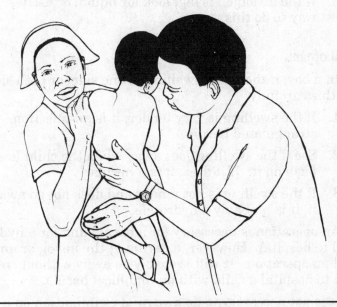

Feeling for the spleen.

The best way to feel for the spleen is with the child lying on his back. See page 107 for the way to examine the spleen in adults. If the child cries, let him sit on his mother's lap. If he keeps on crying, have her put him over her shoulder. Stand behind the child. Feel gently for the spleen with your left hand. The muscles of the abdomen must be soft. If not, you will not be able to feel the spleen. So it is important that the child does not cry.

If the spleen is big, see how big it is. Look at page 108 to see how to make note of the size of the spleen.

5. Feel for other masses in the abdomen. If you feel a mass, make a careful note about it.

   ● Where it is and how big it is.

   ● If is it hard or soft.

   ● If it is smooth or irregular.

   ● If it is tender or not.

   ● If it moves down when the child breathes in. The liver and spleen both move down when the child breathes in. If the child has a mass which does not move with breathing, this is serious. Send the child immediately to hospital.

6. If the abdomen is big, look for liquid, or ascites. See page 110 for the way to do this.

The genital organs

In a boy, if there is a swelling in one side, or both sides, of the scrotum, feel this carefully.

1. If the swelling is very tender, it is an infection. Or it may be a strangulated hernia.

2. See if the swelling goes away when the child lies down, or when you push on it. If it does, it is a hernia.

3. If the swelling is not tender and does not go away when you push on it, it is probably a hydrocele.

An operation is necessary for a hernia and for a hydrocele. Send the child to hospital. However, a hernia at the navel, or umbilicus, does not need an operation. It will probably go away without treatment. So do not send to hospital a child with an umbilical hernia.

It is not necessary to do a vaginal examination on a young girl. Look only to see if the vagina is open. If not, send the girl to hospital.

If there is pus or blood coming from the vagina, do a rectal examination gently. Feel in front of the rectum. There may be an object, or "foreign body," in the vagina. If so, send the girl to hospital. If there is no foreign body, treat the girl for an infection.

Usually it is not necessary to do a rectal examination on a child. Do it only when the child has one of these conditions.

● Has trouble passing fecal matter.

● Has much blood in the stool.

● Has signs of peritonitis, appendicitis, or intestinal obstruction.

To do the rectal examination, tell the mother that it will not be painful. Your finger is about the same size as a normal stool. Put a rubber glove on your hand. Put the child flat on his back or on one side. Have another person hold him and bend his legs forward. Put some oil or vaseline on the end of your finger.

For a small infant, use your fifth finger. For a child, use your index finger. Push the finger slowly and gently into the rectum. See if:

- The anus is open.
- There is fecal matter or not.
- There is an abnormal lump or mass.
- There is much tenderness or not. If so, where is the tenderness?

Look at your finger after you take it out of the rectum. Is there blood on it? Is there fecal matter on it? If so, what does the fecal matter look like?

Questions for study

1. What rules must you follow when you palpate children?
2. How can you tell if a child has tenderness in the abdomen?
3. If a child has a big liver, what must you find out about it?
4. How can you feel for the spleen of a child?
5. What do you look for in the genital organs of a child?
6. How can you tell a hernia from a hydrocele?
7. When should you do a rectal exam in a child?

The arms and legs

Look for swelling and for lumps. Feel carefully each swelling and lump.

1. Diseases of the heart, liver, and kidneys can cause swelling. Malnutrition and anemia can also cause swelling. In this swelling, you can make a small depression or pit when you push on it gently with your finger. We call this "pitting edema."

2. In the swelling of sickle cell anemia, there is no pitting edema. The swelling is usually just on the back of the hands and the tops of the feet.

3. If there is swelling in only one place, look for tenderness and heat. These are signs of infection.

4. A hard swelling is probably a disease of the bone. It may be an infection, a tumor, or an injury. If there is a fracture, there will be swelling, a change in the shape of the arm or leg, and much pain on

movement and on palpation. A hole in the skin over a bone with pus coming from it is a sign of a bone infection (osteomyelitis).

5. Move the arms and legs. Is there pain on movement of the joints? This is a sign of a disease of the joints.

6. Look for paralysis. See if the child can move his arms and legs. If not, which arm(s) or leg(s) are paralyzed?

7. Look for anesthesia. Do this in the same way you look for anesthesia in an adult. See page 139.

8. Examine his reflexes. Do this with a rubber hammer. Do it in the same way you examine the reflexes in an adult. See page 144.

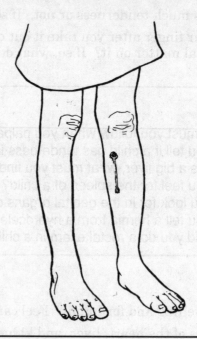

Leg sinus from a bone infection.

The lymph nodes

Feel for big lymph nodes. Feel the neck for big lymph nodes. Feel under the armpits. Feel in the inguinal region and at the top of the legs (the femoral region). Feel also in the abdomen. See page 116 and read about examining lymph nodes in adults.

You can feel small lymph nodes in many places in most infants and children. This is normal. See how big the nodes are. If they are tender, this is a sign of infection. Look for infections on the skin. Big lymph nodes in the abdomen, especially in the very low part of the abdomen, often come from tuberculosis. Send such a child to hospital. See the strategy BIG LYMPH NODES on page 550.

The chest

1. Feel the chest for tender places. If there is a tender place, look for signs of infection - heat, swelling. Ask about an injury. There may be a fracture of a rib. See page 82 for the way to feel for a rib fracture.

2. Feel the heart beat. A very strong heart beat on the chest over a big area can be a sign of heart disease. But if the chest is thin, you can feel even the normal heart beat.

   See where the heart beat is. Normally the "apical pulse" is under the left nipple. If the apical pulse is over on the side of the chest, the heart has become big. This is a sign of heart disease.

3. Percuss softly on the chest. To do this in an infant or child, tap with just one finger on the chest. Keep the finger straight and tap with the whole finger. Do not tap on another finger as you do in percussion on an adult. Listen to the sound. A resonant sound over the lungs is normal. A dull sound over the lungs is a sign of disease, such as liquid in the chest or serious pneumonia.

The neck

1. See if the neck is stiff. Put the child flat on his back on the table or on the bed. Put your hand under his head. Lift your hand slowly.

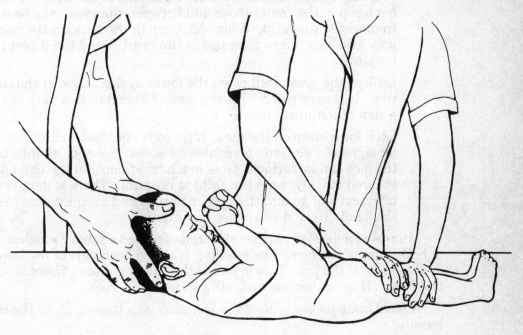

Examining a baby for a stiff neck.

See if the neck bends easily. If not, the neck is stiff. This is a sign of meningitis. In a small infant, if the neck is stiff, see if the fontanel is swollen.

2. Feel for lumps in the neck. If there are lumps, are they big lymph nodes? Or is there a tumor? Look for signs of infection - tenderness, heat. If there are signs of infection, give treatment for an infection. But send the child to hospital in these cases.

  ● There are no signs of infection at all.

  ● The signs of infection do not go away after the treatment.

  The disease may be serious. The doctor must see the child.

The head

1. The fontanel. In an infant under one year, feel the fontanel. This is a small soft place in the top of the head in front. It is between the bones of the head. The fontanel normally becomes small during the first year. It goes away entirely by the age of 18 months. In meningitis, the fontanel becomes big, swollen, and tender. In dehydration, the fontanel becomes deep, or depressed.

2. Feel for lumps. Lumps under the skin at the back of the head are probably lymph nodes. Look for infections of the skin of the head. A big lump in the front, above and between the eyes, may be a tumor from inside the head. A big soft lump in the back, in the middle, may also be a tumor from inside the head. Send the infant to hospital.

3. Look at the eyes. Pull down the lower eyelid. Look at the conjunctiva. Is it very pale? This is a sign of anemia. Is it very red? This is a sign of conjunctivitis.

4. Look for a lump on the face. If there is one, feel it carefully. Look for signs of infection. Look also for sores. Sores or an infection on the face can be serious. Give much treatment. If the child does not get well quickly, send the child to hospital. There is danger that the infection will go into the deeper tissues and even into the inside of the head. Here it can cause meningitis.

Mumps is a disease of older children. It gives a tender swelling on one or both sides of the face. The swelling is at the back part of the lower jaw, on the angle of the jaw. It is in one of the saliva glands. There is some pain and fever. It is not serious and will go away in a week.

A hard lump on one side of the face may be a tumor. Send the child to hospital.

Questions for study

1. What signs of disease can you find in the arms and legs of a child?
2. How can you tell what is causing big lymph nodes in a child?
3. What signs indicate that a small child may have meningitis?

4.3.3 Examine the child with instruments

Instruments often make a child afraid. Let the child see the instrument first. Let him touch it to see that it does not give pain. Show him your stethoscope. Show him the flashlight. Often then he will not be afraid when you use these instruments.

The stethoscope

Listen to the heart

First, listen carefully to the heart. If possible, keep the child from crying. If the child cries, you will not be able to hear signs of disease.

1. Count the heart rate. This is the best way to count the pulse in small infants, when the heart is very fast, or when the pulse is very weak. In small infants, a pulse of 100 to 120 in normal. In older children, a pulse of 80 to 100 is normal.

2. Listen for a heart murmur. A heart murmur comes in diseases of the heart valves. Or it can come in a heart that has a malformation. A severe anemia can also cause a heart murmur. Give such a child treatment for the anemia. If the murmur goes away when the anemia goes away, then the anemia was the cause of the murmur. The heart is probably normal.

3. Look for signs of heart failure. The signs of heart failure in children are not always the same as in adults. Look for these signs.

- A very fast pulse.

- A big tender liver.

- Crackles in the lungs, usually at the bottom of the lungs.

- Swelling, or edema. This sign often comes later, after the other signs.

- Blue lips. This is a sign of serious heart disease. Send such a child to hospital.

Listen to the lungs

Listen carefully to the lungs. Normal breath sounds in a child are like the normal breath sounds of adults. Because the chest of a child is thin, the breath sounds are quite loud.

Crackles are a sign of disease.

- Crackles with fever and difficult breathing are signs of pneumonia. But many times in pneumonia, there may be no crackles. So look for other signs of pneumonia.

- Crackles at the bottom of the lungs may be a sign of heart failure. Look for other signs of heart disease and heart failure.

- Crackles may sometimes come in tuberculosis. But often there are no lung signs in tuberculosis in children.

Rhonchi are loud sounds in the lungs. They sound like air going through water. The rhonchi come when there is water in the bronchial tubes. Air going through this water, or secretions, makes the rhonchi. Rhonchi can come in these cases:

- When a child is crying. This is normal.

- In bronchitis.

- Sometimes in heart failure when there is much edema in the lungs.

Listen to the abdomen

If there is much pain in the abdomen, listen to the abdomen with the stethoscope. Listen for the sounds of peristalsis.

1. In peritonitis, there are no peristaltic waves. The abdomen is silent.
2. In intestinal obstruction, there are strong waves of peristalsis. These make very loud sounds. The sounds go across the abdomen, stop, then start again. The child will cry with pain during these peristaltic waves.

Flashlight

A simple flashlight is very good for examining a child.

Look at the child's eyes.

1. Look for spots on the cornea.
2. Look for a foreign body on the cornea or on the conjunctiva.
3. Look at the pupils. Normally, when you shine a light in the eye, the pupil will immediately become smaller, or contract. It will then become bigger, or dilate, when you remove the light. If this does not happen, a serious disease is present. Send the child to hospital.

Look in the child's mouth.

Often an infant or child does not like this examination. He will cry. Put the child on his back on the table or bed. Have another person hold the child's arms on the sides of his head. In this way, this person can hold the arms and the head of the child together. Have another person, perhaps the mother, hold the child's feet. Use a flat instrument, or the handle of a spoon, to hold down the child's tongue. Look at the child's teeth. How many are there? Are some teeth missing? Look for holes in the teeth. Look for pus at the base of the teeth.

Look for sores inside the mouth, on the gums, on the tongue. Small round sores with a white center and red edges come from a virus infection. We call this "herpes." Often these sores are not serious. But they do cause pain, and they can keep a child from eating. There is no good treatment for them.

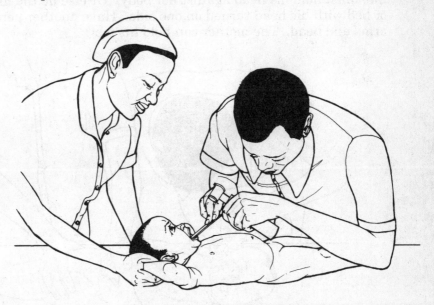

Examining a baby's mouth.

Look at the throat and the tonsils.

This is difficult, so do it slowly and gently. Put the flat instrument or spoon handle on the tongue. Push down. Slowly push the instrument back on the tongue. The throat will open quickly. You can then see the tonsils and the back of the throat. But you must look quickly. The throat will close again immediately and the child will cry.

Often an older child can show you his throat himself. Ask him to open his mouth wide. Tell him to say "AH" and to breathe fast and deeply. In this way the throat may open wide. If not, push down gently on the tongue. Then you will probably be able to see the throat and the tonsils.

Redness of the throat is a sign of infection. Redness alone comes from a virus infection. Redness of the throat and white spots of pus on the throat or on the tonsils are signs of a serious infection. This needs treatment with penicillin.

Otoscope

This is a special flashlight to look in the ears. It is a small light with a glass in front of it. The glass makes things look big. There are also small round plastic cones which go on the light. These help you see inside the ear canal.

To examine the ears of an infant, have the mother hold him on her lap. She must hold his head against her body. Or else lie the infant on the table or bed with his head turned on one side. Have another person hold his arms and head. The mother can hold his feet.

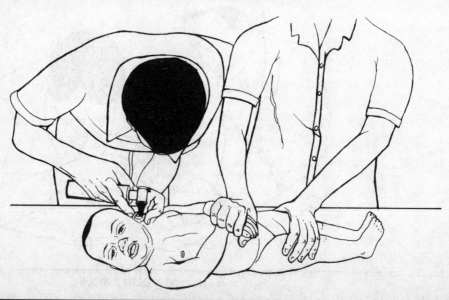

Examining a baby's ear.

An older child will usually let you look in his ears without being afraid. Tell him what you are going to do. Show him the otoscope. Tell him the examination will not hurt. Then do the examination gently. You can usually do it with the child sitting up.

Hold the otoscope in one hand. Pull gently on the top of the ear with the other hand. This will make the ear canal straight. Put the end of the plastic cone gently in the opening of the ear. Look through it, looking through the small glass. In this way, you can see the ear canal and the ear drum at the far end of the canal.

1. Look at the ear drum. A red drum is a sign of infection in the middle ear. Look for a hole in the drum. This is a sign of a chronic and perhaps serious infection in the middle ear.

2. Look for pus in the canal. Pus can come from the middle ear if there is a hole in the ear drum. Or pus can come from an infection of the ear canal. In either case, treatment with an antibiotic is necessary.

Blood pressure machine

It is difficult to take the blood pressure in infants and small children. Often it is not necessary.

In older children over 5 years of age, it is not difficult. Take the blood pressure in the same way you take it in adults. But use a machine with a smaller cuff.

Thermometer

For infants, take the rectal temperature. This will give you the true temperature. A rectal thermometer has a very short, thick bulb of mercury. If you have only a thermometer with a long mercury bulb, do not use it as a rectal thermometer.

Put the infant on his abdomen on the bed, the table, or on his mother's lap. Have the mother or another person hold him.

Look at the thermometer. Make sure the mercury is at $37°$ or below. If it is above $37°$, shake it until the mercury comes down below $37°$.

Put some oil or vaseline on the mercury bulb of the thermometer. Pull the buttocks apart gently. Slowly and gently push the mercury bulb into the rectum. Push it in a little beyond the bulb, but no more. If you push hard, or put it in too far, you can hurt the infant. Wait 3 minutes. Then take out the thermometer and look at it. Read the number of degrees at the end of the mercury line and write this on the child's record. Wipe the thermometer clean with a piece of paper or cloth. Shake the mercury down below $37°$. Put the thermometer back in it's place.

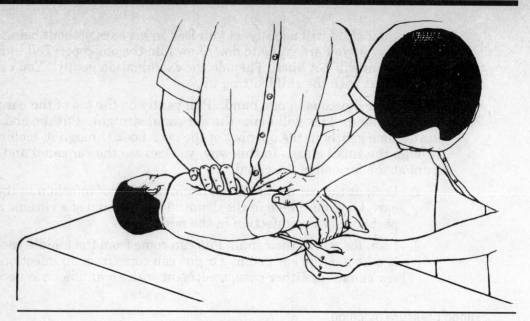

Taking the rectal temperature.

For older children, above the age of 5, you can use an oral thermometer. This has a long mercury bulb. Make sure the mercury is at, or below 37°. Put the bulb in the child's mouth. Make sure the bulb goes under the child's tongue. Tell him to close his lips and keep them closed. But he must not close his teeth. This can break the thermometer and hurt his tongue and mouth. Wait 3 minutes. Then take out the thermometer and read the temperature.

It is also possible to use an axillary thermometer, even for infants. This thermometer has a very long, flat mercury bulb. Be sure the mercury is at, or below 37°.

Have the mother hold the infant or child. Put the mercury bulb under the arm. Press the child's arm to his chest. Have the mother hold the arm against the chest for 3 minutes. Then take the thermometer and read the temperature. But remember that the axillary temperature is about one half degree below the true body temperature.

In sick children, take the temperature at least 3 times each day. Take it in the morning, around 8 o'clock. Take it in the afternoon, around 2 o'clock. Take it again in the evening, around 8 o'clock.

In some chronic infections, like tuberculosis, the temperature is normal during part of the day, usually in the morning. The fever comes only for a few hours, usually in the evening.

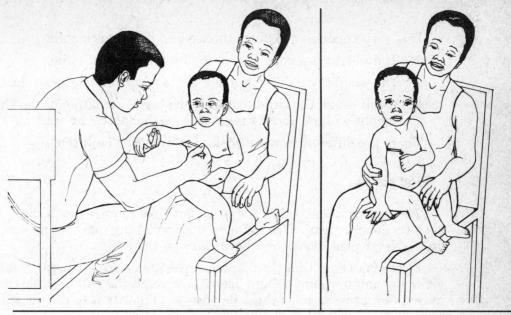

Taking the axillary temperature.

To know if the child has fever or not, you must take the temperature in the morning, in the afternoon, and in the evening. If not, the fever may come at a time when you do not take the temperature. So you will not know that the child does have a fever.

Questions for study

1. What signs in a child indicate heart disease?
2. What diseases can cause crackles in the lungs?
3. How can you find out what disease is causing the crackles?
4. What do you look for in a child's eyes?
5. What do you look for in a child's mouth?
6. What do you look for in a child's ears?
7. Why is it important to take a child's temperature 3 times a day?

Scales

It is very important to know the weight of each sick child.

1. The weight is a good sign of the nutrition of the child.
2. The weight will tell you the doses of medicine to give to the child.
3. If you weigh the child regularly during his treatment, the change in weight will tell you if the child is getting better or not.

There are different sorts of scales for weighing children.

Flat scales

The flat, or "pan", scales are good, but they require much care. You must keep them very clean. Use them only for weighing infants and small children. Never place books or other things on the scales.

First make sure that the pointer of the scales goes to zero. If it does not, make the pointer point to zero before you weigh the child. Different scales have different ways to do this. Be sure you know how to do this with your scales.

To weigh the child, have the mother take off the clothes. Put the child gently on the pan of the scales. Wait until the child stops making movements. Then read the weight on the arm of the scales.

Hanging spring scales

These scales are usually quite strong. They stay strong and accurate for some years if you take good care of them. There are pants that come with the scales. They are made of plastic. If necessary, you can make others of cloth.

Hang the scales from any good strong place, like a door frame, a beam in the ceiling, even a tree branch. Make sure that the needle points to zero. If it does not point to zero, turn the little screw on the top of the scales. Turn it until the needle goes to zero.

Have the mother put the pants on the infant or child. Then lift the child up by the pants. Hang the pants on the hook of the scales. Wait for the child to stop making movements. Do this slowly so that he will not cry. Look at the needle on the scales to see how much the child weighs.

Adult scales

For older children who can stand quietly, you can use an adult scales. Again be sure that the scales read zero when there is nothing on them. If they do not, make them do so before you weigh the child.

You can also use adult scales for weighing infants. Do this if you do not have infant scales. Give the infant to the mother. Have the mother get on the scales. Look at the weight of the mother and the infant together. Write it down.

Now take the infant from her. Look at how much the mother alone weighs. Write this down under the weight of both of them together. Subtract the weight of the mother alone from the weight of both of them together. This will give you the weight of the infant.

To know if the weight of a child is normal or not, you must know his age in months. Ask the mother when the child was born. Then you can find out from the birth date his age now in months.

If the mother does not know the birth date, ask her about what time of the year the child was born. See page 164 for the way to do this. Or else, look at the growth markers of the child as shown on page 162. This can help you know about how old the child is.

The weight is a good sign of the nutrition of a child. Look at the chart on the next page. This chart shows you how much weight a normal child has during the first five years of life. The low line is the low weight line for normal children. A child with a weight below this line is under weight. His nutrition is not good.

The upper line is also normal for children. The weight of most normal children will come between these two lines. But a few children will have a weight just above the top line. This is normal.

Questions for study

1. Why is it important to weigh a child often?
2. How can you be sure the weight is correct?
3. If the mother does not know the birth date of the child, how can you find out about when he was born?

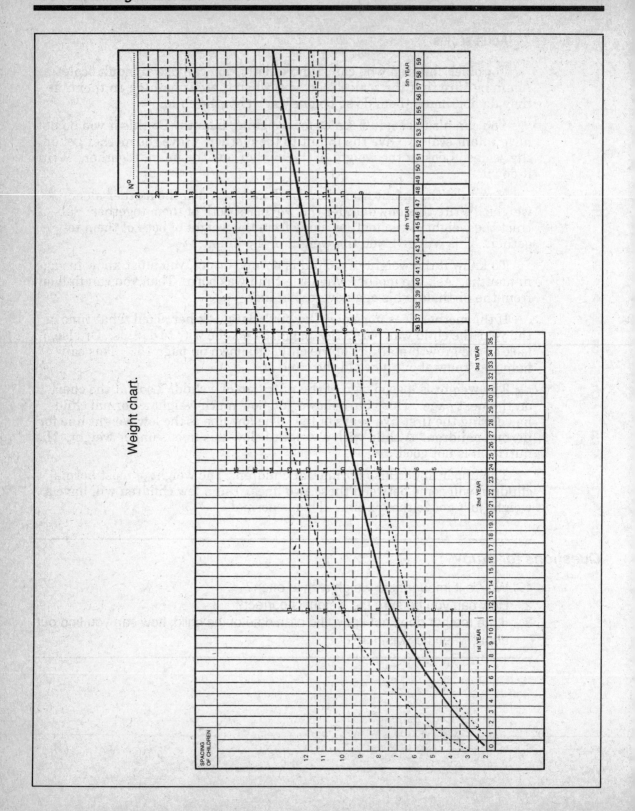

Weight chart.

Chapter 5
UTILISING LABORATORY EXAMINATIONS

5.1 Principles of laboratory examinations

Laboratory examinations (lab exams) can give you much help in making a diagnosis. They can show you important things about the patient and about the disease.

Certain lab exams are very important. Your health center should have the equipment necessary to do them. You must be able to do these exams yourself.

But perhaps someone else in your health center does them regularly. In this case, you must still know how to do the exams yourself. You must be sure that this other person does them correctly. Be sure to supervise regularly the work and the results of your lab helper.

This book will not tell you how to do each examination. There are good laboratory manuals that give specific instructions for each lab exam. One good book is called <u>A Medical Laboratory for Developing Countries</u>. It is by Dr. Maurice King. It comes from the Oxford University Press in London.

5.1.1 Indications for laboratory examinations

It is not necessary to do lab exams on every patient. To do so would waste much time. But you must know when a lab exam will help you make the right diagnosis. Do a lab exam only when you need certain information about the disease, information which you can find only by doing the lab exam. For each lab exam, you will find a list of the indications for doing that exam.

5.1.2 Precision in doing laboratory examinations

It is essential to do every lab exam correctly. An incorrect result leads to an incorrect diagnosis. This in turn leads to incorrect treatment for the patient. It is even possible for a patient to die because of an incorrect result of a lab exam. Be sure to follow these rules in your laboratory.

Keep order

Keep your laboratory in good order. Keep each piece of equipment in a certain place. Make sure the equipment and your work tables are always clean. At the end of each day, clean the equipment. Put each piece of equipment back into its place. Clean the work tables. Clean also the windows and the floor.

Use good solutions

Be sure the solutions you use for the lab exams are good. Keep all solutions in bottles with a tight top or cover. Be sure that no dust, dirt, or insects can get into them. Old solutions can become bad. They can then give incorrect results. So replace old solutions with new ones.

Keep a register

A register for your lab exams is very important. Record in your register each examination you do. Write the date, the name of the patient, the exam done, and the result. This will help you do good work. For every examination you must record certain things in three different places.

1. Write the name of the patient on each specimen. This is very important. If you forget this, you may change one specimen for another. Then you will get an incorrect result for the two patients whose specimens you have marked incorrectly.

2. Record in the register the information noted above about the patient and the exam.

3. Record on the patient's card or chart the date, the exam done, and the result.

Follow instructions

Follow the instructions for each exam correctly. When you get the result, think about it. Does the result seem correct? If the result seems strange, perhaps you have made a mistake. In this case, do the exam again.

Collect specimens correctly

Follow carefully the instructions about how to collect specimens correctly. A poorly collected specimen can give an incorrect result. This is especially true for urine specimens from women. It is also true for sputum specimens and even stool specimens.

Make good preparations

Make each preparation correctly. A poorly made preparation can give incorrect results. Follow very carefully the instructions in your lab manual for the making of the preparation.

SUMMARY

These are the rules to follow in your laboratory.

1. Keep everything clean and in order.

2. Use good solutions.

3. Keep a register.

4. Follow the instructions for doing each examination.

5. Collect specimens correctly. Write the name of the patient on each one.

6. Make good preparations.

7. Record the results of each exam in the register and on the patient's record.

At the end of each day, go to your laboratory. See if it is clean and in good order. Check the register. Look at the equipment to see if it is all clean. Look especially at the microscope and see that all parts of it are clean. In this way, your lab will work well. The lab exams will then help you make the right diagnosis in your patients.

5.1.3 Interpretation of lab results

It is essential to know what the results of lab exams mean. Very often they can make the diagnosis definite. Look at these examples.

1. A patient has a high fever and a headache. You think he has malaria. You do a thick blood film and find malaria parasites in his blood. Now you are certain that the patient has malaria.

2. A baby has a high fever, convulsions, and a stiff neck. You do a lumbar puncture and examine the cerebro-spinal fluid. In the fluid you find many white blood cells. So the diagnosis of meningitis is certain.

3. A man has frequent urination with much urine each time. The urine exam shows sugar in the urine. The diagnosis of diabetes is certain.

4. A small child has colicky pain in the abdomen. The stool exam shows roundworm (ascaris) eggs. So you know the child has roundworms.

In these examples, we say that the result of the lab exam is "positive." It makes the diagnosis certain. If the result is "negative," we must then look for another cause of the illness.

Sometimes a disease is present but the lab sign is absent. That is, the result of the lab exam is negative even though the disease is present. For example:

1. The thick blood film is sometimes negative in malaria.

2. The urine sugar is sometimes negative in diabetes.

3. The stool exam is sometimes negative even when roundworms are present.

4. A sputum exam for tubercle bacilli may be negative even when the patient has tuberculosis.

5. The stool exam can be negative for ameba even when the patient has an amebic infection.

Perhaps you feel strongly that the patient has the disease in question. But do not treat the patient immediately if the lab exam is negative unless the patient is very ill. Do the lab exam again. Do it two or three more times if necessary. Very often, if the disease is really present, the exam will be positive on the second, third, or fourth exam.

If the lab exam is done correctly, a positive result makes the diagnosis certain. A negative result shows that the disease is perhaps not present. However, a negative result may become positive if we repeat the exam. Perhaps we repeat it three or four times and it is still negative. In this case, we are quite certain the disease is not present.

5.1.4 Be complete in your examinations of each patient

It is clear that lab exams can be very helpful. But they are only a small part of the examination of the patient. You must do a complete examination on many of your patients. Do not simply do one or more lab exams and think you have done all that is necessary. First, take a good history and do a complete physical examination.

Do not do the lab exams the first thing. For example, a patient has had a cough for one month. Do not tell him simply to give you a sputum specimen. First, take the history of the illness. Then do the physical examination. After this, ask for the sputum specimen and do any other exams you think will help you.

5.1.5 Protect yourself from infections

In some diseases the microbes causing them are in the blood of the patient or in pus coming from him. This is true in AIDS, in one form of hepatitis, in syphilis, in gonorrhea, and in others. You can get these infections by touching the blood or pus of patients with these diseases. Therefore, it is very important to wear rubber or plastic gloves to protect yourself from these diseases. It is not necessary for the gloves to be sterile.

Always wear gloves:

1. When taking blood or pus from a patient.

2. When putting the blood or pus on a microscope slide or in a tube.

Always throw away, or sterilize by boiling, every needle you use to draw blood, pus, or cerebro-spinal fluid. When you finish drawing the blood or pus and putting it on a slide or in a tube, wash your gloved hands in water. Then take off your gloves and put them in a disinfectant solution for at least a half hour. You can then dry the gloves and use them again.

When the blood or pus is dry on the slide, or is in the tube, it is no longer dangerous. You do not need to wear gloves to examine the preparation.

When you take blood into a pipette for a Hg exam or a white blood cell count, never draw the blood into your mouth. Always have a long rubber or plastic tube on the end of the glass pipette. Put the other end of the tube into your mouth. Watch carefully the blood going up into the pipette. Never let it get into the rubber or plastic tube.

Questions for study

1. How can you decide what lab exams to do in a patient?
2. What must you do to be sure that your lab exams are done correctly?
3. Why is a lab register important? How can it help you?
4. Where must you record the results of each lab exam?
5. How does a positive lab exam help you make a diagnosis?
6. What does a negative lab exam mean?

5.2 Hemoglobin (Hg) examination

We measure hemoglobin in grams per 100 ml of blood. We call this "g%" (grams percent). Some people measure Hg in percent of normal, 100% being normal. However, the normal value is different for different people. So the "percent" method is not very good. The "g%" method is much better.

The normal values for hemoglobin are as follows:

- Babies up to two years have 10g% or more.

- Children from 2 to 12 years have 12g% or more.

- Adult women have 13g% or more.

- Adult men have 14g% or more.

If the patient's Hg is less than the normal value, the blood is thin. We say the patient has anemia. See page 474 for the important causes of anemia and how to find the cause in each case.

5.2.1 The technique

There are two different and simple techniques for doing the Hg exam. The Talquist technique is very simple, but it is not precise. In this technique, you put a drop of the patient's blood on a piece of special paper. You then look at the color of the drop.

The Talquist book of papers has a series of colors on the cover. Look at the color of the drop of the patient's blood. Then find the color on the Talquist book that is most like the color of the patient's blood drop. The number by the color on the Talquist book is then the percent of Hg in the patient's blood.

The other technique is the dilution technique. This gives a better result, because it is more precise. To do this, you need a special instrument called a "hemoglobinometer." There are two kinds:

- Sahli.
- Lovibond.

The Lovibond method is more precise. But the Lovibond hemoglobinometer is expensive. Look at your lab manual for the way to do the hemoglobin exam by this method.

5.2.2 Indications for the hemoglobin exam

Do a Hg exam on any patient with one or more of these indications.

1. A patient with any serious disease. This patient may also have anemia.
2. A patient with a chronic disease. Many chronic diseases cause anemia.
3. A patient with bleeding.
4. A patient who is in shock.
5. A patient who has malaria, hookworm, malnutrition, or sickle cell anemia.
6. A patient who is pale or very weak.
7. A patient who has swelling of the legs, the abdomen or the eyelids.
8. A patient who has heart disease or heart failure.
9. A woman who is pregnant.
10. A patient who needs an operation.
11. A patient who has a severe snake bite.

5.3 Stool examination

The stool exam will show you if the patient has intestinal parasites, such as:

- Helminths: ascaris, ankylostomes, trichuris, strongyloides, enterobius, Schistosoma mansoni, tapeworm (Taenia).
- Protozoa: ameba, Giardia.

5.3.1 Collecting the specimen

Tell the patient to bring a stool specimen on a big leaf, in a small can, or in a piece of aluminium paper. He must bring a small piece of stool. A very small amount from the skin near the anus taken after passing the stool is not enough.

Take a small piece of stool from the middle of the specimen. Use a small stick or a match to do this. Put the specimen on a microscope slide in a drop of saline - salt water at 0.9%. Stir the specimen gently in the saline. Put a cover slip over the drop of saline.

Look at the preparation for at least five minutes under the low power of your microscope. Even if you quickly see the eggs, larva or protozoa of one parasite, continue looking. The patient may have two or more kinds of parasites. Do not consider the result negative until after you have looked for five or more minutes and found no parasites.

If the patient has diarrhea, tell him to bring a stool specimen immediately after passing it. Give him a can or a bedpan to collect the specimen. Look at the stool specimen right away. First, look at it with your eyes. What does the stool look like? Is there blood or pus in it?

Put a drop of liquid stool on a microscope slide. Put a cover slip on the drop. Look at it immediately under the low and then the high power of the microscope. If the patient has ameba, you will see them. They are very small objects which move slowly through the liquid.

5.3.2 Indications for a stool exam

Do a stool exam on all patients who have one or more of the following conditions.

1. Diarrhea.
2. Blood or pus in the stool.
3. Pain in the abdomen, or heart burn.
4. Vomiting.

5. Anemia.

6. Malnutrition, or loss of weight.

7. Chronic liver disease.

5.4 Fresh blood drop examination

This can help you make the diagnosis of filariasis and of sickle cell anemia. In Central Africa it can also help you make the diagnosis of sleeping sickness (trypanosomiasis).

5.4.1 Collecting the blood

With a small sterile needle, make a prick at the side of the end of one of the patient's fingers. Do not prick the tip end of the finger. Put a drop of blood on a slide. Use a small stick or match to spread the drop a little. Put a cover slip on the drop. Look at it under the low power of the microscope.

Look for microfilaria. They are like long, thin worms. Sometimes they move a little.

In Central Africa, look also for trypanosomes. They are very small parasites in the liquid of the blood, or serum. You can see them moving.

If you think the patient has sickle cell anemia, first put a rubber band tightly around one of his fingers. Leave it there for five minutes. Then make a prick at the side of the end of the finger. Put a drop of blood on a slide. Put a cover slip on the blood drop. Put vaseline all around the cover slip to keep out air from the drop.

5.4.2 Looking at the blood for sickle cells

Look at the red blood cells (RBC) under the high dry power of the microscope. Normally the RBC are round with pale thin centers. In sickle cell anemia, they are different. They are crescent shaped, like the new moon.

See how many sickle cells there are. Count 100 RBC. In those 100 RBC, count how many of them are sickle shaped. If 10 are sickle shaped, the patient has 10% immediate sickling. If there are 50, the patient has 50% immediate sickling. Then put the slide away for 24 hours.

Look at the slide again after 24 hours. Again count 100 RBC. Count how many are in sickle shape. This will give you the percentage of sickling after 24 hours.

Immediate sickling is serious. Sickling after 24 hours is less serious. Patients with no immediate sickling, but with sickling after 24 hours, usually do not suffer from the disease. But they can give the disease to their children.

Patients with much immediate sickling suffer from the disease. Those with a very high percentage of sickling suffer very much. These are usually infants or small children.

5.4.3 Indications for a fresh blood drop

Do a fresh blood drop exam on all patients who have:

1. Symptoms or signs of filariasis:
   - Itching, swelling of the eyelids, hands, or other parts of the body.
   - Chronic swelling of the legs or genital organs.
   - Chronic enlarged lymph nodes.
2. Symptoms or signs of sickle cell anemia:
   - Frequent attacks of anemia, of jaundice, or of both.
   - Swelling of the backs of the hands or feet.
   - Frequent pains in the bones of the legs or arms in children.
   - Frequent severe pain in the abdomen in children.
3. Symptoms or signs of African sleeping sickness: see page 551.

Questions for study

1. What are the possible causes of anemia?
2. In a patient with anemia, what other lab exams should you do?
   See the strategy on ANEMIA on page 474.
3. In what patients should you do a stool specimen?
4. What must you do to find ameba in a patient's stool?
5. In what patients should you examine a fresh blood drop?
6. What must you do to find sickle cells?

5.5 Urine examination

5.5.1 Indications

Do a urine exam on all patients who have one or more of the following conditions:

1. Symptoms of disease of the urinary system.
2. Swelling of the legs, of the abdomen, or of the eyelids.
3. High blood pressure or heart disease.
4. Pain in the back or in the lower abdomen.

5. Fever for which you can find no cause.
6. Symptoms of diabetes.
7. Swelling of the legs during pregnancy.
8. Coma.
9. Convulsions.

5.5.2 Collecting the specimen

Give the patient a clean receptacle. If the receptacle is not clean, the exam will not be correct.

If the patient is a woman, she must follow certain instructions very carefully. Explain these to her clearly. First, she must wipe very carefully the opening of the vagina and urethra. This will remove all secretions from these openings. If she does not do this, these secretions may get into the receptacle along with her urine. They will then make the results of the exam incorrect.

Tell each patient, a man or a woman, to start urinating first into the sanitary installation. After the urine has started to come, the patient should put the receptacle into the stream of urine. When the receptacle has a good amount of urine in it, the patient should take it away and finish urinating into the sanitary installation. In this way, you can be sure there is only urine in the receptacle. This urine comes only from the bladder and not from the urethra.

If you need to exam urine from the urethra, have the patient put the first urine into the receptacle. This urine comes from the urethra.

Be sure to exam a urine specimen on every child who has a fever with no evident cause for the fever. The child may have an infection in the kidneys or the bladder.

Getting a urine specimen from a baby or small child can be difficult. Give the mother a small bottle with a big opening. Have her undress the child. She must hold the bottle at the penis or the vagina until the child urinates.

5.5.3 Examining the specimen

Do the urine exam immediately. This is very important. After one hour or more, the urine specimen will no longer be good. Many blood cells, if present, will have disappeared. So do the urine exam right away. Here is what to look for.

1. Look at the color of the urine. Dark urine is normal if the patient has not had much water to drink. It also comes when there is fever, diarrhea, or much sweating.

Dark urine can also be a sign of bile in the urine. This comes in jaundice from liver disease or from some forms of anemia. Put some urine in a test tube. Put your finger over the end of the tube and shake it hard. Look at the foam that comes on top of the urine. If the foam is white, there is no bile in the urine.

If the foam is yellow, this is a sign of bile in the urine. Look for jaundice in the eyes, the fingernails, the mouth, or the skin.

2. Test the urine for sugar. The presence of sugar is a sign of diabetes.

3. Test the urine for protein (albumin). Protein comes in the urine in these diseases.

   - Diseases of the kidneys.
   - Diseases of the bladder or urethra when there are many white blood cells.
   - The disease of pregnancy called "toxemia".
   - Many infections with fever.
   - Some patients with no sign of serious disease.

4. Look at a drop of urine under the microscope. If you have a centrifuge, put some urine in a centrifuge tube. Centrifuge it for 5 minutes. Then put a drop of urine from the bottom of the tube on a microscope slide. Put a cover slip over the drop.

   If you do not have a centrifuge, let the urine stay in the tube for a few minutes. Then put a drop of urine from the bottom of the tube on a slide. Put a cover slip on the drop.

   Look at the drop of urine under the low power of the microscope. Look for:

   - White blood cells (WBC). These are a sign of infection somewhere in the urinary system. See page 560 to find the causes for WBC in the urine.
   - Red blood cells (RBC). These are a sign of a serious disease. See page 562 to find the cause of the hematuria.
   - Long cylinders, called "casts." These are a sign of a serious kidney disease.
   - Eggs of Schistosoma hematobium.
   - Epithelial cells. These often come in normal urine. They are not a sign of disease.

5.6 Sputum examination

The sputum exam is the best way to diagnose tuberculosis of the lungs. Do a sputum exam on all patients who have a cough with sputum for more than two weeks. Do it also on all patients who have blood in their sputum.

5.6.1 Collecting the sputum specimen

It is essential to get a good sputum specimen from the patient. Give him a small jar with a wide opening and with a cover for it. Give him clear instructions about how to get the specimen.

- Tell the patient to get the specimen in the morning when he first wakes up.

- He must cough very hard while sitting on the side of the bed.

- He must cough up sputum from very deep down in his chest.

- He must not put just saliva in the jar.

- He must put the sputum in the jar and place the cover on it.

- He must be careful not to let sputum get on the outside of the jar. This can spread his tuberculosis bacilli to other people, including you.

- He must then bring the jar to you as soon as possible.

If the patient has trouble coughing up real sputum, give him an expectorant 3 times a day. See page 257 for the dose. This will make the sputum become more liquid and easy to cough out.

5.6.2 Examining the sputum

First look at the sputum in the jar. See if there are thick white or yellow pieces of matter in it. See if there is blood. If it is clear liquid, then it is only saliva. It does not come from the lungs. You do not need to examine it.

Make a small loop out of a piece of thin wire. With this wire, take out a piece of yellow or white matter. Put it on a microscope slide and spread it around a little. Let it dry. If possible, hold the slide, specimen side up, over the flame of an alcohol lamp. Then you are sure the sputum will not come off. Pass the loop of wire through the flame. This will kill the bacteria on the loop.

If you do not have a wire, use a small stick to take a piece of sputum. Throw the stick into the fire after using it.

If you can do the Ziehl-Neelsen stain in your health center, do it right away. If you cannot, write the patient's name clearly on the slide. Then send the slide and a note to the nearest health center that can do the examination.

If you find tubercle bacilli in the sputum, you know your patient has tuberculosis of the lungs. You can now start giving treatment - see page 698 for the treatment. But send the slide to your reference hospital for a control in the laboratory there.

Be very sure you know from which patient the positive sputum has come. This is very important. Always put the name of the patient on the specimen jar and on the slide. If you put the wrong name on the specimen, you will give treatment for tuberculosis to someone who does not have it. You also will not treat someone who does have it. So be VERY CAREFUL.

Perhaps you do not find tubercle bacilli in the first specimen. But you think the patient probably has tuberculosis. In this case, repeat the sputum exam each day for 3 days. If after 3 exams the results are negative, the patient probably does not have tuberculosis of the lungs. If you still think he does, send him to hospital for other examinations. Never give treatment for tuberculosis without a positive sputum exam.

Questions for study

1. What are the diseases a urine exam can help you find?
2. What must you do to collect a good urine specimen?
3. How can you get a urine specimen from a baby or a small child?
4. Why must you examine a urine specimen quickly?
5. What do you look for in a urine exam?
6. What instructions do you give a patient about giving a good specimen of sputum?
7. If you think a patient has tuberculosis but the sputum exams are negative, what should you do?

5.7 Thick blood film

The thick blood film can show you the parasites of malaria and of African sleeping sickness. You can also find microfilaria if the patient has filariasis from Loa loa or Wuchereria.

The exam requires a careful technique. It also requires good stains. Talk to your doctor about this. Do not use an old or poorly prepared stain. This will give you an incorrect result.

5.7.1 Indications for a thick blood film

1. A patient with a high fever.
2. A baby or small child with convulsions.
3. A patient with anemia.

4. A patient with a big tender spleen.

5. A patient with fever and watery diarrhea.

6. A patient in Central Africa with a low fever for some days or weeks, or with small lymph nodes in the neck.

5.8 White blood cell count

5.8.1 Changes in white blood cell count

The normal white blood cell (WBC) count in an adult is from 5000 to 10,000 WBC per cubic millimeter of blood (mm3). In infants and young children, the count may go up to 12,000 WBC per mm3.

The white blood cell count can help you find the cause of fever in some patients. The WBC count is high in patients with an acute infection caused by bacteria. The WBC count is not high in the following infections.

- An acute infection from a virus.
- Typhoid fever with no complications.
- A chronic infection like tuberculosis, leprosy, or syphilis.
- An infection from parasites.

A very high WBC count - more than 60,000 per mm3 - is a sign of a very serious blood disease called leukemia. Any patient with a WBC count this high must go immediately to hospital.

5.8.2 Indications for a WBC count

1. A patient with a high fever that does not go away after treatment with chloroquine.

2. A patient who may have appendicitis.

If the WBC count is high, the patient probably has an acute bacterial infection. Look for the source of the infection. Be sure to do a urine exam to look for an infection in the urinary system. The infection will probably respond to a treatment with antibiotics. In case of appendicitis, the patient will need an operation. Send him to hospital immediately.

If the WBC count is normal, the patient probably does not have an acute bacterial infection. He may have a virus infection, typhoid fever, or malaria.

5.9 Cerebro-spinal fluid examination

The cerebro-spinal fluid (CSF) is around the brain and the spinal cord. We can take out a small amount of it to look at or to examine under the microscope. We do this by making a lumbar puncture (LP) with a special spinal needle.

5.9.1 Indications for a CSF examination

Do a CSF examination in these cases.

1. An infant or small child with fever and convulsions.
2. A patient with fever and a stiff neck.
3. An adult with convulsions. But do not do one in a pregnant woman with convulsions. Send her immediately to hospital. She may have toxemia of pregnancy.
4. A patient with a chronic headache and fever.
5. A patient who has, or may have, African sleeping sickness.

5.9.2 Technique for doing a lumbar puncture

The needle must be sterile. The needle goes between the bones of the spinal column into the spinal canal.

Wash your hands well and put on sterile gloves. The patient must lie on his side with his head on a pillow. His knees must be bent and come up to his chest. His head must bend forward. It is good to have someone hold him steady so he will not move.

If the patient is an adult, he can sit on a chair or a bed and bend forward. His back must be bent out. Someone must hold his shoulders so he will not fall.

1. Clean the skin very well with an antiseptic solution.
2. Feel the bones of the spinal column with the fingers of your gloved left hand.
3. Find a spot low in the back between two bones of the spinal column. This should be about the level of the iliac crests.
4. Take the sterile needle with your right hand.
5. Push it through the skin in the middle of the back and between the two bones.
6. Keep pushing it in slowly and steadily.
7. Be sure it is in the middle and that it points a little up toward the patient's head.

8. It must go in about 2 cm in a baby and about 5 cm in an adult.

9. Take out the thin wire (mandarin) inside of the needle. If thin liquid comes out, this is CSF.

10. Put 1 or 2 ml in a small test tube.

11. Put the wire back into the needle and pull the needle out.

12. If no liquid comes through the needle, put the wire back in and push a little further.

13. Again take out the wire and see if there is liquid.

14. If not, pull out the needle and try in a different place.

15. If blood comes out, pull out the needle and get another one. Try again in a different place.

16. If a little blood comes and then liquid, wait until the liquid becomes clear. Then put it in the test tube.

17. When you finish, put the patient in bed. He must lie down flat for several hours.

5.9.3 Examine the CSF

First, look at the liquid. See if it is clear. Or see if it is cloudy or has blood in it.

Take a small dropping pipette or a medicine dropper. Fill it with CSF. Put the CSF in the same slide and chamber you use for the WBC count. Do not use any solution with it. Examine it under the low power of the microscope. Look for small spots. These are white blood cells. Count them to see how many there are. Look in your lab manual to see how to do this.

Normally there are no WBC in the spinal fluid. If WBC are present in the CSF, the patient has a serious disease. The number depends on the disease.

1. Acute bacterial meningitis: too many to count.

2. Meningitis from tuberculosis: from 50 to 1000 per mm3.

3. Viral meningitis: from 10 to 500 per mm3.

4. African sleeping sickness: from 4 to 200 per mm3.

5.10 Pus smear

A pus smear can help you in two ways.

1. It can show you what kind of bacteria are in the pus, if any.

2. It can show you what kind of WBC are in the pus.

5.10.1 Indications for a pus smear

Do a pus smear in any patient who has one of these conditions.

1. Pus draining from a hole in the skin.
2. Pus coming from the urethra.
3. Thick secretions in or from the vagina.
4. Pus in the chest or abdomen.
5. Pus in a joint, like the knee.

5.10.2 Look for bacteria

Put a drop of pus on a slide. Spread it around with a small wire loop or a stick. Let it dry. Then color it with the stains of the Gram stain. Look in your lab manual to see how to do this. Look at the slide under the oil immersion power of your microscope. Look for bacteria. See what kind they are.

1. Small, round, blue or violet bacteria are called "cocci." Penicillin will usually cure them.
2. Small, round, red cocci inside WBC in pus from the urethra or from the vagina or the mouth of the uterus (cervix) are probably the cocci of gonorrhea.
3. Long red rods are called "bacilli." Penicillin will probably not cure them. They will require a "broad spectrum" antibiotic.

5.10.3 Look at the white blood cells

Do a pus smear in a patient with pus in the chest, in the abdomen, or in a joint. Make the preparation as above. Look at the WBC.

1. If they have more than one nucleus, from 2 to 5, they are polynuclear WBC. These come in acute bacterial infections.
2. If the WBC have only one nucleus, they are mononuclear WBC. These come in chronic infections like tuberculosis.
3. If there are no WBC in the pus, there is probably no longer an infection causing the liquid. The bacteria have gone away.

5.11 Blood sedimentation rate

When a specimen of blood which does not clot stands for some time in a thin tube, the red blood cells move down slowly toward the bottom of the tube. Normally they move down very slowly. But in some diseases they move down more rapidly. We call this the blood sedimentation rate, or "sed rate." A fast, or elevated, sed rate is an indication of:

1. A bacterial infection.
2. A chronic infection like tuberculosis.
3. Some parasite infections, like African sleeping sickness.
4. A malignant tumor.
5. Malnutrition.

The sed rate can help you in diagnosing certain diseases. But it does not give you a specific diagnosis. This is because the sed rate is elevated in many different diseases.

The sed rate is very useful in following the progress of certain diseases, like tuberculosis. If the sed rate returns to normal, this is a sign that the patient is getting better.

5.11.1 Indications

Do a sed rate on a patient who has one of these conditions:

1. A fever for some days or weeks.
2. Signs of tuberculosis or African sleeping sickness.
3. Signs of chronic inflammation. If the sed rate is elevated, then the patient probably has a chronic infection.

Look in your lab manual to see how to do the sed rate.

There are other laboratory examinations which can give you much help. But they are difficult to do. These ten examinations will help you make the diagnosis of many diseases. Learn to do them well and to do them without making errors.

Questions for study

1. In what patients can a thick blood drop exam help you?
2. In what patients can a white blood cell count help you?
3. In what patients can a cerebro-spinal fluid exam help you?
4. What do you look for in the CSF?
5. What does the number of WBC in the CSF mean?
6. How can a pus smear help you make a diagnosis?
7. In what patients can a sed rate help you?
8. What does an elevated sed rate mean?

Chapter 6
ANALYSING THE INFORMATION

You have now found out many things about the illness of the patient. You know the symptoms. You know many of the changes which the disease has made in the patient's body. These are the physical signs and laboratory signs of the disease. Now it is time to make the diagnosis. It is time to decide which disease is making the patient ill.

There are five important things to do to make the right diagnosis.

1. Write down in the patient's record all the important information about the disease.
2. Think carefully about this information.
3. Make a decision about the diagnosis and about what you must do.
4. If necessary, look for more information from the patient.
5. Solve any problems about the diagnosis.

6.1 Writing the patient's record

Every patient must have a record of his illness. You can write this on a special form, on a special card, or, if you have no card or form, on ordinary paper. But be sure to write down all the information.

If the patient's illness is simple, the record will be short. If the patient's illness is serious or complicated, the record will be long. Write down these important things on the record for every patient.

1. Today's date.
2. Information about the patient: name, sex, age or birth date, address, whether married or single; if married, the number of children.
3. The history of the present illness.
4. The physical examination (PE): the signs you found of the disease.
5. The results of the laboratory examinations, if any.
6. The definite, probable, or differential diagnosis.
7. The care and treatment you prescribed.
8. Any other exams you must do later.
9. The instructions you gave.

Under history, record all of the patient's symptoms. Record how the illness began, how it developed, and what the symptoms are now. Write down the answers to the questions you asked in the history. Write down also any important information about the health of the patient before the illness. Write down anything important about the health and the condition of the family.

Under PE, write down the physical signs of the disease. Be sure to write down any important signs that are not present. For example, in some cases of anemia there is jaundice. Jaundice is a sign that the anemia comes from a disease that destroys the red blood cells. But in other kinds of anemia there is no jaundice. So in a case of anemia, look for jaundice. Record on the patient's record if there is jaundice. If there is no jaundice, write down that there is no jaundice.

Under lab exams, write down the lab exams that were done and the results of these exams. Perhaps some results are not ready yet. You will write in these results later.

If you are certain of the diagnosis, write it down. Call this the **definite diagnosis**. If you are not certain of the diagnosis, call it the **probable diagnosis**. Perhaps there are two or more possible diagnoses. Write these down as the **differential diagnosis**.

Record all of the things you will do to care for the patient. This includes nursing care, food, medicines, and special instructions.

Perhaps you must do other exams to make the diagnosis clear. If so, write these down. You may need to look for other physical signs in the next few days. You may need to do other lab exams. Write these down so you will remember to do them.

You will give instructions to each of your patients. Often you will talk to the family of the patient. Write down these instructions. When you see the patient again, you will then remember to ask him how well he followed these instructions.

This record is important for several reasons.

1. The record will help you think carefully about the illness. It will help you make the correct diagnosis.

2. The record is a description of the present condition of the patient. It shows the symptoms and signs of the illness at the time the patient comes to you. The record will help you see any changes in his condition as time goes by.

   For example, after one week you will not be able to remember if this patient had trouble breathing or not, or how big the liver was. But if you write down all these things when you examine the patient, you will be able to remember them later.

3. Sometimes you will not know what is the disease of your patient. So you must look at the patient again and again for a number of days. You will see what changes come. These changes in the symptoms and signs, with perhaps new ones coming, will help to show you what disease the patient has. Write down all of these changes. If you do not, you will forget them. Then you will not be able to make the right diagnosis.

4. Sometimes you will consult with the doctor about a patient. The record will show the doctor the condition of the patient.

5. If you send the patient to hospital, send either a copy of the record or a letter with the patient. Then the doctor at the hospital will know what the patient's condition was and what treatment you have given. Never send a patient to hospital without a copy of the record.

6. Keep the record in your health center. If the patient becomes ill later, the first record will help you very much. It will show you what disease the patient had before and what treatment helped him get well. This may give you an idea of what the new disease is now.

7. Sometimes the authorities will want to know about a patient. They may ask you what disease a patient had and what treatment you gave. The record of your patients will help you give the necessary information to the authorities.

6.2 Asking questions about the illness

Now look at the record carefully. Think about the illness. Ask yourself questions about the illness. Look for the answers to these questions in the record and in the patient. The answers to these questions will help you make the right diagnosis.

6.2.1 Is the illness acute or chronic?

Some diseases are acute and last only a few days or two or three weeks. Other diseases are chronic and can last for one or more months or even years. It will help you make the right diagnosis if you know how long the patient has been ill. For example, a cough for three days probably does not come from tuberculosis. An illness that came six months ago is not tetanus.

6.2.2 What sort of illness is this?

There are different sorts of illness. Each sort causes certain symptoms and signs. Often you can tell which sort of illness a patient has. These are the sorts of illness to look for.

Infection

An infection usually causes a fever. There may be signs of inflammation. What sort of infection is it?

- An acute bacterial infection usually causes an increase in the number of white blood cells, or a high WBC count. So a WBC count can help you decide this.

- A virus infection does not cause a high WBC count. The count is normal.

- Tuberculosis does not cause a high WBC count. But it causes fever for many days. It also causes a high sedimentation rate.
- You can find some parasite infections by lab exams: a fresh blood drop, a thick blood film, a stool exam.
- You can find a urinary infection by doing a urine exam.

Ask yourself what organ or system of organs is infected. The symptom review will help you with this. This can help you find where the infection is. Perhaps it will help you find what sort of infection it is.

Accident or injury

In this case the patient will have a history of an accident or injury. Always ask about this. Then try to find out what organ or organs are injured. The symptom review will help you do that.

Allergy

The disease may be a reaction to something the patient has eaten, or to a medicine he is taking. These diseases can cause:

- A skin eruption, like urticaria (see page 150), or an eruption on most of the body with papules, scaling, and much itching.
- A chronic runny nose with sneezing and often red eyes with many tears.
- Attacks of dyspnea of expiration with signs of asthma.
- Very rapid shock.

The history will help you make the diagnosis. Also the signs are usually very easy to recognize.

Congenital disease

The baby is born with the disease. These are some of the common congenital diseases:

- Sickle cell anemia.
- Congenital hernia.
- Malformations of the head, of the mouth, of the feet or hands, of the hips, of the heart, of the intestines, or of the urine system.

The history and the signs will help you make this diagnosis.

Diseases of nutrition

Poor nutrition can cause certain diseases:

- Protein malnutrition from eating too little protein.

- Some anemias, from eating too little iron or too little of certain vitamins.
- Goiter, from getting too little iodine in the diet.

Ask about the patient's food. Try and see how much food with protein and with iron the patient eats each day or each week. Do a good physical exam to look for signs of malnutrition or anemia. Do a Hg exam.

Intoxication

An intoxication, coming from a poison, can cause illness. Sometimes the poison is too much medicine. This can be traditional medicine, or it can be a very big dose of regular medicine. It can come from eating or drinking something that is a poison. The history will often show you if this is the case.

An intoxication can come from drinking too much wine or other alcoholic drinks. It can come from taking drugs like cocaine, marijuana, or heroin. You may have to get the history of this from someone else in the patient's family.

Tumor

Look for a lump or swelling. Look for big hard lymph nodes. Ask about bleeding from the vagina, the rectum, the nose or the throat. Look for an ulcer that does not heal. Ask about chronic diarrhea.

After some weeks or months, a malignant tumor causes loss of appetite and much weight loss. It can cause weakness and anemia. Look for these things.

Change in an organ

The disease may be a change in an organ, such as:

1. High blood pressure, with changes in the arteries.
2. A disease of the heart, with changes in the heart or the heart valves.
3. Diabetes, with changes in the cells in the pancreas that make insulin.
4. A stomach ulcer, from an inflammation of the lining of the stomach.
5. Cirrhosis, from chronic inflammation of the liver.

The review of symptoms will help you find this out. Also, some lab exams can help you: urine exam, Hg exam.

Diseases of old age

Some diseases come because of old age. The body is "wearing out." Cataracts, some kinds of arthritis or of heart disease come with old age.

Mental disease

Many patients are ill because they have problems in their mind. They have much fear, very strong emotions, or much worry. These can cause symptoms in the body. Often, in this case, you can find no physical or laboratory signs of disease. Take a good history to find out about these problems. Ask about the emotions, feelings, and beliefs of the patient.

Learn by heart this list of the different sorts of diseases. It will help you make a good diagnosis in your patients.

1. Infection.
2. Accident or injury.
3. Allergy.
4. Congenital disease.
5. Disease of nutrition.
6. Intoxication, or poisoning.
7. Tumor.
8. Change in an organ.
9. Disease of old age.
10. Mental problem or disease.

Go over this list with every difficult case. Think about all the patient's symptoms and signs. Ask yourself which one of these kinds of disease is probably causing the illness of the patient.

6.2.3 What organ or system is ill, or changed by the disease?

Is it a disease of the stomach, of the liver, of the lungs, or of the heart? Is it a general disease, like malnutrition or diabetes? Or is it a disease that affects one, two, or more organs, like some infections or tumors? The review of symptoms will help you with this. If the patient has one or more symptoms of disease of an organ, that organ may be ill.

6.2.4 What are the possible causes for each of the important symptoms or signs?

Look at these examples.

1. A child has severe diarrhea for 3 days. What are the possible causes for this diarrhea?
2. A man has pain in the low part of his back. What are the possible causes for pain in the low part of the back?

The diagnosis strategies in this book will help you answer this question. There is a strategy for each important symptom and sign. The strategy gives a list of the important causes of each symptom and sign. You will see what to do to find the most probable cause in your patient. We will show you how to use these charts in Chapter 7 of this book.

As you examine each patient, see how many of his symptoms and signs point to the same diagnosis. One sign can come from several different diseases. Another sign can come from other diseases. So look at the diagnosis strategies for all the important symptoms and signs your patient has. Follow the diagnosis strategy for each one. Perhaps there is one disease that can cause each of the symptoms and signs. In that case, it is probably the disease the patient has.

Look at this example. A man has a cough, pain in the chest, and swelling of the legs. Under each symptom or sign is a list of the possible causes of each one. Find the **one** disease which can cause all of the symptoms and signs.

cough	chest pain	swelling of the legs
heart failure	pneumonia	heart failure
pneumonia	heart failure	anemia
tuberculosis	tuberculosis	toxemia of pregnancy
asthma	asthma	malnutrition
bronchitis	chronic bronchitis	chronic kidney disease
	abdominal disease	cirrhosis
	malaria	bad circulation
	chest injury	
	arthritis	
	gastritis	

One disease can cause each of the 3 symptoms or signs. That is heart failure. So this man probably has heart failure. To make sure of your diagnosis, look for the other signs of heart failure - see page 94.

However, the man could have tuberculosis. Tuberculosis can cause cough and chest pain. Tuberculosis, being a chronic infection, can also cause anemia. The anemia, if severe, would cause the swelling of the legs.

So look for all the patient's symptoms and signs. You must think about what disease is **most probably** the cause of them all. Do all the necessary physical and laboratory examinations to find out what disease he really has.

Look in your other books on diseases (books on pathology) for a complete description of this disease. Then see if your patient has the other symptoms and signs of that disease.

6.3 Making the diagnosis

Now you can make the diagnosis. This means answering the question, "What disease does my patient have?" What are the different kinds of diagnoses we make?

6.3.1 Definite diagnosis

Very often the diagnosis is certain. You know the patient has malaria, or high blood pressure, or gastritis, or hookworm. The diagnosis is certain, or **definite**. So you can immediately give the patient the care and treatment needed.

6.3.2 Probable diagnosis

In other cases you are quite certain of the diagnosis. But you are not completely sure. For example, a patient has heart burn that comes after eating a big meal, or when the stomach is empty. He has no tenderness or lump in the abdomen. He has not lost weight. You are quite sure he has gastritis. So you make the **probable diagnosis** of gastritis.

You give him treatment for gastritis and instructions about what to do to get well. You will see him some days later to see if he has gotten well.

If he has gotten well, you are sure of the diagnosis. If he has not gotten well, your diagnosis was probably wrong. You must now look for another disease.

6.3.3 Differential diagnosis

Sometimes you are not certain which one of several diseases is present. For example, the patient has pain in the abdomen, loss of appetite, and loss of weight. You do not find any specific signs of disease. The stool exam is negative. So what is the diagnosis? Several diseases can cause these symptoms.

In this case, there are several things to do.

1. Go through the diagnosis strategy for each symptom. Ask all of the questions listed in each strategy. Do all of the exams listed there.

The strategy will show you the most probable diagnosis of that symptom or sign.

2. Make a list of all of the diseases you think can give an illness like this. This list is called the differential diagnosis. Perhaps there are three or four possible diseases, like gastritis, chronic amebiasis, chronic infection of the liver, a disease of the lymph nodes of the abdomen. You are not certain which one of these diseases your patient has. This list, or differential diagnosis, will show you what diseases to look for.

3. The differential diagnosis will help you think about all of the things you need to do to find out which one of these diseases is causing the patient's illness. Make a list of all of these things. In this case, the list might be:

   ● A fresh stool exam each day to look for ameba and other parasites.

   ● Follow the temperature curve for 5 days.

   ● See the results of 5 days of symptomatic treatment.

4. Look at the result of these things to see if they show you the definite diagnosis. If not, examine the patient again to look for more signs of disease. Examine him as often as necessary to look for more signs of the disease.

5. Give the patient treatment for the symptoms. Give the care and treatment that will help him feel better and will take away his symptoms.

6. If the condition of the patient is serious, or becomes serious, you may have to send him to hospital. Send a letter with him telling what your differential diagnosis is and what care and treatment you have given him.

6.3.4 Helpful clues

While you are taking the history, think about certain possible diseases. For example, a patient has a cough with sputum and a fever. You will quickly think about pneumonia or tuberculosis.

This is good. So ask more questions about other symptoms of pneumonia and tuberculosis, such as how long the patient has been ill, or if he has chest pain, trouble breathing, blood in the sputum, loss of weight, or another member of the family with tuberculosis.

These further questions will help you decide if the patient has pneumonia, tuberculosis, or perhaps another disease. During the physical exam, examine the lungs carefully for signs of these diseases.

Another patient may have diarrhea with blood in the stools. You will think about dysentery or amebiasis. Ask about fever, pain in the abdomen, vomiting. In the physical exam, examine the abdomen for tenderness. Do a stool exam to look for ameba.

However, be careful. A patient may not have the first disease you think about. It may be another disease is causing these symptoms. Or the patient may have two or more diseases.

So even when you feel quite sure a patient has a certain disease, do a careful history and physical exam to make sure. Look also for symptoms and signs of other diseases.

For example, here are some mistakes we often make.

1. A man has blood in the sputum. We quickly decide he must have tuberculosis. We do not look for other diseases. But he could have heart failure, pneumonia, or bronchitis.

2. A child has jaundice, so we think immediately of hepatitis. But the child could have sickle cell anemia or malaria.

3. A woman has much urine and passes urine often. We decide quickly she has diabetes. But she could have a chronic kidney disease, or even kidney disease and diabetes together.

4. A child has a high fever and convulsions. We think immediately of malaria. But he could have meningitis. So we must look carefully for signs of meningitis: loss of consciousness, a stiff neck, a swollen fontanel. If necessary, we must do a lumbar puncture to look at and examine the cerebro-spinal fluid.

It is good to think about certain diseases while you are taking the history and doing the physical exam. This will help you look carefully for all the symptoms and signs of those diseases. Be sure, however, to do a complete history and physical examination. The patient may not have the disease you first think about. Or he may have one or more other diseases.

6.4 Solving problems of diagnosis

In the first chapter we talked briefly about certain things that make it difficult to make the diagnosis. Let us look at these things again. Let us see how to overcome these difficulties.

6.4.1 A poor history

A poor history of the illness can keep you from making the right diagnosis. The history can be poor because you forgot to ask certain important questions. As a result, you did not find out about certain important symptoms. For example, the patient has pain in the abdomen. But you did not ask where the pain is. You did not ask when the pain comes. So you cannot know what is causing the pain.

Sometimes patients do not give a good history. They may forget to tell you about certain symptoms. Or they may not want to tell you about certain things. Or they may not understand the questions you are asking them. As a result, the history is incomplete.

Here is what you must do to take a good, complete history:

1. Try to get the confidence of your patients.

2. Ask questions that are simple and clear.

3. Let patients finish responding before you ask more questions.

4. Do not criticize them, or make them feel badly.

5. For each important symptom, ask all of the questions listed on the diagnosis strategy of that symptom. If there are questions you did not ask but should ask, go back to the patient and ask them.

6.4.2 A poor physical examination

1. Perhaps you did not find certain physical signs of disease. The patient may have a heart murmur, but you did not hear it. He may have a big liver, but you did not feel it. Be sure to do the physical examination very carefully.

2. Perhaps you made an error in your examination. A patient has a hernia, but you thought it was a lymph node. A patient has the skin spots of leprosy, but you thought it was a fungus infection.

3. Perhaps you forgot to do a certain examination. You did not do a rectal exam, or feel for the spleen, or look in the patient's mouth. Look at the diagnosis strategy for each symptom and sign the patient has. Look for all the other signs listed in the strategy. Do all of the exams listed on the strategy. If there are signs you forgot to look for, go back to the patient and look for them.

6.4.3 An incorrect lab exam

This can be very serious. For example, you find tubercle bacilli in the sputum of a patient. You make the diagnosis of tuberculosis and begin giving the care and treatment for tuberculosis. But in reality, the sputum did not come from that patient. The sputum came from another patient. You made an error in writing the name on the sputum specimen. So you give treatment for a disease the patient does not have.

So be sure to do all of your lab exams with much care. Be very careful in writing the patient's name on the specimen and on the preparation. Record the results correctly.

If another person does the lab exams in your health center, check on his work. Be sure he does the exams well. In the case of an important result, like tubercle bacilli in the sputum, make sure no error has been made in the specimen or the preparation.

6.4.4 The absence of certain symptoms and signs

At the beginning of an illness, the first symptoms are often vague or indefinite. The real symptoms and signs of that disease have not come yet. So at the beginning of an illness it is often difficult to know which disease is starting.

In certain infections, the definite signs may come only after some days. For example, in hepatitis, the jaundice comes only after the fourth or the fifth day of the disease. It is usually not possible to make the definite diagnosis of hepatitis until the jaundice comes.

Therefore, it is sometimes necessary to wait a few days to make the definite diagnosis. During those days, look at the patient often to see if definite signs have come. While waiting, give the patient the care he needs and treatment for the symptoms.

In general, a disease gives some, but not every one, of the symptoms and signs of that disease. One or more symptoms or signs may be absent. For example, one can have malaria but not have a big spleen. One can have heart failure but not have edema of the legs. But if you do find several of the symptoms or signs of that disease, then you can make the diagnosis of that disease.

6.4.5 Two diseases that look alike

Two different diseases can look alike. Each disease can give some of the same symptoms and signs. For example, asthma and heart failure both cause difficult breathing and often asthmatic breathing. Pneumonia and tuberculosis can look alike. Both cause fever, cough with sputum, and crackles in the lungs. An acute infection of the inguinal nodes can look like a strangulated hernia.

However, a good history, a careful physical examination, and often some lab exams will usually help you tell which of the two diseases is present. So examine the patient very carefully and look for all the symptoms and signs of each of the two diseases.

6.4.6 No signs of disease at all

Sometimes patients come who have one or more symptoms. But you can find no signs of disease at all. For example, a patient has a severe headache, but your physical and lab exams are all negative. Another patient may have pain in the abdomen, but you can find no physical or lab signs of disease.

We often make an error in this kind of patient. We tell them, "You are not really ill." But this is not true. They have symptoms. They know they are ill. If we tell them they are not ill, they will then feel we do not know our work well. They will not have confidence in us. So avoid that error. Never say, "You are not ill." Say, "We will try to find out what is making you ill."

These are some reasons why a patient may have no signs of disease.

1. The disease is just beginning. The signs have not yet come.

2. You did not do a complete exam, or do all the necessary lab exams.

3. The disease changes the feelings of the patient (causes symptoms), but does not cause changes in the organs. A disease like gastritis can do this.

4. The cause of the symptoms is in the emotions or feelings of the patient. The disease comes from worry, fear, jealousy, anger, or from a problem in the life or the family of the patient. But these feelings often do not make changes in the patient's body.

What must you do if you find no signs of disease in a patient?

1. Take a good history. Do a complete PE. Do any lab exams which can help you find the disease.

2. Ask about problems in the life of the patient. Ask about feelings, emotions, family, work. See if there is much fear, worry, or other problems in the patient's mind.

3. Give symptomatic treatment.

4. Look at the patient again after some days. Ask about new symptoms. Look for signs of disease that may have come.

5. If the disease continues, or becomes more serious, send the patient to hospital. Send also a note describing the treatment you have given.

6.4.7 Poor knowledge of diseases

There is one other serious problem in making a diagnosis. You can make a good diagnosis in your patients only if you have a good knowledge of the common diseases in your area. You must know what tuberculosis is like, cirrhosis, heart failure, malaria, and the other common diseases.

Study your books about these diseases. Learn what each disease does to patients, how to diagnosis that disease, and how to care for patients who have that disease.

6.4.8 No diagnosis possible

In some patients you will not be able to make a diagnosis. Usually they have simple problems, like a headache, pain in the back, in the abdomen, in the leg, or in the knee.

In these patients, look for signs of a serious disease, signs such as loss of weight, anemia, tenderness in the abdomen, a lump or a swelling. If you find signs of a serious disease, send the patient to hospital with a note.

If you find no signs of serious disease, just give symptomatic treatment. Sometimes it is not necessary to give any treatment at all. Just reassure the patient that soon he will be well.

SUMMARY

To avoid errors in diagnosis, do these things:

1. Take a good history.
2. Do a complete physical examination.
3. Do your lab exams correctly.
4. Look at your difficult patients often to look for more symptoms and signs of disease.
5. Have a good knowledge of the common diseases in your area.

Questions for study

1. Why is the patient's record so important?
2. What must you write in the record?
3. Why must the record be complete?
4. How can you tell what kind of disease the patient has?
   - An infection or a tumor?
   - An allergy or an accident?
5. How can this help you make the diagnosis?
6. What must you do if you are not sure of the patient's diagnosis?
7. What errors can lead to a wrong diagnosis?
8. How can you avoid these errors?
9. What other things can make it difficult to make a diagnosis?
10. What must you do if you can find no signs of disease in your patient?

6.5 Caring for the patient

When you have made the diagnosis, you will be able to decide what to do for your patient. The first thing to do is to make a **plan** for the care of the patient. This is important especially for patients with serious illnesses. But it is important even for patients with simple illnesses. How do you make this plan? There are four parts of the plan.

6.5.1 The plan for care

1. What does the patient need? These are the needs patients have:
   - Care.
   - Food.
   - Medicines.
   - Instructions about the illness and the treatment.
   - Education about how to stay healthy after getting well.
2. Who will meet each of these needs?
   - Can the patient care for some of these needs?
   - What must you do for the patient?
   - What can other members of the family do for him?
3. What medicines and equipment are necessary to care for the patient?
   - Do you have all that is necessary?
   - If not, what must you do?
4. How can you tell if the patient is getting better?
   - How can you tell if the disease is going away?
   - How can you tell if the disease is getting worse?
   - How can you tell if the patient needs a different treatment?
   - How can you tell when he has gotten well?

6.5.2 Putting the plan into effect

What care does the patient need?

Most patients who come to your health center will be able to care for themselves. But some patients will need care from you. A patient may have a wound, a sore, or an ulcer that needs to be cleaned and have a dressing. The patient may need to do exercises to help get back strength in an arm or leg after an injury.

Some patients will need to stay in bed at the health center. They will need nursing care. Make a plan for all the nursing care to give to each patient.

Think about all the things each patient may need: bed, mattress, blanket, sheets, water to drink, food, equipment like a bed pan, a urinal, a sputum cup, and others. Think about how to take care of each need. Plan your nursing care so that all of the needs of the patient will be met. Write this plan for nursing care on the patient's record.

If the patient needs special care which you cannot give, send him to hospital.

What treatment does the patient need?

There are two kinds of treatment:

1. Specific treatment to cure the disease, like chloroquine for malaria, penicillin for pneumonia, or metronidazole (*Flagyl) for amebiasis.
2. Symptomatic treatment to make the patient feel better, like aspirin for pain or fever, or belladonna for colicky pain in the abdomen.

Some patients may not need any medicines at all. Perhaps a patient has come who has one or more symptoms and is worried about the illness. Another patient comes with a disease that will quickly go away by itself. In either case, after you examine these patients, tell them there is nothing to worry about. The symptoms will go away soon and need no medicines for treatment. This assurance is the most important treatment you can give these patients.

Who will give the treatment?

1. Can the patient take the treatment himself?
2. Must you give it to him?
3. Will one of your helpers give it to him? If so, be sure to tell the helper what to give and how to give it.
4. Can a family member give it to him? If so, show him or her how to give it.

Must the patient go to hospital?

Send a patient to hospital if:

● The disease is serious and needs hospital care.
● The patient needs a special exam that can be given only in a hospital, like an X-ray, or a special lab exam.

- The patient needs a special treatment that can be given only in a hospital.
- The patient needs an operation.
- You cannot make the diagnosis, and the patient is not getting well.

When you send a patient to hospital, always send a letter of reference. The letter must tell these things.

- The name of your health center.
- The date of the transfer.
- The name, sex and age of the patient.
- The history of the illness of the patient.
- The signs of disease you have found.
- The diagnosis you have made.
- The treatment you have given.
- The reasons for the transfer.
- Your name and signature.

However, in some cases it is difficult to send a patient to hospital. The hospital may be far away. You may not find a way to transport him to hospital. He may not have enough money to go to hospital. In such a case, you will have to care for the patient yourself. Tell him you will do all you can to help him. But tell him and his family to continue to look for a way to go to hospital.

What must you tell the patient about the illness?

There are several things your patients should know.

1. In many cases, the patient should know about the disease. Talk about the cause of the disease. Tell him what the disease is like. Explain about how long the disease will last and how long it will take to get well. This will help him understand what you are doing. He will be able to work with you better. If later he goes to another health center or to hospital, he will know what his disease was.

2. Some diseases go from one person to another. Talk to patients with one of these diseases about avoiding giving the disease to someone else. Tell them what to do and what not to do.

3. Talk to the patient about the treatment. Tell him these things:
   - What it is.
   - How to take it.
   - What the treatment will do.

In some cases, like tuberculosis or diabetes, patients must take medicine for a long time. They should know this. They should know it is important to continue the treatment until you tell them to stop. Tell them about the dangers of stopping the treatment before it is finished.

4. Talk to your patients about food. Tell them what they can eat and what they must not eat. This is important especially in diseases of the stomach and intestines, in malnutrition, and in diabetes. Always talk to the mother of a sick child about the child's food. Be sure she understands what you tell her.

5. Tell your patients what they can do and what they must not do. Must a patient avoid certain things, like lifting a heavy load, or doing hard work? Explain this carefully so the patient can understand.

6. Tell your patients about any signs of danger that may come, like a high fever, severe bleeding, vomiting blood, or a bad skin eruption that can come from the medicines being taken. If a patient has any of these signs, he must come back immediately to the health center.

7. Some diseases come because of bad habits of hygiene. In these cases, talk about the importance of being clean. Talk about the importance of a good sanitary installation, of good drinking water. Help patients avoid getting the same disease again.

8. Some of your patients may be afraid of serious illness, of dying, of an enemy, or of evil spirits. Talk to them about this. Let them talk about these fears. Tell the truth about the illness. This can take away much fear. Perhaps the religious leaders of your community can help you with patients who have much fear.

What must you tell the family of the patient?

Many times the family needs to know what you tell the patient. They must know what they can do to help him get well and stay well. If the members of the family understand this, they can help the patient very much. So take time to talk to the family about the disease of the patient.

Do the patient and the family need health education?

Many diseases can be prevented. If people know what to do, they can keep from getting these diseases. You know what these diseases are: malnutrition, hookworm, roundworm, measles, tuberculosis, severe diarrhea, and others. You know what to do to keep from getting these diseases.

When you have a patient with one of these diseases, this is a good opportunity to give health education. Talk to the patient, and talk also to the family. Tell them how this disease comes. Tell them what to do to keep from getting it themselves or from giving it to other persons. Talk about the things which people can do in the community. Explain carefully the rules about good food, cleanliness, and good hygiene.

Remember this: the time you spend in health education will do more good than the time you spend giving treatment for diseases.

Must you tell the government health authorities about this disease?

The government health authorities must know about every case of certain diseases, like leprosy, tuberculosis, gonorrhea, and typhoid fever. Learn what the diseases are that you must report.

Make a list of every case of each of these diseases you see. Send this list every week, or every month, to your doctor, or directly to the government health authorities.

Remember to write on the record of every patient:

- The diagnosis.
- The care and treatment given.
- The results of all the exams done.
- The instructions given to the patient and to the family.
- The result of the treatment.

6.6 Solving problems of treatment

Most of your patients will get well quickly. But some of them will not. They will come back to you. You must then try to find out why each of them is not getting well. There are several possible reasons for this.

6.6.1 The diagnosis is wrong

You gave the patient treatment for a certain disease. However, he has another disease. Therefore, the treatment did not help him. For example, you treated him for pneumonia, but he has tuberculosis. So examine him again. Look for signs of other diseases. If necessary, do other lab exams. Change your diagnosis and the treatment necessary for the new disease you find.

6.6.2 The treatment is wrong

The diagnosis is correct. But the treatment you gave is not correct. Make sure you know what treatment to give for each disease. Look in Chapter 12 to find out the best treatment for each disease. If you did not give the correct treatment, change the treatment to the correct one.

6.6.3 The dose is insufficient

You gave the right medicine, but you gave only a small dose. Be sure you know the right dose of each medicine to give to the patient.

6.6.4 The medicine did not act in this case

You gave the right medicine. But in this case, the medicine did not act. This is often the case in bacterial infections. The bacteria become resistant to the antibiotics we use. So these antibiotics will not act against them. If the medicine has not acted, change it. If the new medicine does not act either, send the patient to hospital.

6.6.5 The treatment did not act on the real cause of the illness

You gave good treatment. The treatment helped the patient feel better. But it did not take away the cause of the illness. So the illness has come back. Examine the patient again. Sometimes you will find another cause of the disease. In this case, give treatment for that cause. Sometimes the cause is in the emotions or feelings of the patient. If so, talk to the patient about this. Try to help him get rid of these problems.

6.6.6 The length of the treatment was too short

The treatment for each disease must last a certain period of time. If the patient comes back before he has finished the treatment, tell him to complete the treatment. But if you think the medicine is indeed not correct, change it and give the correct medicine.

6.6.7 The patient did not follow your instructions

The patient did not take the medicine as instructed. So he has not gotten well. Ask the patient how he has taken the medicine. If you see he did not follow the instructions, explain them again. Make sure this time that he understands them. Help the patient understand the importance of following the instructions carefully.

6.6.8 The disease has come back

In some cases, the patient did indeed get well. But now the disease has come back. This happens often with diseases like gastritis, gonorrhea, malnutrition, and asthma. Be sure your diagnosis is correct and that the patient does indeed have the same disease. In this case, give again the treatment needed. Explain to the patient what to do to try to avoid getting the same disease again.

6.6.9 We have no specific treatment for this disease

For certain diseases, we have no specific treatment.

- A malignant tumor.
- Cirrhosis of the liver.
- Certain virus infections.

You can give symptomatic treatment for these diseases. But it is not possible to give treatment that will make the patient well. Explain this to the patient. Help the patient understand about this disease. This will help the patient follow your instructions better.

Questions for study

1. Why is it important to make a plan for the care of each patient?
2. What kinds of care does the patient need?
3. What instructions must you give to the patient and to the family?
4. What kinds of care can you give in your health center?
5. How can the patient's family help in this care? What can they do?
6. What kinds of care can a patient receive only in a hospital?
7. What must you do if you send a patient to hospital? Why?
8. What must you do if a patient does not get better after some days of treatment?
   - What questions must you ask?
   - What things must you look for?

Chapter 7
USING THE DIAGNOSIS STRATEGIES

In this section you will find a diagnosis strategy for each of sixty common symptoms and signs of diseases. Each strategy will help you find the disease probably causing the symptom or sign. For each possible cause, or disease, the diagnosis chart will show you the number of the page in this book where you will find the treatment for that disease. In many cases the strategy will also show you how to treat that symptom or sign. Each diagnosis strategy has four parts.

1.1 Possible causes

This is a list of the diseases that can cause this symptom or sign. For each disease, there is a short description of the other important symptoms and signs of that disease. It is a list of the symptoms and signs that will help you see if this disease is present in your patient.

We have underlined the symptoms and signs of each one that are very important. This is not a complete description of the disease. For a complete description you must look in your books on pathology.

1.2 To make the diagnosis

This part of the strategy shows you the things to do to make the diagnosis. There are three lists.

- Questions to ask the patient to make the history clear.
- Signs to look for in the physical examination.
- Lab exams to do.

The answers to these questions, the presence or absence of these physical signs, and the responses to these lab exams will help you find which disease is making your patient ill.

You may want to ask the patient other questions. You may want to look for other signs. There may be other lab exams to do. This is fine. But first be sure to ask the questions on the list. Look for the signs on the list and do the lab exams on the list. Then you will be sure that you have not forgotten anything important.

1.3 Diagnosis chart

This chart is like a road map. It shows you the route to follow to make the diagnosis. Learn how to follow the diagnosis chart. This will be of much help to you in making the diagnosis in your patients.

A list of the the possible causes of the symptom or sign is on the right side of the chart. Under each possible cause, or disease, is the number of the page in this book where you will find the treatment of that disease.

The chart has boxes and arrows. In each box you will find one or two symptoms or signs to look for. You must see if this, or these, symptoms or signs are present in your patient. One or two arrows go from each box. These arrows show you the route to follow.

The patient may have the symptom(s) or sign(s) shown in the first box. In this case, follow the arrow marked YES. In most cases this will lead you to the name of a disease.

This is the disease probably causing the illness of your patient. In some cases, the arrow marked YES will lead you to another box. Look for the symptoms or signs noted in that square.

Perhaps the patient does not have the symptom(s) or sign(s) shown in the first box. In this case, the patient probably does not have the disease indicated by the arrow YES. So follow the arrow marked NO. This will lead you to the next box. Look for the symptom(s) or sign(s) noted in that box.

Follow the arrows down to the bottom of the chart. You may find that the patient has one of the causes, or diseases, listed on the right near the top of the chart. But it is a good idea to continue down the chart until you come to the bottom.

Often a patient has two or even three diseases. You need to find them all.

In some boxes there is a group of symptoms or signs. For example, you may find in a box "signs of heart failure," or "signs of malnutrition." In this case you must look for the signs of heart failure or of malnutrition. If you find some of these signs, follow the arrow YES. If you find no signs, follow the arrow NO.

Two symptoms or signs may be in a box. In some of these boxes the word AND is between the two symptoms or signs. In this case, look for BOTH of the symptoms or signs. If they are BOTH present, follow the arrow YES. If none is present, or only one is present, follow the arrow NO.

In other boxes with two or more symptoms or signs the word OR is between the symptoms or signs. In this case, look for each one of the symptoms or signs. If any one of them is present, follow the arrow YES. If none is present, follow the arrow NO.

In some cases you will find another arrow coming from the right and pointing down and to the left. This arrow comes from a disease and takes you to another box with symptoms or signs to look for. This means that very often another disease is present.

You must continue down the chart to see if other diseases are present. In each chart the serious diseases which can cause that symptom or sign are at the top of the chart. The diseases which are not very serious are farther down the page. In this way, you will always look first for the very serious diseases. If no serious disease is present, continue down the chart. Look for the diseases which are not serious.

Let us look at an example. Look at the diagnosis chart for "Cough in an older child or an adult" on page 260. If the patient has had the cough for less than 2 weeks, start at the top left corner of the chart. Look at the first box. See if the patient has signs of heart failure. If he does, follow the arrow YES. This means he has heart failure. Give him the treatment for heart failure that you find on page 636. Then follow the arrow going back to the left. It will take you to the second box.

Perhaps the patient does not have signs of heart failure. So he probably does not have heart failure. Follow the arrow NO which leads you to the second box.

See if the patient has wheezes on expiration AND a history of asthma in the past. If BOTH are present, follow the arrow YES. The patient has asthma and needs the treatment for asthma shown on page 601.

If the patient does not have wheezes on expiration AND a history of asthma, he does not have asthma. So follow the arrow NO.

This leads you to the third box. See if the patient has difficult breathing OR fever OR crackles in the lungs. If he has ONE or MORE of these, follow the arrow YES. This shows that he has pneumonia. Give him the treatment for pneumonia shown on page 676.

Perhaps the patient has none of the three things listed in the third box. This means he does not have pneumonia. Follow the arrow NO. This leads you to the only other possible cause of an acute cough, bronchitis. So give the patient the treatment for bronchitis shown on page 606.

Make the diagnosis of bronchitis only if the patient DOES NOT HAVE:

- Signs of heart failure.
- Asthmatic breathing AND a history of asthma in the past.
- Difficult breathing OR fever OR crackles in the lungs.

If the cough has been present for more than two weeks, start in the middle of the chart. Look first for signs of heart failure. If you find signs of heart failure, follow the arrow YES.

The patient has heart failure and needs the treatment shown on page 636. Follow also the arrow going back to the left. The patient may also have another disease. If the patient does not have signs of heart failure, follow the arrow NO to the second box. If the patient has sputum, look for tubercle bacilli in the sputum. If tubercle bacilli are present, the patient has tuberculosis. Follow the instructions for tuberculosis on page 698.

If the patient does not have tubercle bacilli in the sputum, follow the arrow NO to the next box. See if the patient has a fever. If so, the patient probably has pneumonia. Give the treatment for pneumonia listed on page 676. If the patient has no fever, follow the arrow NO. This leads you to the diagnosis of bronchitis. Follow the instructions for bronchitis shown on page 606.

In a patient with a chronic cough for more than 2 weeks, you make the diagnosis of bronchitis only if the patient has:

- No signs of heart failure.
- No tubercle bacilli in the sputum.
- No fever.

In some cases you will not find the cause of the patient's symptom or sign. Or perhaps you are not certain that the cause indicated by the strategy is the real cause of the patient's illness. Then see if the patient has other symptoms or signs. Follow the strategies for each of these.

Often each one of the strategies leads you to the same cause. Then you can be quite sure this is indeed the cause of the patient's illness.

In other cases, you will not find a specific cause for the patient's illness. In this case, if the illness seems serious, send the patient to hospital. If the patient is not seriously ill, give symptomatic treatment. But tell the patient to come back to see you:

- If the illness becomes more serious.
- If the illness does not go away.

1.4 Symptomatic treatment

The specific treatment for the cause of the illness of the patient is important. But we must also give symptomatic treatment to help the patient feel better.

In many of the diagnosis strategies you will find instructions for symptomatic treatment. This will show you how to treat that particular symptom or sign. For example, in the strategy on COUGH, you find what treatment to give the patient for the cough. In the strategy on diarrhea, you will find instructions about treating the diarrhea and the dehydration that comes from diarrhea.

Give the symptomatic treatment at the same time you give specific treatment. The symptomatic treatment will help the patient to feel better and to have confidence in you and in the treatment. The specific treatment will help the disease go away. Then the patient will have no more symptoms.

It is difficult to remember all of the information in these strategies. It is not necessary to do so. Keep this book with you in your consultation room. When you have a patient with a difficult illness, use this book to follow the necessary strategies. The book will help you remember all you should do. You will not forget something important.

Do not be embarrassed to use this book in front of your patients. They will not mind. It will show them you really want to find the cause of their illness. They will have more confidence in you. So always keep this book on your table as you talk to patients and examine them. Use it when you need help to make a diagnosis.

Remember that a patient may have more than one disease. So do a complete examination on all of your patients. Follow each diagnosis strategy completely. Look for all possible diseases.

Remember that a symptom or sign of a disease may sometimes be absent. A patient can have heart failure but have no swelling of the feet or legs. A patient can have tuberculosis with no crackles in the lungs. This is another reason why you must take a complete history and do a complete examination on your patients. You will then have all possible information from the patient to help you make the diagnosis.

Chapter 8
STRATEGIES FOR SYMPTOMS

COUGH IN A CHILD LESS THAN 5 YEARS OLD

The possible causes are:

1. Croup
2. Pneumonia
3. Whooping cough
4. Measles

5. Asthma
6. Tuberculosis
7. Sore throat
8. Bronchitis

1. CROUP

- A severe infection of the larynx. The vocal cords become very swollen and thick. Air can enter the lungs only with much difficulty. It makes a very loud sound.

- **Severe dyspnea**, with retraction of the lower ribs and sternum during inspiration.

- Loud noise during inspiration which we call **croup or stridor**.

- **Cyanosis**, a blue color of the lips and mucus membranes.

- Without treatment, death comes quickly.

2. PNEUMONIA

- **Painful cough**.
- **Signs of dyspnea**.
  - Rapid respirations: 40 times per minute, or more.
  - Retraction of the ribs during inspiration.
  - Flaring of the sides of the nose during inspiration.
- **Fever**, often very high. The fever is sometimes absent in a child with malnutrition. It may be absent if the child has already started treatment with an antibiotic.
- Crackles in the lungs. These are sometimes present, but not always. They are difficult to hear if the child is crying.
- Sputum. A baby or small child does not produce sputum. An older child can sometimes produce sputum.

3. WHOOPING COUGH

- **Spasms of coughing**. The spasm is a long series of coughs with no inspiration. The lips become blue. At the end of the spasm, the baby or child takes a deep breath. This makes a loud sound, or "whoop." When you hear this noise, you know the child has whooping cough. The whoop may not be present when you examine the child. So ask the mother if the child does make this loud sound, or whoop, after a spasm of coughing. A baby less than 1 year old often does not make a whoop.
- The baby or child becomes **blue**, and often vomits after the spasm.
- The baby or child has **very thick secretions** in the mouth after coughing. Often the mother must take these secretions out of the child's mouth with her fingers.
- Fever: absent.
- Loss of appetite, usually with loss of weight. This loss of weight can lead to malnutrition.
- No dyspnea: no crackles in the lungs.
- A high fever, dyspnea, or crackles in the lungs mean the child also has pneumonia.

4. MEASLES

- **A dry cough**.
- **Fever**, often up to 40° C.
- Redness of the eyes, without pus.
- **Rash**, or skin eruption, of measles after the 3rd day of fever. The rash is made of very fine bumps on the skin. It comes first on the face, then the chest and arms, then on the whole body. It lasts 7 days. Often fine scales of skin will come off after the rash has gone away. We call this "desquamation."
- Loss of appetite, usually with loss of weight. This can lead quickly to malnutrition.
- Dyspnea or crackles in the lungs mean the child also has pneumonia.

5. ASTHMA

- **Wheezes**. Air goes out of the lungs with difficulty. This makes a special sound called a "wheeze," or "asthmatic breathing."
- A dry cough.
- A **history** of attacks of wheezing in the past.

- High sounds like music in the lungs during expiration.
- No fever.
- No crackles in the lungs during inspiration.
- Fever or crackles in the lungs during inspiration mean the child also has pneumonia.

6. TUBERCULOSIS

- A **chronic cough**. This is often absent in a baby.
- **An irregular fever** going up sometimes to 39° C or 40° C. A child with malnutrition may not have a fever with tuberculosis.
- **Loss of appetite** and **loss of weight**. These can sometimes lead to malnutrition.
- Often there is a **history of another member of the family** with tuberculosis, or with a chronic cough.
- No sputum.
- Crackles: sometimes present, often absent.
- No improvement after treatment with penicillin or another antibiotic.

7. SORE THROAT

- **Pain in the throat** especially during swallowing.
- **Redness of the throat**.
- A dry cough.
- Fever, sometimes quite high.
- Sometimes white spots of pus on the tonsils. In this case, there is usually a high fever, a fast pulse, and tender lymph nodes in the neck.

8. BRONCHITIS

- A **dry cough**.
- Sometimes symptoms of a cold: runny nose, red eyes.
- No fever, or only a very low fever.
- No crackles in the lungs.
- Sometimes "wheezes" on expiration, like the wheezes of asthma. But in this case, there is no history of past attacks of asthma.

TO MAKE THE DIAGNOSIS:

In the history, ask the mother:
- When did the child begin coughing?
- Does the child have difficulty breathing? If so, what kind of difficulty?
- Does the child make a noise while breathing? What kind of a noise?
- Are there spasms of coughing followed by a whoop and vomiting?
- Are there secretions in the mouth?
- Does anyone in the family have tuberculosis, or a chronic cough, or trouble breathing, or blood in the sputum?
- Has the child had attacks of coughing with wheezing in the past?
- Are there other symptoms, like fever, sore throat, pain in the chest?
- Does the child have a cold?
- Does the child eat well? If not, has he lost weight?

In the physical exam, look for:
- Croup with each inspiration. If this is present, start treatment immediately - see page 610. Then send the child **immediately** to hospital. Be sure you can tell the difference between the stridor of croup with inspiration and the wheezing of asthma on expiration.
- Spasms of coughing with cyanosis, followed by a "whoop," and vomiting.
- Signs of dyspnea.
- Dyspnea on expiration, with wheezing.
- Crackles in the lungs. Are they on inspiration or expiration?
- Sounds like music in the lungs on expiration.
- The rash of measles.
- Redness in the throat. Are there white spots on the tonsils?
- Loss of weight.
- Signs of malnutrition.

SYMPTOMATIC TREATMENT OF A COUGH

There are two sorts of medicines for the treatment of a cough:

● An expectorant which helps the patient cough up sputum.

● A cough suppressant which helps the patient stop coughing.

Two common expectorants are:

1. Ammonium chloride.

   ● In a 10% solution, called "cough mixture" or in pills of 0.5 g.

   ● Dose for an adult: 0.5 g (5 ml) 3 or 4 times a day.

   ● Dose for a child: 1 or 2 ml of cough mixture 3 or 4 times a day.

2. Potassium iodide, in a saturated solution.

   ● Dose for an adult: 10 drops in a little water 3 or 4 times a day.

   ● Dose for a child: 1 drop per year of age in a little water 3 or 4 times a day.

   ● Do not use this expectorant if you think the patient has tuberculosis.

There are many suppressant cough mixtures. Usually they have codeine in them. You will find the dose to give written on the bottle.

Give an expectorant to all children who cough. Give it to adults who have a productive cough, that is, a cough with sputum. Give a suppressant cough mixture to adults who have a dry cough, that is, a cough with no sputum.

A patient who coughs, especially an infant or small child, can quickly develop pneumonia. A high fever, dyspnea or crackles in the lungs mean the patient now has pneumonia.

If the patient continues to cough after one week of symptomatic treatment but does not have pneumonia, he may have tuberculosis. Look for tubercle bacilli in the sputum, or else send the patient to hospital.

Larva of certain intestinal worms, like hookworm and roundworm, go through the lungs before they come to the intestines. They cause a dry cough when they go through the lungs. It is not possible to find these larva in the sputum. In a patient, and especially a child, who has a dry cough for a month or more but has no signs of pneumonia or tuberculosis, look for worm larva or eggs in the stool. If present, give a worm treatment. If the stool exam is negative, do it again after another month. If positive, give a worm treatment and talk to the patient and the family about the rules of hygiene. Help them understand how to avoid getting worms in the future.

COUGH IN A CHILD LESS THAN 5 YEARS OLD

Cough for less than 2 weeks   **Possible causes**

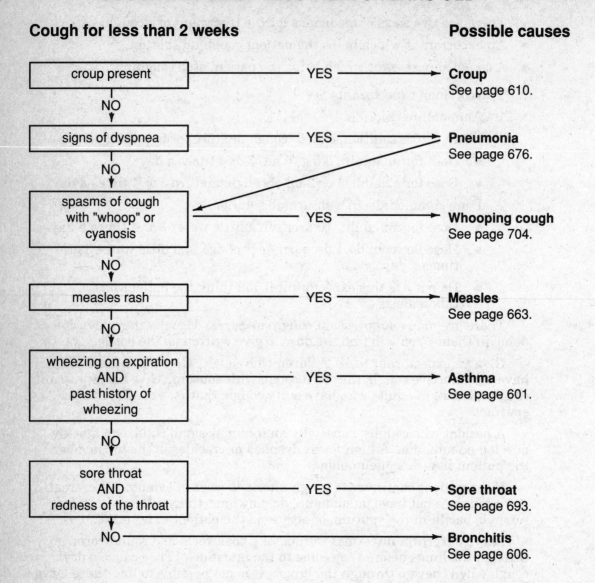

croup present	YES →	**Croup** See page 610.
NO ↓		
signs of dyspnea	YES →	**Pneumonia** See page 676.
NO ↓		
spasms of cough with "whoop" or cyanosis	YES →	**Whooping cough** See page 704.
NO ↓		
measles rash	YES →	**Measles** See page 663.
NO ↓		
wheezing on expiration AND past history of wheezing	YES →	**Asthma** See page 601.
NO ↓		
sore throat AND redness of the throat	YES →	**Sore throat** See page 693.
NO →		**Bronchitis** See page 606.

Cough for more than 2 weeks

Possible causes

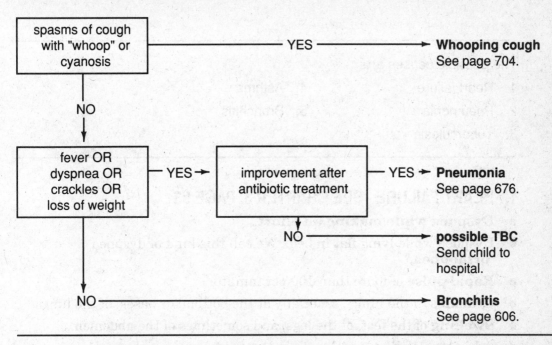

spasms of cough with "whoop" or cyanosis — YES ——→ **Whooping cough** See page 704.

NO

fever OR dyspnea OR crackles OR loss of weight — YES → improvement after antibiotic treatment — YES → **Pneumonia** See page 676.

NO ——→ **possible TBC** Send child to hospital.

NO ——————→ **Bronchitis** See page 606.

SYMPTOMATIC TREATMENT OF A COUGH IN A SMALL CHILD

If there are no signs of a severe disease, like:

- Rapid breathing of more than 40 per minute.
- Retraction of the ribs.
- Flaring of the wings of the nose.
- High fever.
- Noisy breathing: stridor or croup, whoop, or wheezing.
- Cyanosis or crackles in the lungs.
- White spots on the tonsils.
- Loss of weight.

1. Give an expectorant medicine.
2. Explain to the mother that the disease is not serious. But she must bring the child back to the health center if the child develops:
   - Rapid breathing, or noisy breathing.
   - Flaring of the wings of the nose.
   - A blue color of the lips.
   - A high fever.

COUGH IN AN OLDER CHILD OR AN ADULT

The possible causes are:

1. Heart failure
2. Pneumonia
3. Tuberculosis
4. Asthma
5. Bronchitis

1. HEART FAILURE - SEE CHAPTER 3, PAGE 93

- **Dyspnea while making an effort**.
- Dyspnea while lying flat in bed. We call this kind of dyspnea **"orthopnea."**
- **Rapid pulse** of more than 100 per minute.
- **Crackles** in the lungs, especially at the bottom, or bases, of the lungs.
- **Swelling** of the feet, of the legs, and sometimes of the abdomen.
- **A big tender liver**, with pain in the right upper quadrant.
- Swollen veins in the neck.
- Sputum: clear, or with foam, or sometimes with small quantities of brownish blood.

2. PNEUMONIA

- **A painful cough**.
- **Dyspnea**, even while resting. The breathing is rapid and difficult.
- **Fever**, often with chills. The fever may be absent in an older patient, in a patient with malnutrition, or in a patient already on antibiotic treatment.
- **Chest pain**, during the cough, and on deep breathing.
- Sputum: thick, white or yellow. Sometimes there is no sputum.
- Fine crackles in the lungs on one or both sides.

3. TUBERCULOSIS

- **Chronic cough**.
- **Sputum**: white, yellow, or **with blood**. We call sputum with blood "hemoptysis." Sometimes the sputum is pure blood.
- Sometimes dyspnea while making an effort.
- Chest pain.
- Loss of weight, and even signs of malnutrition.
- **TB bacilli** in the sputum.
- Often a **history of a member of the family** who has tuberculosis, who has had tuberculosis, or who has a chronic cough or hemoptysis.
- A low chronic fever usually in the afternoon or evening.
- Cold feelings in the afternoon and sweating at night.
- Sometimes crackles in the lungs, especially at the top.

4. ASTHMA

- **Wheezes** on expiration, or "asthmatic breathing."
- **History** of attacks of wheezing in the past.
- A dry cough, with no sputum.
- High sounds like music in the lungs on expiration.
- No fever. A fever or crackles in the lungs during inspiration mean the patient also has pneumonia.

5. BRONCHITIS

- **Cough**, acute or chronic.
- Often sputum: white, yellow, or green, sometimes with a little blood.
- **No fever**.
- **No crackles**.
- Chronic bronchitis sometimes causes dyspnea while making an effort.

TO MAKE THE DIAGNOSIS

In the history, ask:

- When did the cough begin? How many days ago? Or how many weeks ago?

- Is there sputum? If so, what is it like?

- Is there blood in the sputum?

- Do you have trouble breathing? If so, when? Only while making an effort? Or while lying down? Or all of the time?

- Is there pain in the chest during breathing or coughing?

- Do you feel cold in the afternoon, or have much sweating at night?

- Do you have a fever?

- Is there someone in your family who has tuberculosis, or a chronic cough, or who has blood in the sputum?

- Have you had attacks of wheezing and dyspnea in the past?

- Do you smoke cigarettes? If so, how many in a day?

In the physical exam, look for:

- Fever. If you suspect tuberculosis, take the patient's temperature three times a day: in the morning, in the afternoon, and in the evening. Often the fever comes only during the evening.

- Crackles in the lungs. Where are they? What are they like?

- Signs of heart failure:

  - A rapid pulse: more than 100 per minute.

  - Rapid breathing: more than 30 times per minute.

  - Crackles at the bottom of the lungs.

  - A big tender liver.

  - Swelling of the feet, the legs, or the abdomen.

  - Swollen veins in the neck.

- Musical sounds in the lungs during expiration.

- Signs of loss of weight or of malnutrition.

In the laboratory, do:

- At least 3 sputum exams to look for TB bacilli. Do one exam each day. Use the Ziehl-Neelsen stain. If you cannot do this, make a sputum preparation on a slide. Send at least 3 slides to the nearest center where someone can examine them.

COUGH IN AN OLDER CHILD OR AN ADULT

Cough for less than 2 weeks

Possible causes

| signs of heart failure | ———— YES ————→ | **Heart failure** See page 636. |

NO ↓

| wheezes on expiration AND history of asthma | ———— YES ————→ | **Asthma** See page 601. |

NO ↓

| difficult breathing OR fever OR crackles in lungs | ———— YES ————→ | **Pneumonia** See page 676. |

NO ————————————————————→ **Bronchitis** See page 606.

Cough for more than 2 weeks

Possible causes

| signs of heart failure | ———— YES ————→ | **Heart failure** See page 636. |

NO ↓

| tubercle bacilli in the sputum | ———— YES ————→ | **Tuberculosis** See page 698. |

NO ↓

| signs of dyspnea | ———— YES ————→ | **Pneumonia** See page 676. |

NO ————————————————————→ **Bronchitis** See page 606.

TROUBLE BREATHING (DYSPNEA) IN A CHILD

Dyspnea means breathing that is rapid and difficult. In a small child there are three important signs of dyspnea:

1. Rapid breathing - more than 40 times per minute.

2. Retraction, or "pulling in," of the lower ribs and the upper part of the abdomen during inspiration.

3. "Flaring" of the sides of the nose during breathing. The sides of the nose move out during inspiration and in during expiration.

In the case of asthma, the child has trouble pushing air out of the lungs. We call this "dyspnea of expiration." This makes a noise during expiration which we call a "wheeze."

Dyspnea in a child is always a sign of a serious disease. Look carefully for the cause of the dyspnea. Give the treatment necessary for the disease causing the dyspnea. Send the child to hospital:

- If you cannot find the cause of the dyspnea, or
- If the child does not get better quickly.

The possible causes of dyspnea in a child are:

1. Croup
2. Pneumonia
3. A serious infection
4. A severe anemia
5. Heart failure
6. Dehydration
7. Asthma
8. Asthmatic bronchitis

1. CROUP - A SEVERE INFECTION OF THE LARYNX

- The vocal cords become very swollen and thick. Air can enter the lungs only with much difficulty. It makes a very loud sound.
- **Severe dyspnea**, with retraction of the lower ribs and sternum during inspiration.
- A loud noise during inspiration which we call **croup** or **stridor**.
- **Cyanosis**, a blue color of the lips and mucous membranes.
- Without treatment, death comes quickly.

2. PNEUMONIA

- **Painful cough**.
- **Signs of dyspnea**.
- **Fever**, often very high. But the fever is sometimes absent in a child with malnutrition. It may be absent if the child has already started treatment with an antibiotic.
- Crackles in the lungs. These are sometimes present, but not always. They are difficult to hear if the child is crying.
- Sputum. A baby or small child does not produce sputum. An older child can sometimes produce sputum.

3. A SERIOUS INFECTION - CEREBRAL MALARIA, MENINGITIS, SEPTICEMIA, ETC.

- **A high fever**, rapid breathing, a fast pulse.
- **Signs of the infection**.

4. SEVERE ANEMIA - A HEMOGLOBIN OF LESS THAN 6 G

- **Paleness** of the mucous membranes.
- Rapid and deep breathing.
- With the anemia of malaria, or with sickle cell anemia, there is sometimes jaundice.

5. HEART FAILURE

- **Rapid pulse**.
- **Rapid breathing**.
- **A big tender liver**.
- Sometimes crackles in the lungs.
- Sometimes swelling of the legs.
- Sometimes cyanosis.
- Heart failure can come quickly in a child during an infusion or a transfusion if it is given too rapidly or if too much is given.

6. DEHYDRATION

- From diarrhea, vomiting, a burn, or diabetic coma.
- The loss of water and salt causes much acid to form in the blood. This "acidosis" makes the breathing rapid and deep.
- **Signs of dehydration**.
  - Dryness of the mouth.
  - Skin dry, with many folds.
  - Eyes dry and sunk deep into the eye sockets.
  - Little or no urine.
- In the case of diabetes, sugar in the urine.

7. ASTHMA

- **Wheezes**. Air goes out of the lungs with difficulty. This makes a special sound called a "wheeze," or "asthmatic breathing."
- A dry cough.
- A **history** of attacks of wheezing in the past.
- High sounds like music in the lungs during expiration.
- No fever.
- No crackles in the lungs during inspiration.
- A fever or crackles in the lungs during inspiration mean the child also has pneumonia.

8. ASTHMATIC BRONCHITIS

The symptoms and signs are like those of asthma. But there is no history of asthma in the past. This is the first attack of asthmatic breathing the child has had.

TO MAKE THE DIAGNOSIS:

In the history, ask the mother:
- When does the child have dyspnea? While resting? During expiration?
- Is there a loud croup when the child breathes? Or wheezing?
- Does the child cough? Is there pain with the cough?
- Is there any sputum?
- Has the child had diarrhea, or vomiting, or a severe burn?
- Does the child have diabetes?
- Is there a history of attacks of wheezing in the past?

In the physical exam, look for:
- Croup, wheezing, asthmatic breathing.
- Fever.
- Signs of dyspnea.
  - Retraction of the ribs and the upper abdomen.
  - Flaring of the sides of the nose.
- Signs of serious infection: cerebral malaria, meningitis, septicemia, or another infection.
- Signs of heart failure.
  - Rapid pulse.
  - A big tender liver.
  - Crackles in the lungs.
  - Swelling of the legs.
  - Cyanosis.
- An infusion or transfusion running very fast.
- Signs of dehydration.
  - Dry mouth.
  - Dry skin with many folds.
  - Dry eyes sunk into the eye sockets.
  - Little or no urine.

In the laboratory, do:
- A hemoglobin exam.
- A urine exam for sugar.
- If there is sputum, 3 sputum exams for TB, one each morning.

DYSPNEA IN A CHILD

Possible causes

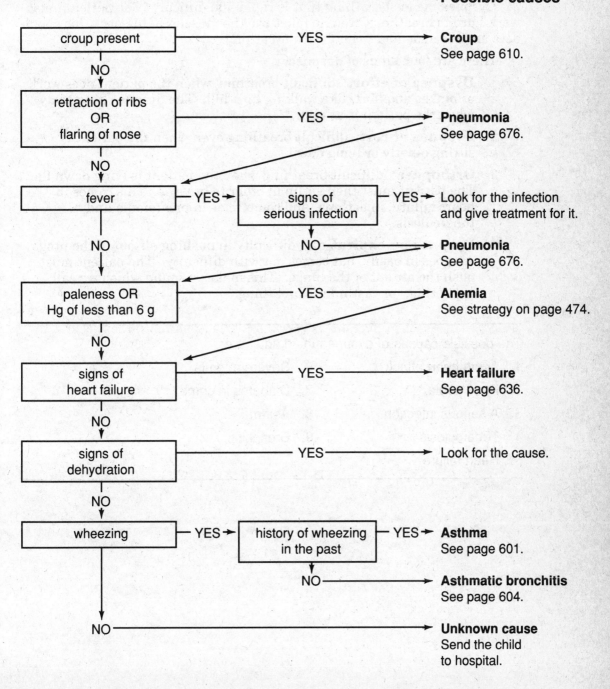

TROUBLE BREATHING (DYSPNEA) IN AN ADULT

Dyspnea means breathing that is rapid and difficult. The patient must work hard to breathe. Often he must use the muscles of his neck, his shoulders and his abdomen to help with breathing.

There are four kinds of dyspnea.

1. **Dyspnea of effort**: difficult breathing when the patient does work or makes an effort, like walking up a hill. The dyspnea goes away when the patient is at rest.

2. **Dyspnea at rest**: difficult breathing even when the patient is sitting quietly or lying down.

3. **Orthopnea**: difficult breathing when the patient is lying down flat. The patient must then sit up in order to breathe. This comes in heart failure, in asthma, and sometimes in pneumonia and tuberculosis.

4. **Dyspnea on expiration**: difficulty in pushing air out of the lungs. Air goes in easily, but comes out with difficulty. The patient must push the air out of the lungs. This makes a sound which we call "wheezing," or "asthmatic breathing."

The possible causes of dyspnea in an adult are:

1. Acute heart attack
2. Pneumonia
3. A serious infection
4. Tuberculosis
5. Heart failure
6. Severe anemia
7. Diabetes in coma
8. Asthma
9. Bronchitis

---

1. ACUTE HEART ATTACK

- **Sudden severe chest pain** which may go to the left shoulder or arm.
- **Much weakness**, or even loss of consciousness.
- **Fast pulse**, often irregular.
- **Low or absent blood pressure**.

2. PNEUMONIA

- **Painful cough**.
- **Dyspnea**, even at rest.
- **Fever**, often with chills. However, the fever may be absent in an older patient, in a patient with malnutrition, or in a patient already on treatment.
- **Chest pain** during the cough and on deep breathing.
- Sputum: thick, white or yellow. Sometimes there is no sputum.
- Fine crackles in the lungs on one or both sides.

3. A SERIOUS INFECTION - PERITONITIS, MENINGITIS, SEPTICEMIA

- **A high fever**, rapid breathing, a fast pulse.
- **Signs of the infection**.

4. TUBERCULOSIS

- **Chronic cough**.
- **Sputum**: white, yellow, or **with blood**. We call sputum with blood "hemoptysis." Sometimes the sputum is pure blood.
- Sometimes dyspnea of effort and orthopnea.
- Chest pain.
- Loss of weight, and even signs of malnutrition.
- **TB bacilli** in the sputum.
- Often a **history of a member of the family** who has tuberculosis, who has had tuberculosis, or who has a chronic cough or hemoptysis.
- A low chronic fever, usually in the afternoon or evening.
- Cold feelings in the afternoon and sweating at night.
- Sometimes crackles in the lungs, especially at the top.

5. HEART FAILURE

- **Dyspnea of effort** and often **orthopnea**.
- **Pain in the chest** made worse by effort.
- **Rapid pulse**, more than 100 per minute.
- **Crackles** in the lungs, especially at the bottom, or bases, of the lungs.
- **Swelling** of the feet, of the legs, and sometimes of the abdomen.
- A **big, tender liver**, with pain in the right upper quadrant.
- Swollen veins in the neck.
- Sputum: clear, or with foam, or sometimes with small quantities of brownish blood.

6. SEVERE ANEMIA - A HEMOGLOBIN OF LESS THAN 6 G

- **Paleness** of the mucus membranes.
- Rapid and deep breathing.
- No cough, unless there is also heart failure or pneumonia.
- In some cases of severe anemia, there is also jaundice.

7. DIABETES IN COMA

- **Rapid and very deep breathing**.
- **Sugar in the urine**.
- Mental confusion (delirium), or coma.

8. ASTHMA

- **Wheezes** on expiration, or "asthmatic breathing."
- **History** of attacks of wheezing in the past.
- A dry cough, with no sputum.
- High sounds like music in the lungs during expiration.
- No fever. A fever or crackles in the lungs during inspiration mean the patient also has pneumonia.

9. BRONCHITIS

- **Cough**, acute or chronic.
- Often sputum: white, yellow, or green, sometimes with a little blood.
- **No fever**.
- **No crackles**.
- Chronic bronchitis sometimes causes dyspnea of effort.

TO MAKE THE DIAGNOSIS

In the history ask:

- How long have you had this trouble breathing?
- When do you have trouble breathing: when making an effort like walking up a hill? When resting? When lying flat in bed?
- Do you have difficulty breathing air out of your lungs?
- Do you have a cough?
- Do you have sputum? If so, what is the sputum like?
- Is there blood in your sputum?
- Do you have pain in your chest? If so, where? When does it come:
  - All the time?
  - When you work or walk up a hill?
  - Only when you cough or take a deep breath?
- Do you feel cold in the afternoon?
- Do you have much sweating at night?
- Have you lost weight? If so, since when?
- Is there someone else in your family who has tuberculosis, or a chronic cough, or who has blood in the sputum?
- Have you had attacks of wheezing in the past?

In the physical exam, look for:

- Fever.
- Pale mucus membranes - conjunctiva, mouth.
- The rate of breathing: how fast is it?
- Crackles: where are they? Do they come on inspiration or expiration?
- Signs of a serious infection, like peritonitis, meningitis, septicemia.
- Signs of heart failure: fast pulse, crackles in the bases of the lungs, a big tender liver, swelling of the feet or legs, swollen neck veins.
- Sounds like music in the lungs during expiration.

In the laboratory, do:

- A hemoglobin exam.
- 3 sputum exams to look for TB bacilli, one exam each morning.
- A urine exam to look for sugar.

DYSPNEA IN AN ADULT

Possible causes

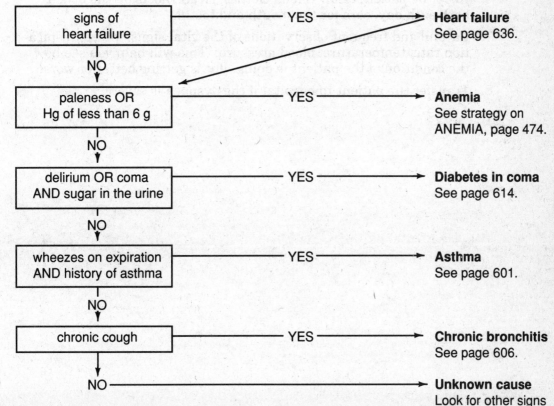

strong pain AND signs of heart attack	— YES →	**Heart attack** Send patient to hospital immediately.

NO ↓

fever	YES → painful cough OR chest pain OR crackles in lungs	YES → **Pneumonia** See page 676.

NO ↓

TB bacilli in the sputum — YES → **Tuberculosis** See page 698.

NO → Look for another infection and give treatment for it.

signs of heart failure	— YES →	**Heart failure** See page 636.

NO ↓

paleness OR Hg of less than 6 g	— YES →	**Anemia** See strategy on ANEMIA, page 474.

NO ↓

delirium OR coma AND sugar in the urine	— YES →	**Diabetes in coma** See page 614.

NO ↓

wheezes on expiration AND history of asthma	— YES →	**Asthma** See page 601.

NO ↓

chronic cough	— YES →	**Chronic bronchitis** See page 606.

NO → **Unknown cause** Look for other signs of disease.

SYMPTOMATIC TREATMENT OF DYSPNEA IN AN ADULT

The most important treatment is the treatment of the cause. Do your best to make a correct diagnosis so that you can give the correct treatment. If the cause of the dyspnea is pneumonia, or heart failure, or asthma, or tuberculosis, the patient will need:

1. Bed rest, with the head elevated, or with the patient sitting up.

2. Good circulation of air. Do not let too many people into the patient's room.

3. If the patient has a cough, give symptomatic treatment for the cough - see page 257.

4. If the patient has sputum, give him a sputum cup with a cover. Show him how to use it, empty it and wash it carefully as often as necessary.

5. Much water to drink. The patient loses much water because of the rapid breathing. Drinking much water will make the patient feel better.

6. Keep the patient clean - clean clothes, clean sheets on the bed, a bath each day, care for the mouth and teeth.

7. Careful and frequent observations of the vital signs: pulse, respiration rate, temperature, blood pressure. This will help you see how the condition of the patient is doing, if it is getting better or worse.

8. Transfer the patient to hospital if the dyspnea is severe.

SPUTUM WITH BLOOD (HEMOPTYSIS)

The possible causes are:

1. Tuberculosis
2. Heart failure
3. Pneumonia
4. Bronchitis

1. TUBERCULOSIS (TBC)

The tubercle bacilli make small abscesses in the lung tissue. Each abscess slowly becomes bigger. Sometimes an abscess makes a hole into a bronchus, or air tube. In this case, the pus in the abscess will go out of the abscess into the bronchus. It will then come out in the sputum. There are usually tubercle bacilli in the pus of the abscess. There will therefore be tubercle bacilli in the pus from the abscess that comes out in the sputum.

In the lining of the abscess there are small blood vessels. The abscess can also make a hole into one of these blood vessels. As a result, there will be bleeding into the abscess. If the abscess makes a hole in a bronchus, there will now be pus and blood coming out in the sputum. If the blood vessel is a big one, much blood will be in the sputum. Sometimes the sputum is pure blood, often with blood clots.

For the other symptoms and signs of tuberculosis, look at the strategy COUGH IN AN ADULT on page 260.

Remember that penicillin and other ordinary antibiotics do not act on the tubercle bacilli. They do not work against tuberculosis. They will not cure a patient with tuberculosis. A patient with hemoptysis may have tuberculosis. If you treat him with penicillin, he will not get well. But pneumonia can also cause hemoptysis. In this case, penicillin will make the patient well. So a cure of penicillin can often help you decide if a patient has tuberculosis or pneumonia.

2. HEART FAILURE

In certain cases of heart failure, edema liquid comes into the alveoli, the tiny air spaces in the lungs. This edema liquid in the alveoli makes the crackles you hear with the stethoscope. The edema liquid also makes the patient cough and produce sputum. Foam is often mixed with the sputum.

In heart failure the pressure of the blood going through the lungs is often increased. This increase in pressure can cause some small blood vessels to break. Blood from these vessels mixes with the edema liquid in the alveoli. The sputum now will have blood in it. The blood mixed with the sputum makes the sputum look red-brown, like coffee.

For the other symptoms and signs of heart failure, see the strategy COUGH IN AN ADULT on page 260. There is no fever. There are no other signs of infection in heart failure, unless the patient also has pneumonia.

3. PNEUMONIA

A severe case of pneumonia can cause blood in the sputum. This is not frequent, however. Usually there are only small amounts of blood in the sputum of a patient with pneumonia.

For the other symptoms and signs of pneumonia, see the strategy COUGH IN AN ADULT on page 260.

Penicillin is the treatment for pneumonia. If the cause of the hemoptysis is pneumonia, penicillin will make the patient well.

4. BRONCHITIS

Bronchitis often causes hemoptysis. The frequent cough in bronchitis can make small wounds in the mucus membrane of the bronchi. These wounds bleed, and the blood comes out in the sputum. Usually there is only a little blood in the sputum. Sometimes, however, there is much blood, even with blood clots.

The sputum in bronchitis is usually white, yellow, or green. Often it is quite thick. There is no fever. There are no crackles in the lungs. In chronic bronchitis, there is sometimes dyspnea of effort.

SYMPTOMATIC TREATMENT FOR HEMOPTYSIS

1. If there is much blood in the sputum:
   - Look for signs of shock: fast pulse, low blood pressure. A transfusion will be necessary if the patient is in shock.
   - Put the patient in bed with the head elevated. Give the patient diazepam (*Valium) 10 mg or phenobarbital 50 mg. If the cough is severe, give codeine 30 to 60 mg.
   - Do a hemoglobin exam. If the hemoglobin is very low, the patient will need a transfusion. Look also for other causes of anemia - see the strategy on ANEMIA on page 474.
   - Send the patient to hospital as soon as his condition will permit.

2. Small quantities of blood in the sputum do not need special treatment. The important thing is to find the cause and give specific treatment for it.

3. Perhaps you cannot do a sputum exam. In this case, either
   - Send the patient to hospital, or
   - Make 3 sputum preparations on slides, one each day for 3 days. Send them to the hospital lab or to a center near you that can do the sputum exam.

4. If the patient has a fever, start giving penicillin. Do not wait for the results of the sputum exams. Then if you find tubercle bacilli in the sputum, you know the patient has tuberculosis. See page 698 for the treatment for tuberculosis.

5. If the sputum exam is negative, finish the penicillin treatment. If the cough, fever and hemoptysis stop, the patient is cured. He may go home. But tell him to come back in one month for a control exam. Tell him to come even before then if he again has a fever, a cough, or hemoptysis.

6. If the cough, fever, or hemoptysis do not go away after 10 days of penicillin treatment, send the patient to hospital for other exams. NEVER start treatment for tuberculosis unless you find tubercle bacilli in the sputum.

7. Give the patient a good sputum cup with a cover. Show him how to use it, how to empty it, and how to wash it well. If you do not have a sputum cup, give him a small can with a cover, or a small bottle with a big opening and a top. He must throw the can or bottle away at the end of the day and use a new one the next day. This is to keep the patient from giving the disease to others, including you.

TO MAKE THE DIAGNOSIS:

In the history, ask:
- How long have you had the cough?
- What does your sputum look like?
- How many times have you had blood in the sputum?
- Do you have other symptoms?
  - Dyspnea, orthopnea, pain in the chest.
  - Pain in the right upper part of the abdomen.
  - Swelling of the feet or legs.
  - A cold feeling in the afternoon, sweating at night, loss of weight.
- Does anyone else in your family have tuberculosis, or a chronic cough, or blood in the sputum?

In the physical exam, look for:
- The type of sputum. Try to look at the patient's sputum yourself.
  - Pure blood comes most often from tuberculosis.
  - Blood clots come from tuberculosis or pneumonia.
  - Small amounts of blood come from bronchitis, but can also come from tuberculosis.
  - Brownish sputum, like coffee, comes probably from heart failure. Often there is much foam in the sputum.
- Fever.
- Crackles in the lungs. Note where they are:
  - At the top?
  - At the bottom?
  - Somewhere else?
- Signs of heart failure.

In the laboratory, do:
- 3 sputum exams to look for TB bacilli, one each morning.
- A hemoglobin exam to see if there is anemia.

HEMOPTYSIS

Possible causes

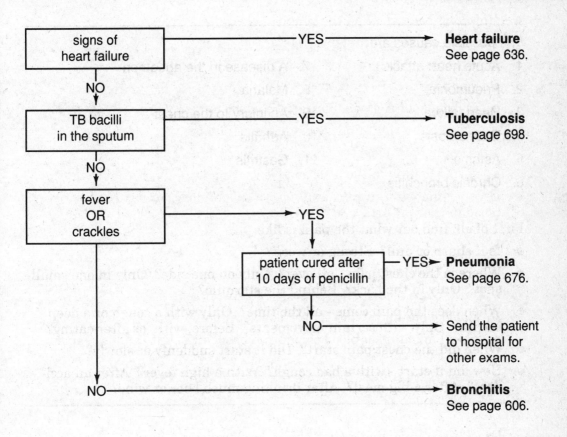

signs of
heart failure
————YES————→ **Heart failure**
See page 636.

NO

TB bacilli
in the sputum
————YES————→ **Tuberculosis**
See page 698.

NO

fever
OR
crackles
————→ YES

patient cured after
10 days of penicillin
—YES► **Pneumonia**
See page 676.

NO————————→ Send the patient
to hospital for
other exams.

NO————————————→ **Bronchitis**
See page 606.

PAIN IN THE CHEST

The possible causes are:

1. Acute heart attack
2. Pneumonia
3. Heart failure
4. Tuberculosis
5. Asthma
6. Chronic bronchitis
7. A disease in the abdomen
8. Malaria
9. An injury to the chest
10. Arthritis
11. Gastritis

First of all, find out what the pain is like.

- Is it sharp or dull? Strong or weak?
- Where is the chest pain - all over? Only on one side? Only in one small spot? Only in the back? Behind the sternum?
- When does the pain come - all the time? Only with a cough or a deep breath? Only with certain movements? Before, with, or after eating?
- When did the chest pain start? Did it start suddenly or slowly?
- How did it start - with a bad cough? With a high fever? After an accident? After a big meal? After drinking much beer or wine?

---

1. ACUTE HEART ATTACK

- **Sudden severe pain in the chest.**
- **Dyspnea at rest.**
- **Much weakness**, or even loss of consciousness.
- **Fast pulse**, often irregular.
- **Low or absent blood pressure.**

2. PNEUMONIA

- **Pain in the ribs** during a cough or when taking a deep breath. To make the pain go away, the patient lies on the side which has pain.
- **Painful cough**.
- **Dyspnea**, even at rest.

- **Fever**, often with chills. However, the fever may be absent in an older patient, in a patient with malnutrition, or in a patient already on treatment.
- Sputum: thick, white or yellow. Sometimes there is no sputum.
- Fine crackles in the lungs on one or both sides.

3. HEART FAILURE

- **Pain** behind the sternum, on the left side, or on both sides. **The pain is made worse by effort**.
- **Dyspnea of effort**.
- Often **orthopnea**.
- **Rapid pulse**, more than 100 per minute.
- **Crackles** in the lungs, especially at the bottom of the lungs.
- **Swelling** of the feet, of the legs, and sometimes of the abdomen.
- **A big**, **tender liver**, with pain in the right upper quadrant.
- Swollen veins in the neck.
- Sputum: clear, or with foam, or sometimes with small quantities of brownish blood.

4. TUBERCULOSIS

- Chest pain, acute or chronic, made worse by effort, by coughing, or by taking a deep breath.
- **Chronic cough**.
- **Sputum**: white, yellow, or **with blood**. Sometimes the sputum is pure blood.
- **Tubercle bacilli** in the sputum.
- Often a **history of a member of the family** who has tuberculosis, who has had tuberculosis, or who has a chronic cough or hemoptysis.
- Sometimes dyspnea of effort.
- Loss of weight, and even signs of malnutrition.
- A low chronic fever, usually in the afternoon or evening.
- Cold feelings in the afternoon and sweating at night.
- Sometimes crackles in the lungs, especially at the top.

5. ASTHMA

- Pain in both sides of the chest during the attack of dyspnea. The pain is in the muscles of the chest and comes because the muscles are tired.
- **Wheezes** on expiration, or "asthmatic breathing."
- **History** of attacks of wheezing in the past.
- A dry cough, with no sputum.
- High sounds like music in the lungs during expiration.
- No fever. A fever or crackles in the lungs during inspiration mean that the patient also has pneumonia.

6. CHRONIC BRONCHITIS

- Chronic chest pain made worse by effort.
- **Chronic cough**.
- Sputum: white, yellow or green, sometimes with a little blood.
- Sometimes dyspnea of effort.
- **No fever, no crackles in the lungs**.

7. A DISEASE IN THE ABDOMEN - PERITONITIS, HEPATITIS, OTHER INFECTIONS.

- The infection is in the abdomen, but the patient feels the pain in the chest.
- **A tender abdomen** and often fever.

8. MALARIA

- Pain behind the sternum or in the lower left side of the chest.
- **Fever and headache**.
- Often a big tender spleen.
- The fever goes away after 1 or 2 days of treatment with chloroquine.

9. INJURY OF THE CHEST - FRACTURE, CONTUSION.

- **History of an accident**.
- **Pain at the site of the injury** often made worse by coughing or by movements of the chest, the arms, or the shoulders.
- No signs of infection or of other diseases.

10. ARTHRITIS OF THE RIBS OR BACK

- **Pain made worse by movements** of the back or by deep breathing.
- Pain present many days, weeks, or months.
- Tenderness made worse by pressing on the chest.
- No history of an accident or injury.
- No fever or signs of other diseases.

11. GASTRITIS

- Pain behind the sternum going to the back between the shoulders.
- **Pain associated with eating**, before, during, or after eating, or after drinking alcoholic drinks.
- No tenderness in the abdomen.
- No signs of other diseases.

TO MAKE THE DIAGNOSIS

In the history, ask:
- What is the pain like?
- Where is the pain? Does it go to the left shoulder or left arm?
- When does the pain come - with coughing? With breathing? With effort? Before, during, or after eating?
- Do certain movements make the pain worse or better?
- When did the pain start?
- Did you fall? Or have an accident or injury?
- Are there other symptoms like a cough, sputum (what is the sputum like?), trouble breathing, cold feelings in the afternoon and sweating at night, loss of weight?
- Does someone else in the family have tuberculosis, or a chronic cough, or blood in the sputum?
- Have you had attacks of wheezing in the past?

In the physical exam, look for:
- Fever.
- Tenderness when pressing on the chest. Note carefully where the tenderness is.
- Crackles in the lungs. Where are they? What are they like?
- Signs of heart attack, such as a fast irregular pulse, a low or absent blood pressure.
- Signs of heart failure:
  - Fast pulse, rapid breathing, crackles in the bases of the lungs, a big tender liver, swelling of the feet or legs, swollen veins in the neck.
- Sounds like music in the lungs during expiration.
- Tenderness in the abdomen.
- A big spleen.

In the laboratory, do:
- 3 sputum exams to look for tubercle bacilli, one exam each morning.

CHEST PAIN

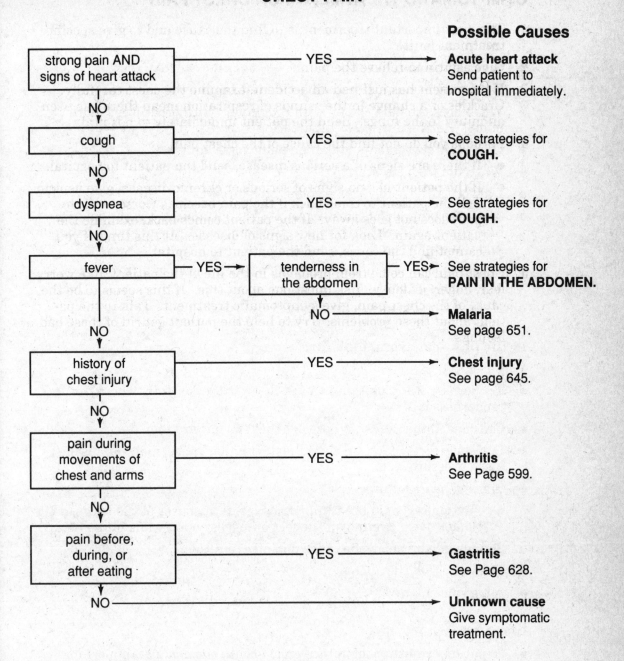

Possible Causes

strong pain AND signs of heart attack — YES → **Acute heart attack**
Send patient to hospital immediately.

NO ↓

cough — YES → See strategies for **COUGH.**

NO ↓

dyspnea — YES → See strategies for **COUGH.**

NO ↓

fever — YES → tenderness in the abdomen — YES → See strategies for **PAIN IN THE ABDOMEN.**

NO → **Malaria**
See page 651.

NO ↓

history of chest injury — YES → **Chest injury**
See page 645.

NO ↓

pain during movements of chest and arms — YES → **Arthritis**
See Page 599.

NO ↓

pain before, during, or after eating — YES → **Gastritis**
See Page 628.

NO → **Unknown cause**
Give symptomatic treatment.

SYMPTOMATIC TREATMENT FOR CHEST PAIN

1. The most important treatment is to find the cause and to give specific treatment for it.

2. Give aspirin to relieve the pain.

3. If the patient has just had an accident, examine the chest carefully. Crackles or a change in the sounds of respiration mean there has been an injury to the lungs. Send the patient immediately to hospital.

4. Perhaps you do not find the cause of the chest pain.

   ● If there are signs of a serious disease, send the patient to hospital.

   ● If the patient has no signs of serious or chronic disease, give aspirin. Tell the patient to come back if the pain becomes worse, or if the pain does not goes away. If the patient comes back, examine the patient again. Look for new signs of disease. At this time, if you cannot find the cause, send the patient to hospital.

5. Chest pain can come from problems in the life of the patient, like worry, fear, anger, jealousy. Ask questions about this. If this seems to be the cause of the chest pain, give symptomatic treatment. Talk to the patient about these problems. Try to help the patient get rid of these bad feelings.

HEART BURN

Heart burn is a feeling of burning in the upper middle part of the stomach. We call this the "epigastric region." The heart burn may be in the low middle part of the chest. In this case, the patient feels the heart burn behind the sternum.

The possible causes are:

1. Heart failure
2. Liver disease
3. Abdominal tumor
4. Intestinal worms
5. Peptic ulcer
6. Gastritis
7. Nervousness

1. HEART FAILURE

The edema of heart failure often affects the liver. The liver becomes big and tender. The swelling of the liver comes from the edema. It causes a feeling of heat, or burning, in the right upper quadrant or in the epigastric region.

For the other symptoms and signs of heart failure, see the strategy on COUGH IN AN OLDER CHILD OR AN ADULT on page 260.

2. LIVER DISEASE

- Hepatitis: fever, vomiting, a tender liver, jaundice.
- Cirrhosis: a big, hard, irregular liver, loss of weight, sometimes ascites, sometimes swelling of the feet and legs, rarely jaundice.
- Liver tumor: a big, hard, irregular liver, often with one large mass in the liver. Usually it is impossible to know if the cause of a big, hard, irregular liver is cirrhosis or a liver tumor.

3. ABDOMINAL TUMOR

- An **abdominal mass**, fixed or mobile.
- Loss of weight.
- Sometimes vomiting, constipation or diarrhea.

4. INTESTINAL WORMS

- **Worm eggs or larva in the stools.**
- Usually it is ankylostomes, ascaris or strongyloides.

5. PEPTIC ULCER

- **Severe burning or pain in a small area** in the epigastric region or in the right upper quadrant. The patient can point to this area with one finger. Often the pain comes during the night, or when the patient has not eaten for some hours.
- Spices, alcoholic drinks and smoking usually **make the pain worse**.
- Food, milk, or antacid medicines usually **make the pain better**.
- **Tenderness in the spot** where the patient feels pain.
- Sometimes loss of weight, vomiting, vomiting of blood, dark or black stools.

6. GASTRITIS

- **Diffuse burning** in the upper abdomen. Often this goes through to the back between the shoulders.
- **The burning usually comes during or soon after a meal**.
- Alcoholic drinks and spices often make the burning worse.
- Gastritis is frequent during the first three months of pregnancy.
- Gastritis can come in a patient with diabetes, with cirrhosis, or with another chronic disease.
- Often the abdomen is not tender.
- Often there are no physical signs of disease.

7. NERVOUSNESS

- **Diffuse and vague burning** in the upper abdomen or the lower chest.
- No association between meals and the heart burn.
- There is often an **association between the heart burn and the emotions**. Worry, anger, jealousy, fear, family or social problems can cause the heart burn.

SYMPTOMATIC TREATMENT FOR HEART BURN

See the treatment for gastritis on page 628.

TO MAKE THE DIAGNOSIS

In the history, ask:
- When did you first start having heart burn? What does it feel like?
- Where do you feel the heart burn? Does it go to your back or shoulder?
- When does the heart burn come:
  - Before eating? During the meal? After eating?
  - During the night?
  - When you are very hungry?
- Does eating make the pain worse or better?
- Do certain things: spices, alcoholic drinks, or smoking make it worse?
- Have you lost weight?
- Are there other symptoms, like:
  - Vomiting, vomiting of blood?
  - Diarrhea, blood in the stools, or black stools? Jaundice?
  - Cough, dyspnea, swelling of the feet, the legs, or the abdomen?
- Do you have worries or problems like anger, fear, jealousy, or sadness?
- If so, do these worries or problems make the heart burn worse?
- Do you suffer from diabetes? If so, for how long?
- In a woman who is pregnant, ask for how many months.

In the physical exam, look for:
- Fever, jaundice.
- A tender spot in the upper abdomen.
- Signs of heart failure:
  - Fast pulse, rapid breathing, crackles at the base of the lungs.
  - Swelling of the feet, the legs, or the abdomen, a big tender liver.
  - Swollen veins in the neck.
- A big liver. If so, note what the liver is like. Is it tender?
- An abdominal mass.
- In a woman, a mass in the lower abdomen may be a pregnancy.

In the laboratory, do:
- A stool exam to look for worm eggs or larva.
- In someone who may have diabetes, a urine exam to look for sugar.

HEART BURN

Possible causes

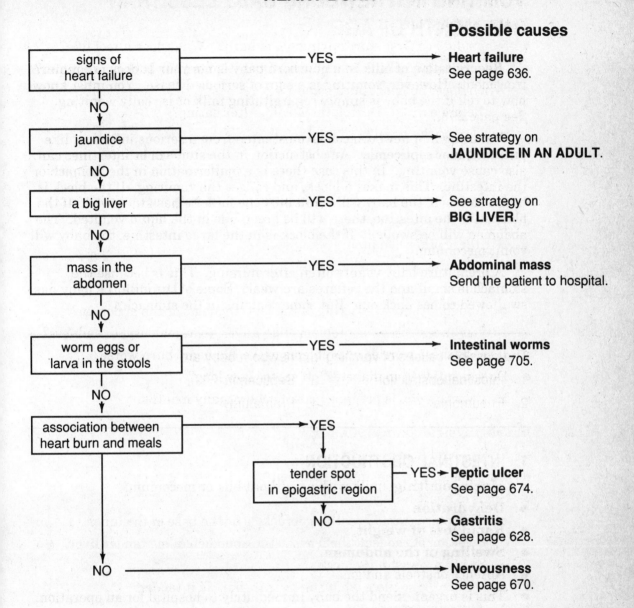

signs of heart failure — YES → **Heart failure**
See page 636.

NO

jaundice — YES → See strategy on **JAUNDICE IN AN ADULT**.

NO

a big liver — YES → See strategy on **BIG LIVER**.

NO

mass in the abdomen — YES → **Abdominal mass**
Send the patient to hospital.

NO

worm eggs or larva in the stools — YES → **Intestinal worms**
See page 705.

NO

association between heart burn and meals — YES →

tender spot in epigastric region — YES → **Peptic ulcer**
See page 674.

NO → **Gastritis**
See page 628.

NO → **Nervousness**
See page 670.

VOMITING IN A NEWBORN BABY LESS THAN ONE MONTH OF AGE

Regurgitation of milk in a new born baby is normal. It does not require treatment. However, vomiting is a sign of serious disease. You must know how to tell if the baby is simply regurgitating milk or is really vomiting. See page 298.

Vomiting in a newborn comes most often from a serious infection, like pneumonia or septicemia. An obstruction in the stomach or intestines can also cause vomiting. In this case there is a malformation in the stomach or the intestine. This makes a block, and causes the vomiting. If the block is in the stomach, the baby will vomit only the milk he has swallowed. If the block is in the intestine, there will be green bile in the liquid vomited. The abdomen will be swollen. If the block is in the large intestine, the baby will vomit meconium.

A premature baby vomits often after nursing. This is because the stomach is small and the reflexes are weak. Some of the milk the baby has swallowed comes back out. But some remains in the stomach.

The possible causes of vomiting in a newborn baby are:

1. Intestinal obstruction
2. Pneumonia
3. Septicemia
4. Prematurity

---

1. INTESTINAL OBSTRUCTION

- **Much vomiting**: milk with or without bile or meconium.
- **Dehydration**.
- **Rapid loss of weight**.
- **Swelling of the abdomen**.
- Absence of stools and gas.
- This is urgent. Send the baby immediately to hospital for an operation.

2. PNEUMONIA

- This is a difficult diagnosis to make in a newborn baby.
- **Signs of dyspnea**: often present, but sometimes absent.
- **Cyanosis of the lips**: often present, but sometimes absent.
- Fever: often present, but sometimes absent.

3. SEPTICEMIA

- **An infection somewhere**: umbiculus, skin, circumcision, abscess.
- **Often the baby was born at home** and not at the maternity. The parents have put unclean cloths or medicine on the umbilicus.
- Fever: often present, but sometimes absent.
- Often jaundice: sometimes a big liver.

4. PREMATURITY

- **Birth weight of less than 2 kg**.
- Vomiting of milk without bile.
- No fever, and no swelling of the abdomen.
- Often a loss of weight.

SYMPTOMATIC TREATMENT OF VOMITING IN A NEWBORN

1. The most important treatment is the treatment of the disease causing the vomiting. The vomiting will stop when the disease has been cured.

2. If you cannot find the cause and the baby seems very ill, start giving treatment for pneumonia. But send the child to hospital as quickly as possible.

3. If you cannot find the cause and the baby does not seem very ill, tell the mother how to help the baby nurse well.

    - The baby must nurse often, at least every two hours.
    - The mother must be calm and relaxed while the baby is nursing.
    - Once or twice during the nursing, the mother must remove the baby from her breast. She must hold the baby upright and tap the baby's back gently between the shoulders. This will permit any swallowed air to come up out of the stomach. Then the baby will not vomit.
    - If the vomiting continues for 3 days, or becomes more severe, the mother must come back with the baby. If you still can find no cause, send the baby to hospital.

4. If the baby is premature, tell the mother how to help the baby nurse well, as above. When the baby has gained some weight, the vomiting will stop. But if the baby does not gain weight, or loses weight, send the baby to hospital.

TO MAKE THE DIAGNOSIS:

In the history, ask the mother:

- Since when has the baby vomited? since birth? or since some days after birth?
- What does the baby vomit: milk? green liquid? meconium?
- Does the baby vomit each time after nursing?
- Has the baby passed meconium? If not, the anus is probably closed.
- Does the baby have stools now? If so, how many times a day? What are the stools like?
- Does the baby have trouble breathing?
- Has the baby lost weight?
- Was the baby born at home or in a maternity?
- How much did the baby weigh at birth?
- What was put on the umbilical cord after the birth?
- Has there been pus or a bad odor around the umbilicus?
- Has the baby had an infection or swelling somewhere?

In the physical exam, look for:

- The kind of liquid vomited. Try to see this liquid yourself.
- Swelling of the abdomen.
- The anus. Is it open? Try to put your fifth finger into the anus. First put on a glove. Put a little vaseline on the end of your fifth finger. Push it gently into the anus. If the anus is closed, send the baby immediately to hospital.
- Signs of weight loss or dehydration.
- Fever.
- Dyspnea.
- Cyanosis.
- An infection of the umbilicus, of the skin, of the penis, or elsewhere.
- An abscess.

VOMITING IN A NEWBORN BABY LESS THAN ONE MONTH OF AGE

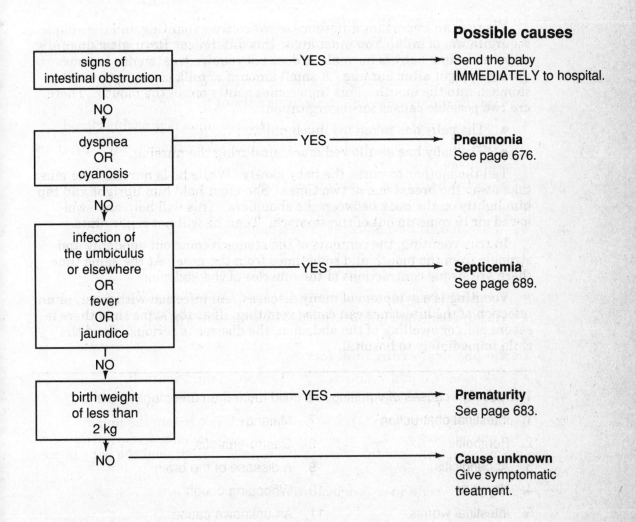

Possible causes

signs of intestinal obstruction — YES → Send the baby IMMEDIATELY to hospital.

NO

dyspnea OR cyanosis — YES → **Pneumonia** See page 676.

NO

infection of the umbiculus or elsewhere OR fever OR jaundice — YES → **Septicemia** See page 689.

NO

birth weight of less than 2 kg — YES → **Prematurity** See page 683.

NO → **Cause unknown** Give symptomatic treatment.

VOMITING IN A CHILD MORE THAN ONE MONTH OF AGE

There is an important difference between true vomiting and the simple regurgitation of milk. You must know this difference. Regurgitation of milk in a young baby is normal. It does not require treatment. It comes during or right after nursing. A small amount of milk comes up from the stomach into the mouth. This then comes gently out of the mouth. There are two possible causes for regurgitation:

- The baby has taken too much milk.

- The baby has swallowed much air during the nursing.

Tell the mother to nurse the baby slowly. While he is nursing, she must take away the breast one or two times. She must hold him upright and tap him lightly on the back between the shoulders. This will help any swallowed air to come up out of the stomach. Then he will not regurgitate.

In true vomiting, the contents of the stomach come out suddenly and strongly from the mouth and sometimes from the nose. At the same time there are strong contractions of the muscles of the abdomen.

Vomiting is a symptom of many diseases. An infection with fever, or an infection of the intestines can cause vomiting. If at the same time there is severe pain or swelling of the abdomen, the disease is serious. Send the child immediately to hospital.

The possible causes of vomiting in a child more than one month old are:

1. Intestinal obstruction
2. Peritonitis
3. Appendicitis
4. Hepatitis
5. Intestinal worms
6. An infection with fever
7. Malaria
8. Gastro-enteritis
9. A disease of the brain
10. Whooping cough
11. An unknown cause

---

1. INTESTINAL OBSTRUCTION

- **Vomiting with force** of food, of bile, or sometimes of brown liquid that has an odor like fecal matter.
- **Swelling of the abdomen**.
- **No stools, no gas** for more than 12 hours.
- Often **waves of peristaltic contractions** going across the abdomen.
- Dehydration.
- Send the child immediately to hospital.

2. PERITONITIS

- **High fever and rapid pulse**.
- **Swelling of the abdomen**.
- **Rebound pain**.
- Rapid breathing limited to the chest. The abdomen does not move with respirations.
- No sounds of peristalsis. The abdomen is silent.
- A high white blood cell count.

3. APPENDICITIS

- **Pain in the right lower quadrant (RLQ)**, with tenderness.
- Fever, vomiting, constipation.
- A high white blood cell count.
- Send the child immediately to hospital for an operation.

4. HEPATITIS

- **Pain in the right upper quadrant (RUQ)**.
- Fever, loss of appetite.
- Often **jaundice**.
- Liver tender, smooth, and often a little bigger than normal.

5. INTESTINAL WORMS

- **Worm eggs in the stools.**

6. INFECTION WITH FEVER

- Meningitis, septicemia, pneumonia, measles, tonsillitis, otitis, urinary infection.
- Fever.
- **Signs typical of the infection.**
- Follow the strategies of the other signs found.

7. MALARIA

- **High fever**, often with convulsions.
- Plasmodium in the thick blood film.
- Sometimes anemia, sometimes jaundice, sometimes diarrhea.
- Often a big spleen.

8. GASTRO-ENTERITIS

- **Much diarrhea**.
- Dehydration.
- Fever, often present, but sometimes absent.

9. BRAIN DISEASE

- Head injury, abscess, or tumor in the brain.
- **Projectile vomiting**: with very much force.
- Changes in the consciousness, in talking, in equilibrium.
- Often a paralysis.
- In case of a head injury, a history of an accident.

10. WHOOPING COUGH

● **Spasms of coughing following by a noisy inspiration, or "whoop**," and often vomiting.

● No fever.

● For other symptoms and signs of whooping cough, see the strategy on COUGH IN A CHILD LESS THAN 5 YEARS OLD, on page 253.

11. UNKNOWN CAUSE

● Send the child to hospital if there is severe vomiting, dehydration, loss of weight.

● If he does not seem very ill, give symptomatic treatment. But if the vomiting continues or becomes worse, send him to hospital.

TO MAKE THE DIAGNOSIS:

In the history, ask the mother:

- Since when does the child vomit?
- What does he vomit?
- Does he seem to have pain in the abdomen? Where is the pain?
- Does his abdomen seem swollen?
- Has he passed stools or gas during the past 12 hours? If not, when was the last time he passed stools or gas?
- Does he have a fever?
- Has he had convulsions?
- Has he had other symptoms?
    - Pain in the neck?
    - Dyspnea, cough?
    - Pain in the throat or in the ear?
- Does he have diarrhea? Jaundice? A skin rash?
- Has he had an accident with an injury to the head?
- Does he have spasms of coughing followed by a "whoop" and vomiting?

In the physical exam, look for:

- The kind of liquid vomited. Try to see this liquid yourself.
- Fever.
- Swelling of the abdomen.
- Visible waves of peristaltic contractions moving across the abdomen.
- Tenderness in the abdomen. If so, where is it?
- Rebound pain.
- Sounds of peristalsis. If the abdomen is silent, this is a sign of peritonitis.
- Signs of an infection with fever:
    - Meningitis: stiff neck, swollen fontanel, convulsions.
    - Pneumonia: signs of dyspnea, crackles in the lungs.
    - Measles: typical skin rash.
    - Tonsillitis: redness in the throat, with white spots on the tonsils.
    - Otitis: pulling on the ear, or pus coming from the ear.
    - Urinary infection: white blood cells in the urine.

- Jaundice. This is a sign of either hepatitis or malaria.
- A tender or swollen liver.
- A big spleen.
- Anemia: from malaria or hookworm.
- Delirium, coma, or paralysis.
- Signs of dehydration:
  - Dry mouth, dry skin with many folds, dry eyes without tears, little or no urine during the past 6 hours or more.
  - If the child is dehydrated, he will need rehydration. See page 322.

In the laboratory, do:
- A thick blood film to look for Plasmodium.
- A white blood cell count to see if there is an infection.
- A stool exam to look for worm eggs.
- A urine exam to look for albumin and white blood cells.
- A lumbar puncture in case of:
  - A child with a stiff neck.
  - A child with a swollen fontanel.
  - A child with fever and convulsions.
  - A child with fever and vomiting with no cause found.

VOMITING IN A CHILD MORE THAN ONE MONTH OF AGE

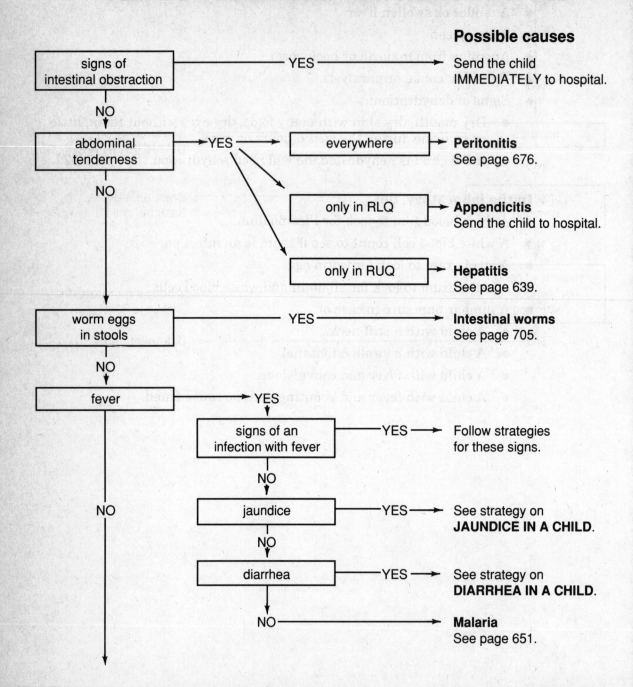

Possible causes

signs of intestinal obstraction — YES → Send the child IMMEDIATELY to hospital.

NO

abdominal tenderness — YES →
- everywhere → **Peritonitis** See page 676.
- only in RLQ → **Appendicitis** Send the child to hospital.
- only in RUQ → **Hepatitis** See page 639.

NO

worm eggs in stools — YES → **Intestinal worms** See page 705.

NO

fever — YES →
- signs of an infection with fever — YES → Follow strategies for these signs.

  NO

- jaundice — YES → See strategy on **JAUNDICE IN A CHILD**.

  NO

- diarrhea — YES → See strategy on **DIARRHEA IN A CHILD**.

  NO → **Malaria** See page 651.

NO

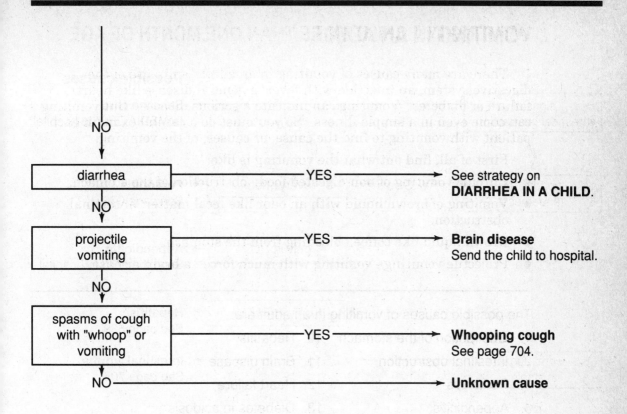

NO

| diarrhea | ——YES—→ | See strategy on **DIARRHEA IN A CHILD**. |

NO

| projectile vomiting | ——YES—→ | **Brain disease** Send the child to hospital. |

NO

| spasms of cough with "whoop" or vomiting | ——YES—→ | **Whooping cough** See page 704. |

NO ————————————————————→ **Unknown cause**

VOMITING IN AN ADULT

There are many causes of vomiting in an adult: a disease of the digestive system, an infection with fever, a general disease like heart failure or diabetes. Vomiting can indicate a serious disease. But vomiting can come even in a simple illness. So you must do a careful exam in each patient with vomiting to find the cause, or causes, of the vomiting.

First of all, find out what the vomiting is like:

- Chronic vomiting of non-digested food: obstruction of the stomach.
- Vomiting of brown liquid with an odor like fecal matter: intestinal obstruction.
- Brown liquid like coffee: bleeding from the stomach.
- Projectile vomiting - vomiting with much force: a brain disease.

The possible causes of vomiting in an adult are:

1. Obstruction of the stomach
2. Intestinal obstruction
3. Peritonitis
4. Appendicitis
5. Gall bladder disease
6. Kidney disease
7. Malaria
8. Gastritis or peptic ulcer
9. Infection with fever
10. Hepatitis
11. Brain disease
12. Heart failure
13. Diabetes in acidosis
14. Food poisoning
15. Gastro - enteritis
16. Pregnancy, especially during the first three months of pregnancy

---

1. OBSTRUCTION OF THE STOMACH

- **Chronic vomiting** of non-digested food.
- Little or no swelling of the abdomen.
- **Visible waves of peristalsis in the left upper quadrant**, moving from the left side to the right side.
- Loss of weight.

2. INTESTINAL OBSTRUCTION

- Vomiting for only some hours or a few days.
- **Vomiting** of green liquid, sometimes brown, and sometimes with an odor of fecal matter.
- **Swelling of the abdomen**.
- **Abdominal pain that comes and goes**, coming with the waves of peristalsis.
- **No stools or gas** for many hours or even days.
- **Visible waves of peristalsis** moving across the abdomen.
- **Loud sounds of peristalsis** heard through the stethoscope. First there is a period of silence. Then come loud, rapid sounds when the patient feels pain and when you see the wave of peristalsis.

3. PERITONITIS

- **Fever**, rapid pulse, breathing rapid and only with the chest muscles.
- **Swelling of the abdomen**.
- **Severe pain** everywhere in the abdomen.
- **Rebound pain**.
- No sounds of peristalsis. The abdomen is silent.
- A high white blood cell count.

4. APPENDICITIS

- **Pain and tenderness in the right lower quadrant** (RLQ).
- Moderate fever, vomiting, constipation.
- A high white blood cell count.

5. GALL BLADDER DISEASE

- **Severe pain and tenderness in the right upper quadrant**.
- Often a **small tender mass** just below the middle of the liver edge that moves down with the liver when the patient breathes in.
- Often fever.
- Often a high white blood cell count.
- Sometimes jaundice.

6. KIDNEY DISEASE - STONE OR INFECTION

- **Severe pain in the flank** which often goes down to the lower quadrant.
- **Tenderness in the flank**.
- Often **red or white blood cells in the urine**.

7. MALARIA

- High fever, severe headache, and much vomiting.
- **Plasmodium in the thick blood film**.

8. GASTRITIS OR PEPTIC ULCER

- Chronic vomiting: liquid clear, yellow, green, or brown.
- Much heart burn.
- No visible waves of peristalsis.

9. INFECTION WITH FEVER

- Fever.
- **Signs typical of the infection**.
- Follow the strategies of these other signs.

10. HEPATITIS

- **Pain in the right upper quadrant (RUQ)**.
- **Jaundice** and often fever.
- **Liver tender** and often a little swollen.

11. BRAIN DISEASE - INJURY, ABSCESS OR TUMOR IN THE BRAIN

- **Projectile vomiting**.
- Often a **change in consciousness**, in talking, in equilibrium.
- Sometimes a paralysis.
- The history of an accident with an injury to the head indicates a hemorrhage inside the skull. Send the patient IMMEDIATELY to hospital.

12. HEART FAILURE

- **Signs of heart failure**: rapid pulse, rapid breathing, crackles at the bases of the lungs, swelling of the feet or legs, a big tender liver, swollen veins in the neck.

13. DIABETES IN COMA

- **Breathing rapid and very deep**.
- Delirium or coma.
- **Much sugar in the urine**.
- Often heart burn.

14. FOOD POISONING

- Much vomiting during the past few hours.
- Often a **history of other members of the family** with vomiting and diarrhea.
- Often diarrhea and much weakness.

15. GASTRO-ENTERITIS

- **Diarrhea**.
- Fever: sometimes present, often absent.

16. PREGNANCY - ESPECIALLY IN THE FIRST THREE MONTHS

- **Vomiting especially in the morning**.
- Signs of pregnancy: amenorrhea, mass in the lower abdomen.

TO MAKE THE DIAGNOSIS:

In the history, ask:

- Since when have you been vomiting?
- What do you vomit? What is the liquid like?
- Have you vomited blood? If so, look at the strategy on VOMITING BLOOD on page 314.
- Do you have pain in the abdomen? If so, where is the pain?
- Is your abdomen swollen, or bigger?
- Are you passing stools and gas? Even today?
- Do you have fever? Diarrhea? Heart burn?
- Have you lost weight?
- Do you have other symptoms, like headache, pain on urination, back pain?
- Have your eyes become yellow?
- What did you eat just before the vomiting started? Have other persons who ate with you also been vomiting?
- Have you ever had heart failure or diabetes in the past?
- Have you just had an accident or an injury to the head?
- If your patient is a woman: are you pregnant? If so, for how many months?

In the physical exam, look for:

- The kind of liquid vomited. Try to see this liquid yourself.
- Fever.
- Swelling of the abdomen.
- Visible waves of peristaltic contractions moving across the abdomen. Note carefully where they start and in which direction they move.
- Loud sounds of peristalsis coming with the waves and with the attacks of pain.

- Tenderness in the abdomen: Where is it? Is there rebound pain?
- Tenderness in the flank.
- Jaundice, a tender or swollen liver.
- A small tender mass in the middle of the liver edge.
- Signs of heart failure.
- Signs of an infection with fever.
- Rapid and deep breathing.
- Delirium, coma, paralysis.
- In a woman, a mass in the lower abdomen typical of a pregnancy.

In the laboratory, do:
- A urine exam to look for sugar (diabetes) and red or white blood cells (kidney disease).
- A white blood cell count to see if there is an infection.
- A thick blood film to look for Plasmodium.

SYMPTOMATIC TREATMENT

If you do not find the cause of the vomiting, send the patient to hospital if:
- The vomiting is severe.
- The patient has vomited for more than 3 days.
- There is dehydration or loss of weight.

Give symptomatic treatment if the patient does not seem very ill.
- Promethazine, 25 mg 2 or 3 times a day, or
- Chlorpromazine, 25 mg 3 times a day.

Tell the patient to drink only liquids until the vomiting stops. Then he may start eating soft foods for 2 days. If there is no more vomiting, he may then eat whatever he wants to eat. He must not drink alcoholic drinks.

VOMITING IN AN ADULT

Possible causes

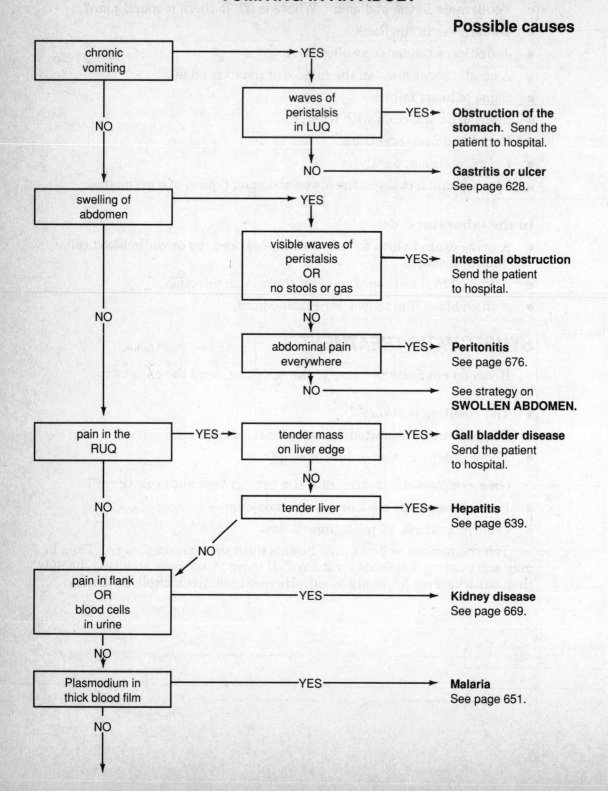

chronic vomiting → YES → waves of peristalsis in LUQ → YES→ **Obstruction of the stomach**. Send the patient to hospital.

waves of peristalsis in LUQ → NO → **Gastritis or ulcer** See page 628.

chronic vomiting → NO → swelling of abdomen → YES → visible waves of peristalsis OR no stools or gas → YES→ **Intestinal obstruction** Send the patient to hospital.

visible waves of peristalsis OR no stools or gas → NO → abdominal pain everywhere → YES→ **Peritonitis** See page 676.

abdominal pain everywhere → NO → See strategy on **SWOLLEN ABDOMEN.**

swelling of abdomen → NO → pain in the RUQ → YES → tender mass on liver edge → YES→ **Gall bladder disease** Send the patient to hospital.

tender mass on liver edge → NO → tender liver → YES→ **Hepatitis** See page 639.

tender liver → NO →

pain in the RUQ → NO → pain in flank OR blood cells in urine → YES → **Kidney disease** See page 669.

pain in flank OR blood cells in urine → NO → Plasmodium in thick blood film → YES → **Malaria** See page 651.

Plasmodium in thick blood film → NO →

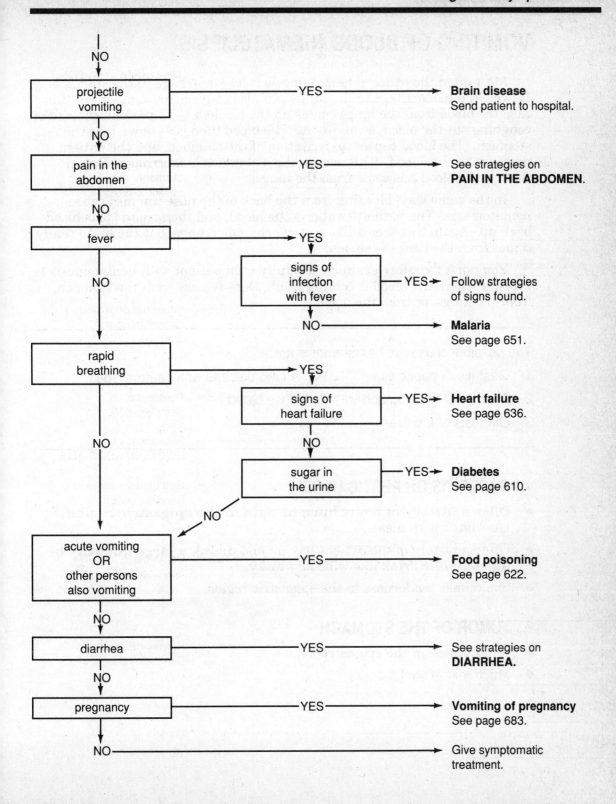

NO

| projectile vomiting | —YES— | **Brain disease**
 Send patient to hospital. |

NO

| pain in the abdomen | —YES— | See strategies on
 PAIN IN THE ABDOMEN. |

NO

fever —→ YES

| signs of infection with fever | —YES→ | Follow strategies <br> of signs found. |

NO—————→ **Malaria**
 See page 651.

rapid breathing —→ YES

| signs of heart failure | —YES→ | **Heart failure**
 See page 636. |

NO

| sugar in the urine | —YES→ | **Diabetes**
 See page 610. |

NO

| acute vomiting
 OR <br> other persons also vomiting | —YES— | **Food poisoning**
 See page 622. |

NO

| diarrhea | —YES— | See strategies on
 DIARRHEA. |

NO

| pregnancy | —YES— | **Vomiting of pregnancy**
 See page 683. |

NO—————————→ Give symptomatic <br> treatment.

VOMITING OF BLOOD (HEMATEMESIS)

Most often the cause of hematemesis is a hemorrhage in the stomach. However, a hemorrhage in the lungs can also cause hematemesis. In this case the blood from the lungs comes up the trachea. The patient, instead of coughing out the blood, swallows it. The blood then goes down into the stomach. The blood causes an irritation of the stomach, and the patient now vomits this blood. This seems like a stomach hemorrhage. But in reality, the blood has come from the lungs.

In the same way, bleeding from the back of the nose can also cause hematemesis. The patient swallows the blood, and then vomits this blood back up. Again this seems like a stomach hemorrhage, but the blood really comes from the back of the nose.

You must therefore examine carefully each patient with hematemesis to find out where the blood is coming from. Does it come from the stomach, from the lungs, or from the nose?

The possible causes of hematemesis are:

1. Gastritis or peptic ulcer
2. A tumor of the stomach
3. Cirrhosis of the liver
4. A lung disease with hemorrhage
5. Nose bleed

---

1. GASTRITIS OR PEPTIC ULCER

- Often **a history of heart burn or pain in the epigastric region** associated with meals.
- Often a history of the patient having just **drunk a large quantity of an alcoholic** drink like wine or whisky.
- Sometimes tenderness in the epigastric region.

2. TUMOR OF THE STOMACH

- A hard mass in the epigastric region.
- Much loss of weight.

3. CIRRHOSIS

- Often a **big, hard, irregular liver** which may be tender.
- Sometimes the liver is very small (atrophic) and impossible to feel.
- Sometimes edema, ascites, jaundice, weight loss.

4. LUNG DISEASE

- History of a cough, dyspnea, or pain in the chest.
- See the strategy SPUTUM WITH BLOOD on page 277.

5. NOSE BLEED

- **Blood in the nose or in the back of the throat**.
- Sometimes a history of an injury to the nose, or of high blood pressure.

SYMPTOMATIC TREATMENT

1. Determine first the general condition of the patient. If there are signs of shock, the patient will need a transfusion.
2. Put the patient in bed. Start an IV infusion of physiological saline.
3. If possible, send the patient to hospital as soon as the patient's condition will permit it. If this is not possible, treat the patient in your health center.
4. The patient must eat or drink nothing for 24 hours, or until the hematemesis has stopped.
5. Give the patient:
    - Diazepam, 5 mg every 6 hours, or
    - Phenobarbital, 50 mg every 6 hours.
6. Give atropine IM, 0.5 mg every 8 hours.
7. After 24 hours with no vomiting, the patient can begin to drink water and milk. After another 24 hours with no vomiting, he can begin eating soft foods.
8. If the vomiting continues, or comes back again, or if the condition of the patient becomes worse, send him to hospital.
9. At the end of the treatment, send the patient to the doctor for more examinations. Tell him not to drink alcoholic drinks.

TO MAKE THE DIAGNOSIS

In the history, ask:
- When did you start to vomit blood?
- Have you ever vomited blood in the past?
- What did you eat or drink just before you started vomiting blood?
- How much alcoholic drinks do you drink regularly?
- Have you had indigestion, gastritis, heart burn, or liver disease in the past? If so, when? What treatment have you had?
- Have your eyes ever been yellow?
- Have you had swelling of the feet, of the legs, or of the abdomen in the past?
- Have you had a cough, sputum, dyspnea, or chest pain?
- Do you often have nose bleeds?
- Have you had an injury to your nose recently?

In the physical exam, look for:
- Signs of shock: a fast weak pulse or no pulse at all, a low blood pressure, or no blood pressure at all.
- Tenderness in the epigastric region.
- A big liver. What is it like?
- Swelling of the feet, the legs, or the abdomen.
- Jaundice.
- Crackles in the lungs.
- Fresh blood in the nose or in the back of the throat.

In the laboratory, do:
- Hemoglobin exam.
- Sputum exam for tubercle bacilli if the patient has a cough with sputum.

VOMITING OF BLOOD (HEMATEMESIS)

Possible causes

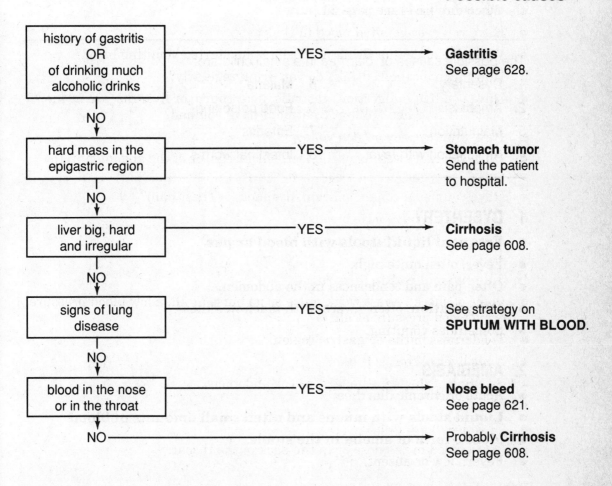

history of gastritis OR of drinking much alcoholic drinks	—YES→	**Gastritis** See page 628.
NO ↓		
hard mass in the epigastric region	—YES→	**Stomach tumor** Send the patient to hospital.
NO ↓		
liver big, hard and irregular	—YES→	**Cirrhosis** See page 608.
NO ↓		
signs of lung disease	—YES→	See strategy on **SPUTUM WITH BLOOD**.
NO ↓		
blood in the nose or in the throat	—YES→	**Nose bleed** See page 621.
NO————————→		Probably **Cirrhosis** See page 608.

DIARRHEA IN A CHILD LESS THAN 5 YEARS OLD

Diarrhea means more than three liquid stools per day. Find out what the stools are like - see page 31.

The possible causes of diarrhea in a small child are:

1. Dysentery
2. Amebiasis
3. Malnutrition
4. An infection with fever
5. Malaria
6. Food poisoning
7. Enteritis
8. Intestinal worms

---

1. DYSENTERY

- **Frequent liquid stools with blood or pus**.
- Fever, often quite high.
- Often pain and tenderness in the abdomen.
- **Dehydration**, often severe, with much weakness.
- Sometimes vomiting.

2. AMEBIASIS

- Acute or chronic diarrhea.
- **Liquid stools with mucus and often small amounts of blood**.
- **Mobile form of ameba in the stools**.
- Fever: low or absent.

3. MALNUTRITION

- **Liquid stools with no blood or pus and with very little fecal matter**.
- **Signs of malnutrition**.
  - Weight loss.
  - Weakness and loss of interest in living.
  - Swelling of the legs, arms, and abdomen.
  - Changes in the color of hair and skin.

4. AN INFECTION WITH FEVER - MEASLES, PNEUMONIA, OTITIS

- **Liquid stools with no blood or pus**.
- Fever.
    - **Signs of the infection**.
    - Measles: the typical rash.
    - Pneumonia: cough, dyspnea, crackles in the lungs.
    - Otitis: pulling on the ear, pus coming from the ear.

5. MALARIA

- **Liquid stools with no blood or pus**.
- **Fever**.
- Sometimes convulsions, vomiting, anemia, jaundice, a big spleen.
- **Plasmodium in the thick blood film**.
- The diarrhea and fever stop quickly after a cure of chloroquine.

6. FOOD POISONING

- **Liquid stools, often with pus or blood**.
- Vomiting.
- **Other members of the family who have diarrhea**.
- Fever: often present, sometimes absent.

7. ENTERITIS

- **Liquid stools with no blood or pus**.
- Dehydration.
- Fever: low or absent.
- Sometimes vomiting.
- Sometimes a history of nursing by bottle.

8. INTESTINAL WORMS

Except for strongyloides and trichuris, intestinal worms do not often cause diarrhea in small children. However, a stool exam will often show worm eggs or larva. This is because most children already have intestinal worms. So, if you find worm eggs in the child's stool, treat first the cause of the diarrhea. When the diarrhea has stopped, then give him the right worm cure.

TO MAKE THE DIAGNOSIS

In the history, ask the mother:

- When did the child start having diarrhea?
- What are the stools like?
- Are there other symptoms, such as: Fever, vomiting, pain in the abdomen, convulsions, cough, dyspnea, pulling on the ear or pus coming from the ear canal?
- Are there other persons in the family who also have diarrhea?
- Is the child nursing by bottle?
- What water does the child drink? Do you do anything to the water to make it safe for drinking?
- Is there a good sanitary installation at home?

In the physical exam, look for:

- Signs of dehydration:
    - Dry mouth and lips.
    - Skin dry with many folds.
    - Eyes dry, with no tears, and sunk back into the eye sockets.
    - Little or no urine for the last 12 hours.
- The aspect of the stools. Try to see the stools yourself.
- Fever.
- Tenderness in the abdomen.
- Signs of malnutrition.
- Signs of an infection with fever.
    - Measles: the typical rash.
    - Pneumonia: dyspnea, crackles.
    - Otitis: pus coming from the ear.
- A big spleen.
- Jaundice, anemia.

In the laboratory, do:

- A fresh stool exam to look for moving ameba. Look also for worm eggs.
- A thick blood film to look for Plasmodium.

DIARRHEA IN A CHILD LESS THAN 5 YEARS OLD

Possible causes

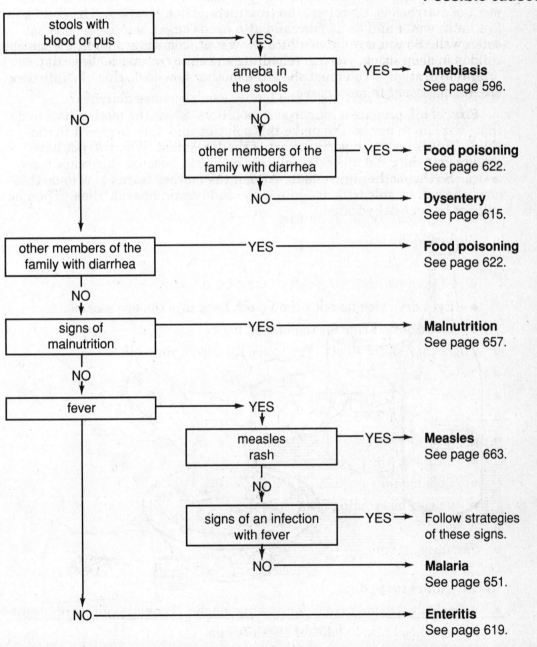

stools with blood or pus — YES →

    ameba in the stools — YES → **Amebiasis** See page 596.

    NO ↓

    other members of the family with diarrhea — YES → **Food poisoning** See page 622.

    NO → **Dysentery** See page 615.

NO ↓

other members of the family with diarrhea — YES → **Food poisoning** See page 622.

NO ↓

signs of malnutrition — YES → **Malnutrition** See page 657.

NO ↓

fever — YES →

    measles rash — YES → **Measles** See page 663.

    NO ↓

    signs of an infection with fever — YES → Follow strategies of these signs.

    NO → **Malaria** See page 651.

NO → **Enteritis** See page 619.

THE TREATMENT OF DEHYDRATION IN CHILDREN

Children do not die of diarrhea. Instead, they die because of the dehydration caused by the diarrhea. The most important part of the treatment of diarrhea is, therefore, the treatment of dehydration. The child has lost much water and salt. The child also needs sugar because he has not eaten well. So you must give all three: water, salt, sugar. Except when the child is in deep shock, you can rehydrate the child by mouth. We call this "oral rehydration." You must show the mother how to do this. IV infusions are not necessary in most cases.

First of all, prepare a "sugar-salt" solution. Show the mother how to do this. Explain to her how to make this solution and how to give it to the child. This is a very important part of the treatment. You will not have time to give the child all of the solution he needs, because this takes many hours. So the mother must do it. Also, if the mother learns how to do this now, she will be able to do it again if the child again has diarrhea. Then he will not become dehydrated.

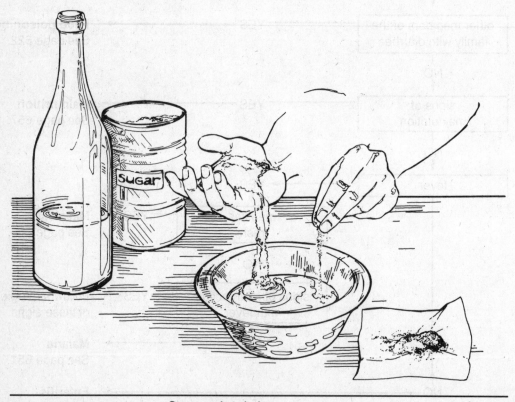

Sugar-salt solution.

1. THE SOLUTION

You need table salt, sugar, water safe for drinking, a cooking pan or bowl, and a bottle. An empty beer bottle is a good one to use. This holds about 750 ml of solution. Make the solution in this way:

- 2 pinches of salt: between your thumb, index, and middle fingers.
- A handful of sugar: in your whole hand.
- A bottle full of water safe for drinking.
- If possible, juice from an orange or lemon. This will give the child the potassium he has lost in the stools.
- Mix the water, salt, and sugar in the pan or bowl. Stir it well. Then put it in the bottle.
- Taste the solution. If it is very salty, do not use it. Too much salt will make the dehydration worse. The solution should taste like normal tears.

2. THE QUANTITY TO GIVE

1. To a child with **no signs of dehydration**.
   - A baby less than 6 months old: 2 bottles of solution per day.
   - A child from 6 months to 2 years: 3 bottles of solution per day.
   - A child from 2 to 5 years old: 4 bottles of solution per day.

2. To a child with **signs of dehydration**.
   - A baby less than 6 months old: 2 1/2 bottles of solution per day.
   - A child from 6 months to 2 years: 4 bottles of solution per day.
   - A child from 2 to 5 years: 6 bottles of solution per day.

Give the solution until the diarrhea stops.

3. HOW TO GIVE THE SOLUTION

- Give the solution slowly, but continuously.
- Use a cup and a small spoon.
- Give one spoonful of solution each time.
- Wait one or two minutes between each spoonful.
- If the child vomits, wait five minutes and then continue. Even if the child vomits, he will not vomit all he has taken. Some will remain in the stomach and be absorbed. So vomiting does not mean you must stop the oral rehydration.

4. A CHILD IN SHOCK, WITH GREAT WEAKNESS

● Prepare immediately a bottle of sugar-salt solution.

● Show the mother how to give it to the child.

● If the hospital is near by, send the child to hospital. Tell the mother to give the sugar-salt solution during the trip.

● If the hospital is far away (more than one hour away), do not send the child. He will probably die on the way. Simply continue with the oral rehydration in your health center. You may be able to save the child's life anyway.

Medicines to stop the diarrhea, like kaolin, paregoric, and others, are of no use. **Do not use them**. Give only oral rehydration and treatment for the cause of the diarrhea.

5. INSTRUCTIONS TO GIVE TO THE PARENTS

1. The child must always drink water that is safe for drinking:

   ● Water from a protected source or well, or

   ● Water that has been boiled for at least 5 minutes.

2. If the mother is nursing the child with a bottle, explain to her the dangers of this causing enteritis. Suggest that she stop doing this. If it is abso-lutely necessary for her to continue giving the child a bottle, explain to her very carefully how to do this properly. She must make the milk with water safe for drinking. She must make it according to the instructions on the milk can. The baby must drink the milk **within two hours**. After this time the milk becomes bad and can cause enteritis. She must wash and boil the bottle and the rubber nipple in water between each feeding.

3. The water in which rice has been boiled is good for simple enteritis and for the diarrhea of malnutrition. Tell the mother that, if the child has diarrhea again, she should cook rice and give the water to the child to drink.

4. Do not put strong spices into food for a small baby.

5. When the mother starts giving a food the child has not eaten before, she should first give only a small amount. If this does not give the child diarrhea, she can then give more. But if the new food does give diarrhea, she should not give this food again for some days or weeks.

6. Talk to the parents about how to protect their water source or well.

7. Water from swamps, ponds, streams, or a river is dirty. It is not safe for drinking. It can cause diarrhea.

8. The home must have a well-built latrine. Talk to the parents about this. The hole must be at least 3 meters deep. Every member of the family must use the latrine. No one should pass stools on the ground.

SUMMARY OF THE TREATMENT OF DIARRHEA IN SMALL CHILDREN

1. Liquid stools with no blood or pus.

   - With no fever: oral rehydration only.

   - With fever: oral rehydration and chloroquine.

   - With fever and signs of another infection: oral rehydration, chloroquine, and treatment for the other infection.

   - With signs of malnutrition: oral rehydration, chloroquine, and treatment for malnutrition - see page 657.

2. Liquid stools with blood or pus.

   - With mobile ameba: oral rehydration and treatment for amebiasis.

   - With no moving ameba: oral rehydration and treatment for dysentery - see page 615.

   - With vomiting, and when other members of the family have diarrhea: oral rehydration and treatment for food poisoning - see page 622.

ACUTE DIARRHEA IN AN OLDER CHILD OR AN ADULT

This means more than three liquids stools per day for less than two weeks. Find out what the stools are like - see page 31.

The possible causes are:

1. Dysentery
2. Amebiasis
3. Food poisoning
4. Malnutrition
5. Malaria
6. Intestinal worms
7. Enteritis

1. DYSENTERY

- **Liquid stools with blood or pus**.
- Fever, often quite high.
- Often abdominal pain and tenderness.
- **Dehydration**, often severe, with much weakness.
- Sometimes vomiting.

2. AMEBIASIS

- Acute or chronic diarrhea.
- **Liquid stools with mucus and often small amounts of blood**.
- **Mobile form of ameba in the stools**.
- Fever: low, or absent.

3. FOOD POISONING

- **Liquid stools, often with blood or pus**.
- Vomiting.
- Often **other members of the family have eaten the same food and also have diarrhea**.
- Fever: often present, sometimes absent.

4. MALNUTRITION
- **Liquid stools with no blood or pus, and with little or no fecal matter**.
- **Signs of malnutrition**.
  - Weight loss.
  - Weakness.
  - Swelling of feet, legs, arms, and abdomen.
  - Changes in the color of skin and hair.

5. MALARIA
- **Liquid stools with no blood or pus**.
- **Fever**.
- Sometimes anemia, jaundice, convulsions.
- Often a big spleen.
- **Plasmodium in the thick blood film**.
- The diarrhea and fever stop quickly after a cure of chloroquine.

6. INTESTINAL WORMS - HOOKWORM, STRONGYLOIDES, TRICHURIS
- **Liquid stools, sometimes with blood**.
- Often pain in the abdomen.
- Sometimes anemia and signs of malnutrition.
- **Worm eggs or larva in the stools**.

7. ENTERITIS
- **Liquid stools with no blood or pus**.
- Fever: low or absent.
- Sometimes dehydration.

TO MAKE THE DIAGNOSIS

In the history, ask:

- When did the diarrhea start?
- What do the stools look like?
- Is there blood or pus in the stools?
- How many times a day do you pass stools?
- Do you have other symptoms, like fever, vomiting, pain in the abdomen?
- Are there other members of your family who have diarrhea?
- What water do you normally drink? Where does it come from? What do you do to make it safe for drinking?
- Do you have a good latrine at your house?

In the physical exam, look for:

- Signs of dehydration:
  - Dry mouth and lips.
  - Skin dry with many folds.
  - Eyes dry with no tears and sunk back into the eye sockets.
  - Little or no urine for 12 hours or more.
- The aspect of the stools. Try to see the stools yourself.
- Fever.
- Tenderness in the abdomen. Where is it?
- Signs of malnutrition.
- A big spleen.
- Anemia, jaundice.

In the laboratory, do:

- A fresh stool exam to look for mobile ameba.
- An ordinary stool exam to look for worm eggs or larva.
- A thick blood film to look for Plasmodium.

ACUTE DIARRHEA IN AN OLDER CHILD OR AN ADULT

Possible causes

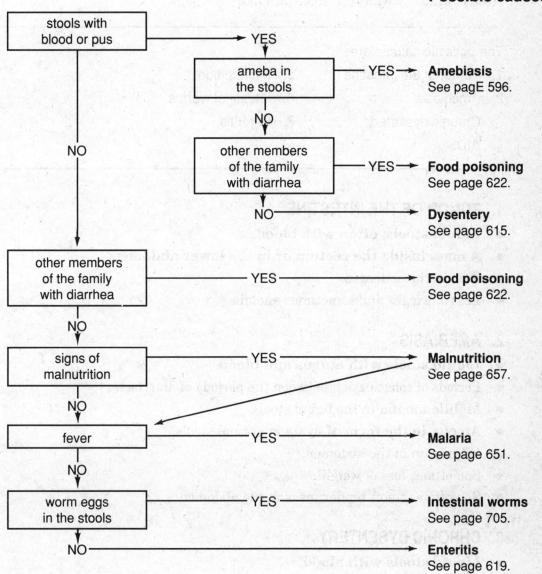

CHRONIC DIARRHEA IN AN ADULT

This means more than three liquid stools per day for more than two weeks. Find out what the stools are like - see page 31.

The possible causes are:

1. Tumor of the intestine
2. Amebiasis
3. Chronic dysentery
4. AIDS
5. Malnutrition
6. Intestinal worms
7. Enteritis

1. TUMOR OF THE INTESTINE

- **Liquid stools, often with blood**.
- **A mass inside the rectum or in the lower abdomen**.
- Pain in the abdomen.
- Loss of weight and sometimes anemia.

2. AMEBIASIS

- **Liquid stools with mucus and blood**.
- Periods of constipation between the periods of diarrhea.
- **Mobile ameba** in the liquid stools.
- **Ameba in the form of cysts** in normal stools.
- Often pain in the abdomen.
- Sometimes loss of weight.
- Sometimes a soft tender mass in the abdomen.

3. CHRONIC DYSENTERY

- **Liquid stools with blood**.
- Often a low or moderate fever, with cold feelings during the afternoon and sweating during the night.

- Pain and tenderness in the abdomen.
- Loss of weight.
- Sometimes signs of malnutrition.

4. AIDS

- **Much weight loss**.
- Often big lymph nodes all over.
- Often a **low fever** for some weeks.
- Sometimes a fungus infection in the mouth and throat: a white film covering the tongue and the mucus membranes of the mouth and throat.

5. MALNUTRITION

- **Liquid stools with no blood or pus, and with very little fecal matter**.
- **Signs of malnutrition**.
  - Loss of weight.
  - Weakness.
  - Swelling of the feet, legs, abdomen, and even the face.
  - Changes in the color of the skin and hair.
- In malnutrition, the signs of malnutrition come before the diarrhea starts. If the malnutrition is caused by a chronic dysentery, the diarrhea comes first and the signs of malnutrition come later.

6. INTESTINAL WORMS

- **Liquid stools, sometimes with blood**.
- **Worm eggs or larva in the stools**.
- Often pain in the abdomen.
- Sometimes anemia and sometimes signs of malnutrition.

7. ENTERITIS

- **Liquid stools with no blood or pus**.
- No fever, no weight loss.
- Little or no pain in the abdomen.

TO MAKE THE DIAGNOSIS

In the history, ask:

- When did you start having diarrhea?
- What do the stools look like? Do they have blood or pus?
- How many times a day do you pass stools?
- Do you have fever, or pain in the abdomen?
- What water do you drink? Where does it come from? What do you do to make it safe to drink?
- Do you have a good latrine at your house?

In the physical exam, look for:

- The aspect of the stools. Try to see them yourself.
- A mass in the abdomen, or inside the rectum.
- Fever, anemia, signs of malnutrition or of loss of weight.
- Tenderness in the abdomen.
- Big lymph nodes in the neck, armpits, and inguinal regions.
- Fungus infection in the mouth.

In the laboratory, do:

- A fresh stool exam to look for mobile ameba and also for worm eggs and larva.

TREATMENT OF THE DEHYDRATION IN ADULTS

Prepare a sugar-salt solution. See the instructions for this on page 323. The formula is the same for adults as for children.

If the patient has no signs of dehydration, give up to six bottles of solution per day. If the patient does have signs of dehydration, give up to eight bottles of solution per day. Keep giving the solution until the diarrhea stops. If the patient vomits, keep on giving the oral solution. But give it more slowly for a few minutes. Even if the patient is very dehydrated, or in shock, you will be able to save his life with oral rehydration.

Medicines to stop diarrhea, like kaolin, paregoric, etc. are useless. **Do not use them**. Give only treatment for the cause of the diarrhea and the oral rehydration solution.

CHRONIC DIARRHEA IN AN ADULT

Possible causes

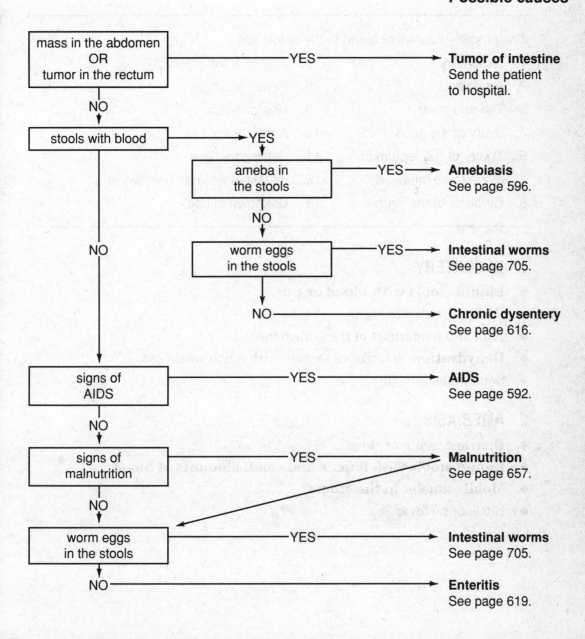

BLOOD IN THE STOOLS - MELENA

Blood in the stools is a sign of danger. This blood comes often from a serious illness. Examine your patient carefully to find the cause.

The possible causes of blood in the stools are:

1. Dysentery
2. Amebiasis
3. Typhoid fever
4. Injury of the anus
5. Tumor of the rectum or of the large intestine
6. Cirrhosis of the liver
7. Tumor of the stomach
8. Peptic ulcer
9. Hemorrhoids
10. Anal fissure
11. Schistosomiasis
12. Intestinal worms: hookworm
13. Unknown cause

1. DYSENTERY

- **Liquid stools with blood or pus**.
- Fever, often quite high.
- Pain and tenderness of the abdomen.
- **Dehydration**, sometimes severe, with much weakness.
- Sometimes vomiting.

2. AMEBIASIS

- Diarrhea, acute or chronic.
- **Liquid stools with mucus and small amounts of blood.**
- **Mobile ameba in the stools**.
- Little or no fever.

3. TYPHOID FEVER

- **High fever, remaining very high**.
- **Delirium, severe headache**.
- No diarrhea.
- **Rectal hemorrhage, with much blood and little or no stools**.
- Often a big spleen.
- Little or no pain in the abdomen.
- Much tenderness in the abdomen with signs of peritonitis indicates a perforation of the intestines. This is very serious. Send the patient immediately to hospital.

4. INJURY OF THE ANUS

- **A fall on the buttocks**. This permits a piece of wood or a sharp stone to cut the anus or even go up inside.
- Blood, often with clots, coming from the rectum.
- Often there is a wound on the skin outside the anus. But sometimes there is no wound. The object has gone inside the rectum, and the only wound is up inside. You cannot see it.
- Look for signs of peritonitis: tenderness of the abdomen, rebound pain, rigid muscles. If you find signs of peritonitis, send the patient immediately to hospital.

5. TUMOR OF THE RECTUM OR OF THE LARGE INTESTINE

- Stools: pure blood, or clots of blood, or stools mixed with blood, or with a small amount of red blood on the outside of the stool.
- **A hard mass in the rectum** found by rectal examination.
- Sometimes a mass in the lower abdomen.
- Often constipation, but sometimes chronic diarrhea.
- Often pain in the abdomen, coming when the patient passes stools.
- Loss of weight, and sometimes anemia.

6. CIRRHOSIS OF THE LIVER

- **Liver big, hard, and irregular**.
- Loss of weight.
- Often liquid in the abdomen (ascites).
- Sometimes swelling of the legs.
- **Black stools** indicate bleeding from the stomach caused by the cirrhosis.

7. TUMOR OF THE STOMACH

- **A hard mass in the epigastric region**.
- Often vomiting and loss of weight.
- **Black stools** coming from bleeding from the tumor in the stomach.

8. PEPTIC ULCER

- **A feeling of burning or intense pain** in a small spot in the upper abdomen coming often at night.
- Tenderness in the right upper quadrant or in the epigastric region.
- **Black stools** coming from bleeding from the ulcer.

9. HEMORRHOIDS

- **Painful swellings at the edge of the anus**.
- Pain when passing stools.
- Often constipation.
- Traces of blood on the outside of the stools or bleeding after the stools have come out.

10. ANAL FISSURE

- **Pain at the anus when passing stools**.
- Often constipation.
- Traces of blood on the outside of the stools or bleeding after the stools have come out.
- Tenderness at the anus during the rectal exam.
- Often the fissure is very small and difficult to see.

11. SCHISTOSOMIASIS

- Stools mixed with blood, often with diarrhea.
- Abdominal pain, often when passing stools.
- **Schistosome eggs** in the stools.

12. INTESTINAL WORMS

- Hookworm.
- Stools mixed with blood, and sometimes diarrhea.
- Often abdominal pain.
- Sometimes anemia, and often malnutrition.
- **Worm eggs, usually hookworm, in the stools**.

TO MAKE THE DIAGNOSIS:

In the history, ask:
- When did you first have blood in your stools?
- What are your stools like: liquid, normal, or very hard?
- How much blood is there in your stools?
- Is the blood red, or is it almost black?
- Where is the blood in your stools: mixed all through the stool, or only on the outside of the stool?
- Do you have pain at the anus when you pass your stools?
- What other symptoms do you have?
  - Fever, pain in the abdomen, vomiting.
  - Headache, heart burn.
  - Loss of weight.
- Have you just had an injury to the anal region?

In the physical exam, look for:
- What do the stools look like? Try to see a stool yourself.
  - Pure blood: this means a real hemorrhage.
    - Red blood: from the large intestine or the rectum.
    - Black stools: bleeding from the stomach or small intestines.
  - Liquid stools mixed with blood: dysentery or amebiasis.
  - Normal stools with traces of blood on the outside: hemorrhoids or an anal fissure.
  - Normal stools mixed with blood: hookworm or schistosomiasis.
  - A few drops of blood coming after passage of the stools: hemorrhoids, or an anal fissure.

- Fever.
- Dehydration.
- In case of an anal injury or typhoid fever, look for signs of peritonitis.
- A wound, or a swelling at the anus.
- A tumor inside the rectum felt by rectal exam.
- A mass in the abdomen.
- A big liver or a big spleen.
- Tenderness in the epigastric region.
- Loss of weight.

In the laboratory, do:
- A stool exam to look for eggs of hookworm or Schistosoma mansoni.
- A fresh stool exam to look for mobile ameba.
- A hemoglobin exam if there has been much bleeding.

BLOOD IN THE STOOLS

Possible causes

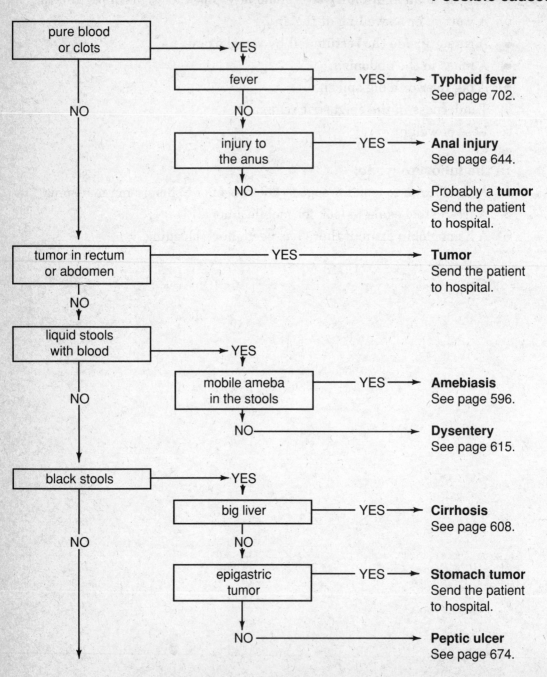

pure blood or clots — YES →
- fever — YES → **Typhoid fever** See page 702.
- NO → injury to the anus — YES → **Anal injury** See page 644.
  - NO → Probably a **tumor** Send the patient to hospital.

NO →

tumor in rectum or abdomen — YES → **Tumor** Send the patient to hospital.

NO →

liquid stools with blood — YES →
- mobile ameba in the stools — YES → **Amebiasis** See page 596.
  - NO → **Dysentery** See page 615.

NO →

black stools — YES →
- big liver — YES → **Cirrhosis** See page 608.
  - NO → epigastric tumor — YES → **Stomach tumor** Send the patient to hospital.
    - NO → **Peptic ulcer** See page 674.

NO

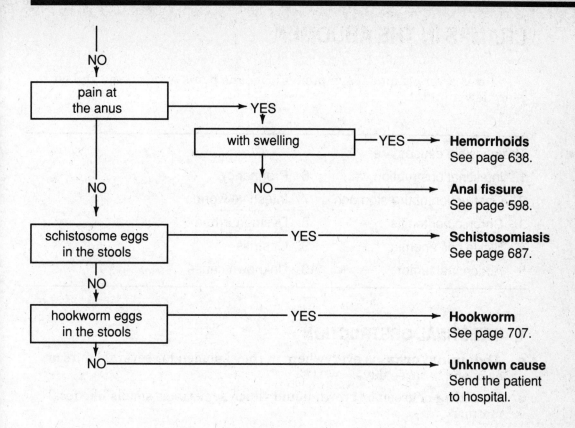

CRAMPS IN THE ABDOMEN

This is a very common symptom. It means pains which come and go every few minutes.

The possible causes are:

1. Intestinal obstruction
2. Obstruction of the stomach
3. Chronic peritonitis
4. Sickle cell anemia
5. Abdominal tumor

6. Pregnancy
7. Intestinal worms
8. Dysmenorrhea
9. Gastritis
10. Unknown cause

---

1. INTESTINAL OBSTRUCTION

- **Abdominal cramps** everywhere in the abdomen for several hours or even one to three days.
- **Vomiting** of green or brown liquid which sometimes smells like fecal matter.
- **Swelling of the abdomen**.
- **No stools or gas** for many hours or even days.
- **Visible waves of peristalsis** moving across the abdomen.
- **Loud sounds of peristalsis** heard through the stethoscope. First there is a period of silence. Then come loud, rapid sounds when the patient feels pain and when you see a wave of peristalsis.

2. OBSTRUCTION OF THE STOMACH

- **Cramps for several weeks** in the upper part of the abdomen.
- **Chronic vomiting** of non-digested food.
- Little or no swelling of the abdomen.
- **Visible waves of peristalsis in the left upper quadrant**, moving from the left side to the right side.
- Much loss of weight.

3. CHRONIC PERITONITIS

- **Irregular fever** for days or weeks.
- **Tenderness in the abdomen** but no rigidity of muscles or rebound pain.
- Loss of weight.
- Sometimes diarrhea, sometimes constipation.

4. SICKLE CELL ANEMIA

- This comes most often in children and young adults.
- **History of repeated attacks of anemia and jaundice**.
- Frequent pains in the arms, legs, and abdomen.
- Often **anemia**, with weakness, a pale color, a hemoglobin below 10 g and sometimes jaundice.
- **Sickle cells** in a drop of fresh blood.

5. ABDOMINAL TUMOR

- **One or more hard masses in the abdomen**. They may be fixed in one place, or mobile.
- Loss of weight.
- Sometimes vomiting.
- Sometimes constipation, sometimes diarrhea.

6. PREGNANCY

- **Absence of periods** for one or more months.
- **Round, soft mass in the lower abdomen** typical of a pregnancy.
- Cramps in the lower abdomen. If the cramps become very strong, or if there is bleeding from the vagina, send the woman to hospital.

7. INTESTINAL WORMS

- Cramps in the lower abdomen or around the umbilicus.
- **Worm eggs in the stools**.
- No tenderness, no fever.

8. DYSMENORRHEA

- Cramps in the lower abdomen that **come before or during menstrual periods**.
- No tenderness or fever.

9. GASTRITIS

- **Heart burn in the upper abdomen.** This often goes up into the chest and through to the back between the shoulders.
- **Cramps in the upper abdomen coming soon after eating**.
- No tenderness or mass.

SYMPTOMATIC TREATMENT

1. The symptomatic treatment depends on the cause of the cramps.
2. Antispasmodic medicines, like belladonna, can calm the cramps.

TO MAKE THE DIAGNOSIS:

In the history, ask:
- When did these cramps start?
- Where do you feel the cramps?
- When do the cramps come? How often do they come?
- Are the cramps worse after eating?
- Do you vomit? If so, what is it like?
- Do you have diarrhea or constipation?
- Do you have heart burn frequently?
- Have you lost weight?
- Have you passed stools or gas today? If not, when did you last pass stools or gas?
- Have you often had attacks of anemia, or jaundice, or pains in the arms or legs?
- If the patient is a woman, ask her:
    - Are you pregnant? Have you missed one or more periods?
    - Do you often have cramps with your periods?

In the physical exam, look for:
- Swelling of the abdomen.
- Strong waves of peristalsis that you can see going across the abdomen.
- Very loud sounds of peristalsis that come when you see the wave and when the patient has a strong cramp.
- Tenderness in the abdomen. Where is it?
- Fever.
- Masses in the abdomen.
- A pregnancy.

In the laboratory, do:
- An exam of a fresh drop of blood to look for sickle cells. If there are sickle cells, do a hemoglobin exam.
- A stool exam to look for worm eggs.

CRAMPS IN THE ABDOMEN

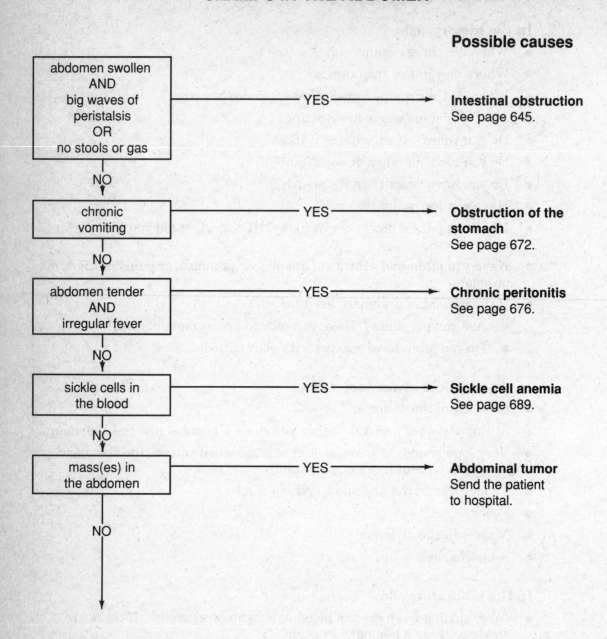

Possible causes

abdomen swollen AND big waves of peristalsis OR no stools or gas → YES →	**Intestinal obstruction** See page 645.
chronic vomiting → YES →	**Obstruction of the stomach** See page 672.
abdomen tender AND irregular fever → YES →	**Chronic peritonitis** See page 676.
sickle cells in the blood → YES →	**Sickle cell anemia** See page 689.
mass(es) in the abdomen → YES →	**Abdominal tumor** Send the patient to hospital.

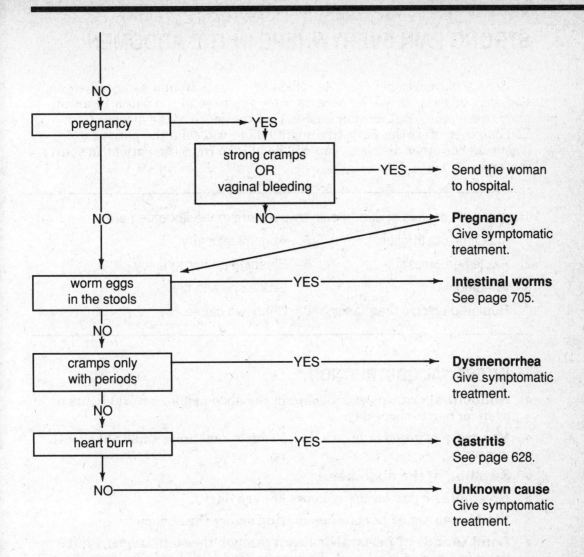

STRONG PAIN EVERYWHERE IN THE ABDOMEN

Strong pain everywhere in the abdomen comes from a serious disease. For some diseases it will be necessary for you to send the patient immediately to hospital. But do your best to find the cause of the disease first. You can then start the right treatment before you send the patient to hospital. For other diseases, you will be able to treat the patient in your center.

The possible causes of strong pain everywhere in the abdomen are:

1. Intestinal obstruction
2. Acute peritonitis
3. Pneumonia
4. Ruptured ectopic pregnancy
5. Abdominal injury
6. Bleeding in a pregnancy
7. Sickle cell anemia
8. Unknown cause

1. INTESTINAL OBSTRUCTION

- **Abdominal cramps** everywhere in the abdomen for several hours or even for one to three days.
- **Vomiting** of green or brown liquid which sometimes smells like fecal matter.
- **Swelling of the abdomen**.
- **No stools or gas** for many hours or even days.
- **Visible waves of peristalsis** moving across the abdomen.
- **Loud sounds of peristalsis** heard through the stethoscope. First there is a period of silence. Then come loud, rapid sounds when the patient feels pain and when you see a wave of peristalsis.

2. ACUTE PERITONITIS

- **Continuous strong pain** everywhere in the abdomen.
- **High fever**, rapid pulse, rapid breathing. The patient breathes only with the chest muscles. The abdomen moves very little with breathing.
- **Swelling of the abdomen**.
- **Much tenderness, with rigid muscles** everywhere in the abdomen.

- **Rebound tenderness**.
- No sounds of peristalsis. The abdomen is "silent."
- No stools or gas.
- High white blood cell count.

3. PNEUMONIA

- Pain in the upper abdomen **made worse by coughing and breathing**.
- **Painful cough**.
- **Dyspnea, even at rest**.
- **Fever**, often accompanied by chills. The fever may be absent in an old person, a patient with malnutrition, or a patient who has already had treatment.
- Sputum: thick and white, or yellow. Sometimes there is no sputum.
- Crackles in the lungs, on one or both sides.
- No rebound tenderness or muscle rigidity.
- High white blood cell count.

4. RUPTURED ECTOPIC PREGNANCY

- The pregnancy develops outside of the uterus: in the tube, inside the abdomen, or in the wall of the uterus. At some time during the first three months, the pregnancy ruptures. There is then much bleeding inside the abdomen. This blood in the abdomen causes signs of peritonitis, but with no fever or other signs of infection.
- **History of amenorrhea** for one or two months. But this history is often not clear. The woman may think she has had normal periods. So you must suspect a ruptured ectopic pregnancy in any woman during her reproductive years who has strong abdominal pain.
- **Rebound tenderness in the abdomen**, especially in the lower abdomen.
- **Signs of anemia**: rapid pulse, pale color, weakness, low blood pressure, low hemoglobin.
- **No fever** or other signs of infection.
- Swelling of the abdomen.
- Normal white blood cell count.

5. ABDOMINAL INJURY

- **History of a recent accident** with injury to the abdomen.
- **Rebound tenderness**.
- Often signs of shock: rapid pulse, low blood pressure, weakness, thirst.
- There has been either bleeding inside the abdomen, or else rupture of an abdominal organ. Give treatment for shock and start giving antibiotics. Then send the patient immediately to hospital.

6. BLEEDING IN A PREGNANCY

- The hemorrhage comes during the last three months of the pregnancy. The bleeding is inside the uterus. Often there is no bleeding from the vagina.
- **Sudden strong pain in the lower abdomen**.
- **Uterus very tender and hard**.
- Signs of anemia: rapid pulse, pale color, weakness, low blood pressure, low hemoglobin.
- No fetal heart sounds; no movements of the fetus.

7. SICKLE CELL ANEMIA

- This comes in children and young adults. A sickle cell crisis can cause strong pain in the abdomen.
- **Rebound tenderness**.
- **Anemia**: rapid pulse, pale color, weakness, low hemoglobin.
- Often **jaundice**.
- **Sickle cells in a fresh drop of blood**.
- History of attacks of anemia and sometimes jaundice in the past.

8. UNKNOWN CAUSE

- Follow the strategies of other symptoms and signs.
- If you are not sure of the cause, start an infusion of normal saline. If the patient has fever, start giving antibiotics. Then send the patient immediately to hospital.

TO MAKE THE DIAGNOSIS

In the history, ask:

- When did the pain start?
- How did the pain start?
- What is the pain like: continuous, or cramps?
- Where is the pain? Where was the pain when it started?
- Have you vomited? If so, what did you vomit?
- Have you been passing stools and gas? If not, when did you stop passing stools and gas?
- Have you had a cough, trouble breathing, sputum?
- Do breathing or coughing make the pain worse?
- In a woman patient, ask her:
  - Are you pregnant? If so, for how many months?
  - Have you missed one or more periods?
  - Have you had bleeding from the vagina?
- Have you had attacks of anemia or jaundice in the past?
- Have you just had an accident, or a blow to your abdomen?

In the physical exam, look for:

- Fever.
- Swelling of the abdomen.
- Signs of intestinal obstruction: visible waves of peristalsis, and loud sounds of peristalsis coming with the waves and with the pain.
- Tenderness in the abdomen. Where is it? Are the muscles rigid?
- Rebound tenderness.
- Crackles in the lungs.
- Signs of anemia: rapid pulse, pale color, low blood pressure.
- A mass in the lower abdomen like a pregnancy.
- Jaundice.

In the laboratory, do:

- An exam of a fresh drop of blood to look for sickle cells.
- A hemoglobin exam.
- A white blood cell count.

STRONG PAIN EVERYWHERE IN THE ABDOMEN

Possible causes

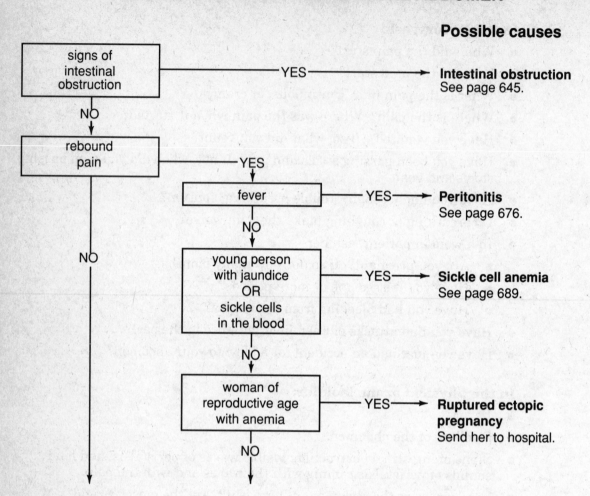

signs of intestinal obstruction

— YES ——→ **Intestinal obstruction**
See page 645.

NO

rebound pain

— YES —

fever

— YES —→ **Peritonitis**
See page 676.

NO

young person with jaundice OR sickle cells in the blood

— YES —→ **Sickle cell anemia**
See page 689.

NO

woman of reproductive age with anemia

— YES —→ **Ruptured ectopic pregnancy**
Send her to hospital.

NO

NO

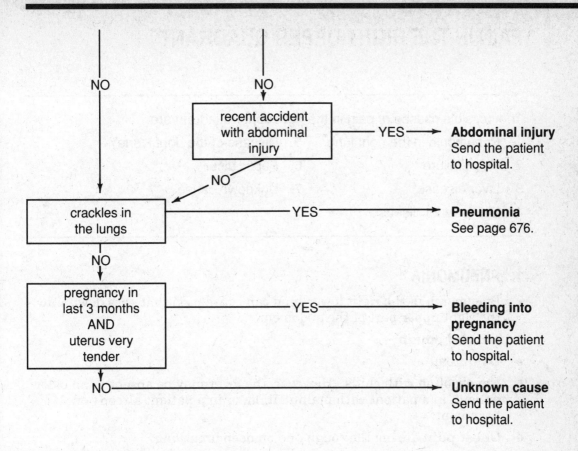

NO

NO

recent accident
with abdominal
injury

——YES——→ **Abdominal injury**
Send the patient
to hospital.

NO

crackles in
the lungs

——————YES————————→ **Pneumonia**
See page 676.

NO

pregnancy in
last 3 months
AND
uterus very
tender

——————YES————————→ **Bleeding into
pregnancy**
Send the patient
to hospital.

NO————————————————————→ **Unknown cause**
Send the patient
to hospital.

PAIN IN THE RIGHT UPPER QUADRANT

The possible causes of pain in the right upper quadrant are:

1. Pneumonia in the right lung
2. Heart failure
3. Liver disease
4. Gall bladder disease
5. Disease of the right kidney
6. Peptic ulcer
7. Unknown cause

1. PNEUMONIA

- Pneumonia in the right lower lung can cause pain that goes down into the right upper part of the abdomen.
- **Painful cough**.
- **Dyspnea**.
- **Fever**, often with chills. However, the fever may be absent in an older patient, in a patient with malnutrition, or in a patient already on treatment.
- **Chest pain** during the cough and on deep breathing.
- Sputum: thick, white or yellow. Sometimes there is no sputum.
- Crackles in the lungs in the right lower chest.
- No tenderness in the abdomen.

2. HEART FAILURE

- Heart failure can cause swelling of the liver. This causes pain in the right upper quadrant.
- **Big, tender liver**.
- For other signs of heart failure, see page 93.

3. LIVER DISEASE

- **Big, tender liver**.
- See the strategy on BIG LIVER on page 512.

4. GALL BLADDER DISEASE

- **Severe pain and tenderness in the RUQ**.
- Often a **small tender mass** just below the middle of the liver edge that moves down with the liver.
- **Vomiting**.
- Often fever.
- Sometimes jaundice.
- High white blood cell count.

5. DISEASE OF THE RIGHT KIDNEY

- **Much vomiting**.
- **Severe pain in the right flank** often going down into the RLQ.
- **Tenderness in the right flank**.
- Often red or white blood cells or albumin in the urine.

6. PEPTIC ULCER

- **Severe burning or pain in a small area** in the epigastric region or in the right upper quadrant. The patient can point to this area with one finger. Often the pain comes during the night, or when the patient has not eaten for several hours.
- Spices, alcoholic drinks, and smoking usually **make the pain worse**.
- Food, milk, or antacid medicines usually **make the pain better**.
- **Tenderness in the spot** where the patient feels pain.
- Sometimes loss of weight, vomiting, vomiting of blood, dark or black stools.

SYMPTOMATIC TREATMENT

1. Send the patient to hospital if the pain is severe.
2. If not, give antacids for heart burn, or aspirin for other pain.

TO MAKE THE DIAGNOSIS

In the history, ask:

- When did the pain start? How did it start?
- What does the pain feel like? Does it go anywhere else?
- Does the pain get worse or better after you eat something? Or drink milk?
- Do you have a cough, trouble breathing, or pain in the chest?
- Do you have swelling of the legs or much urine at night?
- Have you ever had liver disease? Or jaundice?
- Have you vomited? If so, what did you vomit?
- Do you have pain in your back or in your right side?
- Have you had pain on urinating? Or a change in the color of your urine?

In the physical exam, look for:

- Fever.
- Crackles in the lungs.
- Signs of heart failure.
- A big liver. What is it like? Is it tender?
- A small tender mass in the lower edge of the liver.
- Tenderness in the right flank.
- Tenderness in a small spot in the RUQ below the liver.

In the laboratory, do:

- A white blood cell count.
- A urine exam to look for blood cells or albumin.

PAIN IN THE RIGHT UPPER QUADRANT

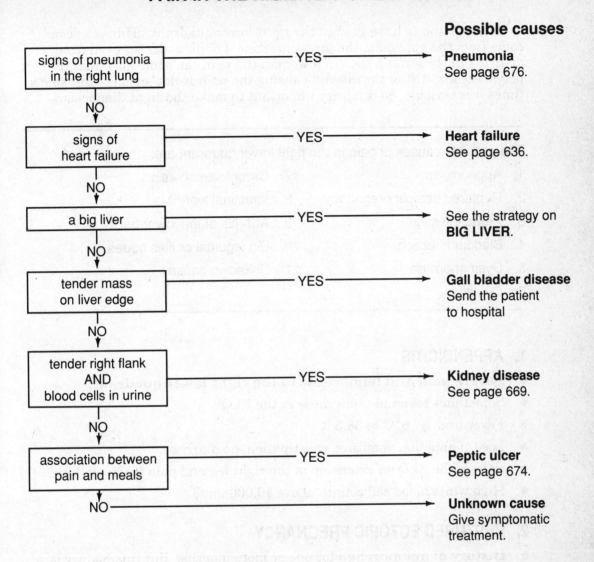

Possible causes

signs of pneumonia in the right lung —— YES ——→ **Pneumonia**
See page 676.

↓ NO

signs of heart failure —— YES ——→ **Heart failure**
See page 636.

↓ NO

a big liver —— YES ——→ See the strategy on **BIG LIVER**.

↓ NO

tender mass on liver edge —— YES ——→ **Gall bladder disease**
Send the patient to hospital

↓ NO

tender right flank AND blood cells in urine —— YES ——→ **Kidney disease**
See page 669.

↓ NO

association between pain and meals —— YES ——→ **Peptic ulcer**
See page 674.

↓ NO —————————————————→ **Unknown cause**
Give symptomatic treatment.

PAIN IN THE RIGHT LOWER QUADRANT

Many patients have pain in the right lower quadrant. This pain can come from the appendix, the large intestine, lymph nodes, or even from arthritis in the lower back. In a woman the pain can come also from the pelvic organs. Often the disease causing the pain is not serious. But sometimes it is serious. So it is very important to make the right diagnosis.

The possible causes of pain in the right lower quadrant are:

1. Appendicitis
2. Ruptured ectopic pregnancy
3. Pelvic infection
4. Bladder infection
5. Dysmenorrhea
6. Ovulation
7. Chronic amebiasis
8. Intestinal worms
9. Arthritis of the lower back
10. Big inguinal or iliac nodes
11. Unknown cause

---

1. APPENDICITIS

- **Severe pain and tenderness in the right lower quadrant**.
- Sometimes rebound tenderness in the RLQ.
- Fever from 37.5°C to 38.5°C.
- Loss of appetite, vomiting, constipation, no diarrhea.
- Pain in the RLQ on extension of the right leg and pain when walking.
- High white blood cell count: above 10,000/mm3.

2. RUPTURED ECTOPIC PREGNANCY

- **History of amenorrhea** for one or more months. But this history is not always clear. The woman may think she has had normal periods. So you must suspect a ruptured ectopic pregnancy in any woman during her reproductive years who has pain in the lower abdomen.

- **Pain and tenderness in the RLQ** which soon go to the whole lower abdomen, often with rebound tenderness.
- **Signs of anemia**: rapid pulse, pale color, weakness, low blood pressure, low hemoglobin.
- No fever or other signs of infection.

3. PELVIC INFECTION

- **Pain and tenderness in the lower abdomen**.
- **Fever** and other signs of infection.
- No rebound tenderness, no swelling of the abdomen.

4. BLADDER INFECTION

- **Pain when passing urine**.
- **Frequent urination**.
- **White blood cells** and often albumin in the urine.

5. DYSMENORRHEA

- Cramps in the lower abdomen that **come before or during each menstrual period**. Ask the woman if she often has pain like this with her periods.
- No tenderness or fever.

6. OVULATION

- Pain in the RLQ that comes **ten days to two weeks after the last period**. This pain can come at this same time after each period. So always ask the woman if she often has pain like this between her periods.

7. INTESTINAL WORMS

- Pain but no tenderness in the lower abdomen.
- **Worm eggs in the stools**.

8. CHRONIC AMEBIASIS

- Ameba live in the cecum, at the beginning of the large intestine. The cecum is in the RLQ.
- **Pain in the RLQ**.
- Often the cecum is tender. You can feel it as a soft mass in the RLQ.
- Often a history of attacks of diarrhea with blood in the past.
- **Ameba in the stools**.

9. ARTHRITIS IN THE LOWER BACK

- Arthritis in the bones of the lower back can affect the nerves going to the lower abdomen. The patient feels the pain in the lower abdomen. There may be little or no pain in the back.
- **Pain in the RLQ made worse by movements of the back** such as bending forward or lifting a heavy load.
- No tenderness or mass in the lower abdomen.

10. BIG INGUINAL OR ILIAC LYMPH NODES

- **Big tender lymph nodes in the inguinal or iliac regions**.

11. UNKNOWN CAUSE

- Sometimes you cannot find the cause of the pain. If the patient does not seem seriously ill, give symptomatic treatment: aspirin or an antispasmodic medicine. But a patient who seems seriously ill should go to hospital.

TO MAKE THE DIAGNOSIS

In the history, ask:
- When did the pain start?
- What does it feel like?
- Have you had pain like this before? If so, when? What did you do about it?
- In a woman, ask:
  - Does pain like this come with each period? Or between your periods?
  - Are you pregnant? Have you missed any periods? If so, how many?
- Do you have fever?
- Do you have vomiting? or constipation? or diarrhea?
- Does it hurt to move your right leg, or to walk on it?
- Does it hurt when you bend forward? Or when you lift something heavy?
- Do you have pain when you pass urine?

In the physical exam, look for:
- Tenderness or rebound tenderness in the RLQ.
- Fever and other signs of infection.
- A mass in the RLQ.
- Signs of anemia: rapid pulse, pale color, low blood pressure.
- Big tender nodes in the inguinal or iliac regions.
- Pain on movements of the right leg or of the back.
- Do a rectal exam. Is there tenderness up high on the right side?

In the laboratory, do:
- A hemoglobin exam.
- A urine exam to look for albumin and white blood cells.
- A white blood cell count.
- A stool exam to look for worm eggs or for ameba.

PAIN IN THE RIGHT LOWER QUADRANT

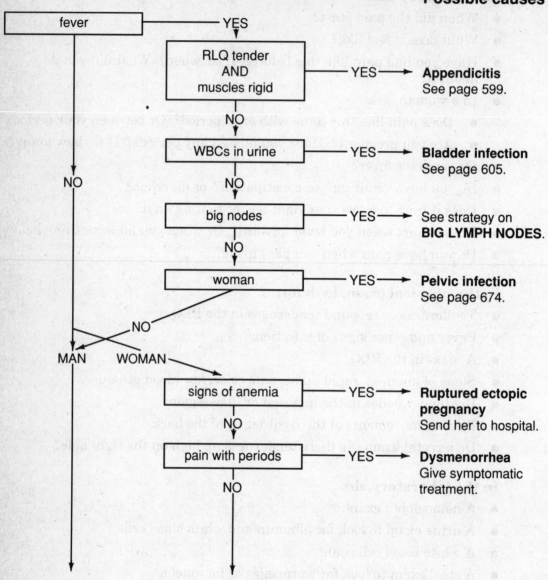

Possible causes

fever — YES

RLQ tender
AND
muscles rigid — YES → **Appendicitis**
See page 599.

NO

WBCs in urine — YES → **Bladder infection**
See page 605.

NO

big nodes — YES → See strategy on
BIG LYMPH NODES.

NO

woman — YES → **Pelvic infection**
See page 674.

NO

NO

MAN   WOMAN

signs of anemia — YES → **Ruptured ectopic
pregnancy**
Send her to hospital.

NO

pain with periods — YES → **Dysmenorrhea**
Give symptomatic
treatment.

NO

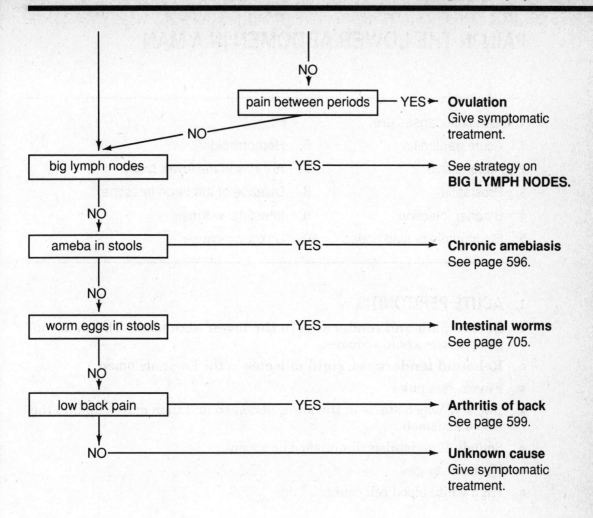

NO

pain between periods —— YES➤ **Ovulation**
Give symptomatic
treatment.

NO

big lymph nodes ———————— YES ————————→ See strategy on
BIG LYMPH NODES.

NO

ameba in stools ———————— YES ————————→ **Chronic amebiasis**
See page 596.

NO

worm eggs in stools ———————— YES ————————→ **Intestinal worms**
See page 705.

NO

low back pain ———————— YES ————————→ **Arthritis of back**
See page 599.

NO ———————————————————→ **Unknown cause**
Give symptomatic
treatment.

PAIN IN THE LOWER ABDOMEN IN A MAN

The possible causes are:

1. Acute peritonitis
2. Appendicitis
3. Prostatitis
4. Bladder infection
5. Big inguinal or iliac nodes
6. Hemorrhoids
7. Arthritis in the lower back
8. Disease of the large intestine
9. Intestinal worms
10. Unknown cause

1. ACUTE PERITONITIS

- **Severe pain and tenderness in the lower abdomen**. This pain can go up to the whole abdomen.
- **Rebound tenderness**, **rigid muscles** in the lower abdomen.
- **Fever**, fast pulse.
- Swelling which starts in the lower abdomen and then moves up into the whole abdomen.
- Sounds of peristalsis diminished or absent.
- No stools or gas.
- High white blood cell count.

2. APPENDICITIS

- **Severe pain and tenderness in the right lower quadrant**.
- Sometimes rebound tenderness in the RLQ.
- **Fever** of $37.5°$ C to $38.5°$ C.
- Loss of appetite, vomiting, constipation; no diarrhea.
- Pain in the RLQ on extension of the right leg and pain when walking.
- High white blood cell count: above 10,000/mm3.

3. PROSTATITIS

- Acute or chronic pain in the lower abdomen, below the umbilicus, in the perineum, or in the lower back.
- **Prostate very tender** on rectal examination. Do a rectal exam on any man who has pain in the lower abdomen, the perineum, or the lower back.
- Sometimes pain when urinating.

4. BLADDER INFECTION

- **Pain and tenderness in the middle of the lower abdomen**.
- **Pain when urinating**.
- **Frequent urination**.
- **White blood cells** and sometimes red blood cells in the urine.

5. BIG INGUINAL OR ILIAC LYMPH NODES

- **Big tender nodes in the iliac or inguinal regions**.

6. HEMORRHOIDS

- **Pain at the anus when passing stools**.
- **Small tender swellings at the edge of the anus**.
- Often constipation; sometimes diarrhea.
- Sometimes blood in or on the outside of the stools.

7. ARTHRITIS IN THE LOWER BACK

- Arthritis in the bones of the lower back can affect the nerves going to the lower abdomen. The patient feels the pain in the lower abdomen. There may be little or no pain in the back.
- **Pain in the lower abdomen made worse by movements of the back** such as bending forward or lifting a heavy weight.
- No tenderness in the lower abdomen.

8. DISEASE OF THE LARGE INTESTINE - TUMOR, INFECTION

- **Pain in the lower abdomen made worse by passing stools**.
- Sometimes a tender mass in the lower abdomen.
- Sometimes blood in the stools.
- Always do a rectal exam on a man with these symptoms to feel for a tumor in the rectum.

9. INTESTINAL WORMS

- Intermittent pain in the lower abdomen.
- **Worm eggs in the stools**.
- No tenderness, no fever.

TO MAKE THE DIAGNOSIS

In the history, ask:

- When did you start having pain in the lower abdomen?
- How did the pain first start? What were you doing at that time?
- Exactly where do you feel the pain?
- Is the pain made worse by urinating, by passing stools, by bending forward, by lifting something heavy?
- Do you have other symptoms, like:
  - Vomiting, constipation, pain at the anus, blood in your stools?
  - Pain when urinating, frequent urination?

In the physical exam, look for:

- Fever.
- Tenderness in the lower abdomen. If there is, where is it?
- Rebound tenderness.
- A mass in the lower abdomen.
- Big lymph nodes in the iliac or inguinal regions.
- Do a rectal exam. Feel for:
  - A tender prostate.
  - Little swellings at the edge of the anus: hemorrhoids.
  - A mass in the rectum: tumor? fecal matter?
- Pain in the lower back when the patient bends forward or does other movements.

In the laboratory, do:

- A urine exam to look for white and red blood cells.
- A stool exam to look for worm eggs.
- A white blood cell count.

PAIN IN THE LOWER ABDOMEN IN A MAN

Possible causes

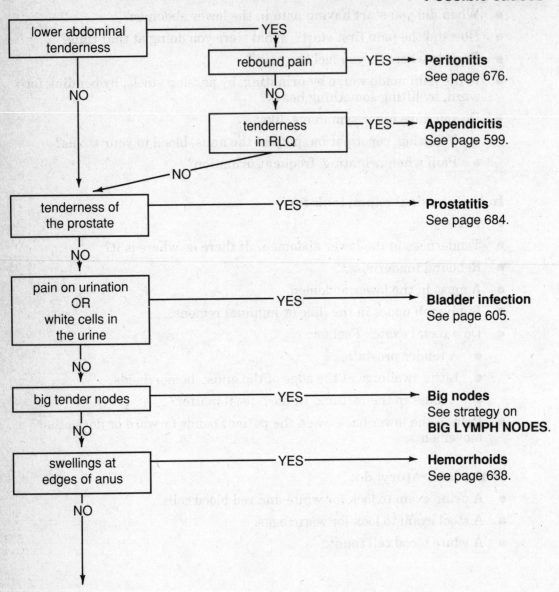

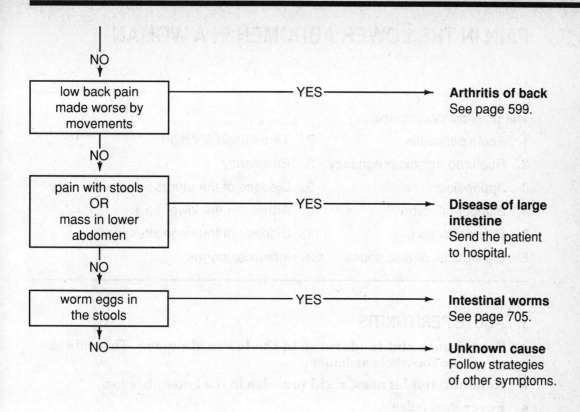

NO

low back pain
made worse by
movements ──────YES──────▶ **Arthritis of back**
See page 599.

NO

pain with stools
OR
mass in lower
abdomen ──────YES──────▶ **Disease of large
intestine**
Send the patient
to hospital.

NO

worm eggs in
the stools ──────YES──────▶ **Intestinal worms**
See page 705.

NO──────────────────────▶ **Unknown cause**
Follow strategies
of other symptoms.

PAIN IN THE LOWER ABDOMEN IN A WOMAN

The possible causes are:

1. Acute peritonitis
2. Ruptured ectopic pregnancy
3. Appendicitis
4. Bladder infection
5. Pelvic infection
6. Big inguinal or iliac nodes
7. Threatened abortion
8. Pregnancy
9. Disease of the uterus
10. Arthritis in the lower back
11. Disease of the large intestine
12. Intestinal worms

1. ACUTE PERITONITIS

- **Severe pain and tenderness in the lower abdomen**. This pain can go up into the whole abdomen.
- **Rebound tenderness**, **rigid muscles** in the lower abdomen.
- **Fever**, fast pulse.
- Swelling which starts in the lower abdomen and can move up into the whole abdomen.
- Sounds of peristalsis diminished or absent, no stools or gas.
- High white blood cell count.

2. RUPTURED ECTOPIC PREGNANCY

- **History of amenorrhea** for one or two months. But this history is often not clear. The woman may think she has had normal periods. So you must suspect a ruptured ectopic pregnancy in any woman during her reproductive years who has strong pain in the lower abdomen.
- **Rebound tenderness**.
- **Signs of anemia**: rapid pulse, pale color, weakness, low blood pressure, low hemoglobin.
- **No fever** or other signs of infection.
- Swelling of the lower abdomen which can go up into the whole abdomen.
- Normal white blood cell count.

3. APPENDICITIS

- **Severe pain and tenderness in the right lower quadrant**.
- Sometimes rebound tenderness in the RLQ.
- **Fever** of 37.5^{0} C to 38.5^{0} C.
- Loss of appetite, vomiting, constipation; no diarrhea.
- Pain in the RLQ on extension of the right leg and pain when walking.
- High white blood cell count: above 10,000/mm3.

4. BLADDER INFECTION

- **Pain and tenderness in the middle of the lower abdomen**.
- **Pain when urinating**.
- **Frequent urination**.
- **White blood cells** and sometimes red blood cells in the urine.

5. PELVIC INFECTION

- **Pain and tenderness in the lower abdomen**.
- **Fever** and other signs of infection.
- No rebound tenderness, no swelling of the abdomen.

6. BIG INGUINAL OR ILIAC LYMPH NODES

- **Big tender lymph nodes in the iliac or inguinal regions**.

7. THREATENED ABORTION

- **Absence of periods** for one or more months.
- **Intermittent pain** in the lower abdomen or in the lower back.
- **Mass in the lower abdomen** typical of a pregnancy.
- No rebound tenderness.
- Sometimes vaginal bleeding.

8. PREGNANCY

- **Absence of periods** for one or more months.
- Vague pain in the lower abdomen.
- **Mass in the lower abdomen** typical of a pregnancy.
- No strong pain; no vaginal bleeding.

9. DISEASE OF THE UTERUS

- Pain during menstrual periods.
- Sometimes an irregular mass in the lower abdomen.
- Sometimes a mass coming out of the vagina: prolapse of the uterus.

10. ARTHRITIS OF THE LOWER BACK

- Arthritis in the bones of the lower back can affect the nerves going to the lower abdomen. The patient feels the pain in the lower abdomen. There may be little or no pain in the back.
- **Pain in the lower abdomen made worse by movements of the back** such as bending forward, or lifting a heavy load.
- No tenderness in the lower abdomen.

11. DISEASE OF THE LARGE INTESTINE - TUMOR, INFECTION, HEMORRHOIDS

- **Pain in the lower abdomen or at the anus made worse by passing stools**.
- Sometimes a tender mass in the lower abdomen which is not a pregnancy.
- Sometimes swellings at the edge of the anus: hemorrhoids.
- Sometimes blood in or on the outside of the stools.

12. INTESTINAL WORMS

- Intermittent pain in the lower abdomen.
- **Worm eggs in the stools**.
- No tenderness, no fever.

TO MAKE THE DIAGNOSIS

In the history, ask:
- When did the pain in the lower abdomen start?
- How did the pain start? What were you doing at that time?
- Exactly where do you feel the pain?
- Is the pain made worse by urinating, by your periods, by passing stools, by bending forward or lifting something heavy?
- Do you have normal periods each month? If not, when was your last normal period?
- Do you have other symptoms, like vomiting, constipation, pain on urinating, frequent urination, bleeding from the vagina, pain at the anus or when passing stools, blood in the stools?

In the physical exam, look for:
- Fever.
- Tenderness in the lower abdomen. If there is, where is it?
- Rebound tenderness.
- Swelling of the abdomen.
- Signs of anemia: fast pulse, pale color, low blood pressure.
- Big lymph nodes in the iliac or the inguinal regions.
- A mass in the lower abdomen. Is it a pregnancy? Is it a tumor?
- A mass coming out of the vagina.
- Pain in the back on bending forward or doing other movements.
- Little swellings at the edge of the anus: hemorrhoids.

In the laboratory, do:
- A hemoglobin exam.
- A urine exam to look for white or red blood cells.
- A white blood cell count.
- A stool exam to look for worm eggs.

PAIN IN THE LOWER ABDOMEN IN A WOMAN

Possible causes

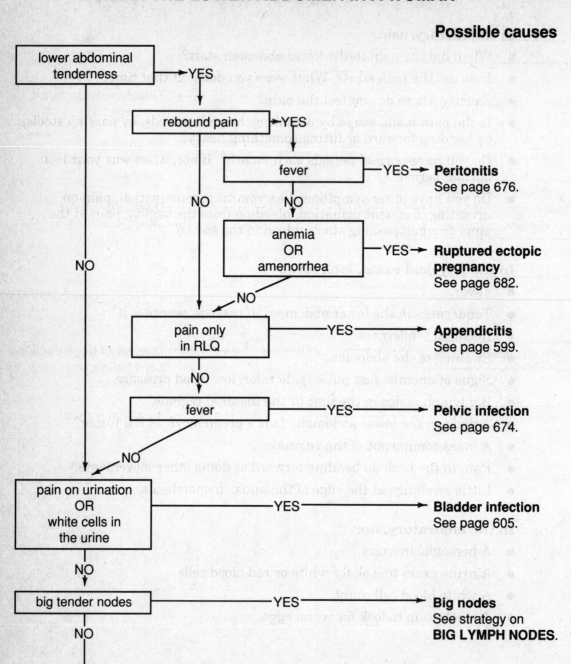

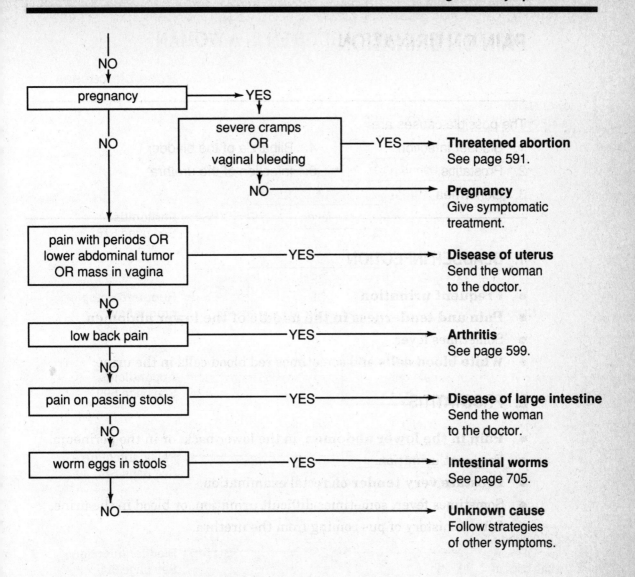

NO

pregnancy ────────► YES
                      ▼
NO   severe cramps
                OR ──────── YES────► **Threatened abortion**
                vaginal bleeding   See page 591.
                      ▼
                     NO ──────────────────► **Pregnancy**
                                            Give symptomatic
                                            treatment.

pain with periods OR
lower abdominal tumor ──────YES────────► **Disease of uterus**
OR mass in vagina   Send the woman
                                         to the doctor.
NO

low back pain ──────────────YES────────► **Arthritis**
                                         See page 599.
NO

pain on passing stools ─────YES────────► **Disease of large intestine**
                                         Send the woman
NO   to the doctor.

worm eggs in stools ────────YES────────► **Intestinal worms**
                                         See page 705.
NO ──────────────────────────────────► **Unknown cause**
                                         Follow strategies
                                         of other symptoms.

PAIN ON URINATION

The possible causes are:
1. Bladder infection
2. Prostatitis
3. Gonorrhea
4. Bilharzia of the bladder
5. Infection of the urethra

1. BLADDER INFECTION

- **Frequent urination**.
- **Pain and tenderness in the middle of the lower abdomen**.
- Sometimes fever.
- **White blood cells** and sometimes red blood cells in the urine.

2. PROSTATITIS

- **Pain in the lower abdomen**, in the lower back, or in the perineum.
- Frequent urination.
- **Prostate very tender** on rectal examination.
- Sometimes fever, sometimes difficult urination, or blood in the urine.
- Often a history of pus coming from the urethra.

3. GONORRHEA

- **Pus coming out of the urethral opening**.
- **Gram negative intra-cellular diplococci**, seen inside white blood cells on a Gram stain of pus coming from the urethra.

4. BILHARZIA OF THE BLADDER - SCHISTOSOMA HEMATOBIUM

- **Frequent painful urination**.
- Desire to urinate even when the bladder is empty - "tenesmus."
- Often blood in the urine.
- **Eggs of Schistosoma hematobium** in the urine.

5. INFECTION OF THE URETHRA

- Often a history of gonorrhea in the past.
- No urinary frequency.
- Often small amounts of pus coming from the urethral opening.
- **No gram negative intra-cellular diplococci** seen in the pus from the urethra.

TO MAKE THE DIAGNOSIS

In the history, ask:

- When did the pain on urination start?
- Do you have to pass urine very often? Even at night? If so, how many times during the night?
- Do you have pain in the abdomen? In the back? In the perineal area?
- Is there liquid or pus coming out of your penis?
- Do you have blood in your urine?
- Have you had a fever?
- Have you ever had gonorrhea? If so, what treatment did you receive?

In the physical exam, look for:

- Fever.
- Pus coming from the urethral opening in a man. You do not see this in a woman.
- Tenderness in the lower abdomen.
- Tenderness of the prostate on rectal exam.

In the laboratory, do:

- A urine exam to look for white and red blood cells. In an area where Schistosoma hematobium is frequent, look for S. hematobium eggs.
- If possible, a smear and a Gram stain of any pus coming from the urethral opening. Look carefully for Gram negative (red) diplococci inside the white blood cells. If there are no Gram negative (red) diplococci inside the white blood cells, the patient does not have gonorrhea.

SYMPTOMATIC TREATMENT OF PAIN ON URINATION

1. Tell the patient to drink much water. This will make him have much urine. It will help make the pain and infection go away.
2. Phenazopyridine (*Pyridium) will take away the pain on urination.

PAIN ON URINATION

Possible causes

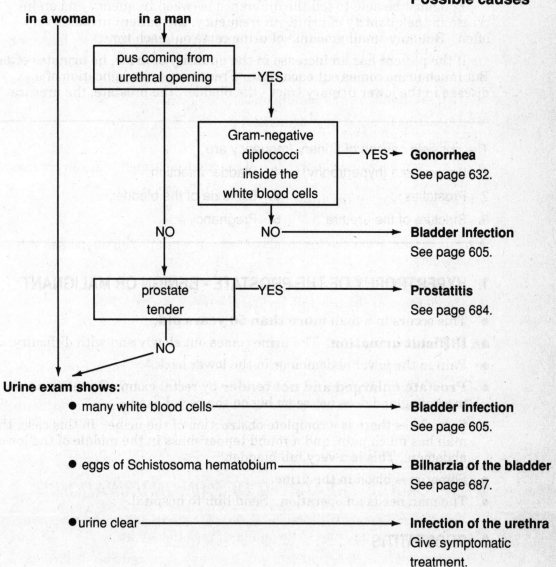

in a woman   **in a man**

pus coming from
urethral opening — YES

Gram-negative
diplococci
inside the
white blood cells — YES → **Gonorrhea**
See page 632.

NO   NO ————————→ **Bladder Infection**
See page 605.

prostate
tender — YES ————————→ **Prostatitis**
See page 684.

NO

Urine exam shows:

● many white blood cells ————————→ **Bladder infection**
See page 605.

● eggs of Schistosoma hematobium ————→ **Bilharzia of the bladder**
See page 687.

● urine clear ————————————————→ **Infection of the urethra**
Give symptomatic
treatment.

FREQUENT URINATION - "FREQUENCY"

You must be able to tell the difference between frequency and an increase in the quantity of urine. In frequency, the patient urinates very often. But only small amounts of urine come out each time.

If the patient has an increase in the quantity of urine, he urinates often. But much urine comes out each time. Frequency is an indication of a disease in the lower urinary tract - the bladder, the prostate, the urethra.

The possible causes of urinary frequency are:

1. Big prostate (hypertrophy)   4. Bladder infection
2. Prostatitis   5. Bilharzia of the bladder
3. Stricture of the urethra   6. Pregnancy

1. HYPERTROPHY OF THE PROSTATE - BENIGN OR MALIGNANT

- This occurs in a man **more than 50 years old**.
- **Difficult urination**. The urine comes out slowly and with difficulty.
- Pain in the lower abdomen or in the lower back.
- **Prostate enlarged and not tender** by rectal exam. Sometimes the prostate gland does not seem big on the rectal exam.
- Sometimes there is a complete obstruction of the urine. In this case, the man has much pain, and a round tender mass in the middle of the lower abdomen. This is a very full bladder.
- Sometimes blood in the urine.
- The man needs an operation. Send him to hospital.

2. PROSTATITIS

- A disease that can come in a man **at any adult age**.
- **Pain in the lower abdomen**, the lower back, or in the perineum.
- **Prostate very tender** on rectal exam. Often it is big.
- Sometimes fever, sometimes difficult urination.
- Sometimes pain on urination.
- Sometimes blood in the urine.

3. STRICTURE OF THE URETHRA

- This is scar tissue in the urethra. It makes the urethra very narrow.
- It can come in a man **at any age**.
- Often a history of gonorrhea or of an injury to the urethra.
- **Difficult urination**.
- Prostate not tender, not big.
- Sometimes there is a complete obstruction of the urine. In this case, there will be a tender round mass in the lower abdomen. This is a very full bladder.
- A catheter will not pass into the bladder.
- Sometimes there are one or several urinary fistulas in the perineum, or signs of infection in the perineum: swelling, tenderness.
- The man needs an operation. Send him to hospital.

4. BLADDER INFECTION

- **Pain on urination**.
- **Tenderness in the middle of the lower abdomen**.
- Sometimes fever.
- **White blood cells** and sometimes red blood cells in the urine.

5. BILHARZIA OF THE BLADDER

- **Pain on urination**.
- Desire to urinate even when the bladder is empty - "tenesmus."
- Often blood in the urine.
- **Eggs of Schistosoma hematobium in the urine**.

6. PREGNANCY

- The pressure of the large uterus on the bladder causes the frequency.
- No pain on urination.
- No white or red blood cells in the urine.
- A round soft mass in the middle of the lower abdomen typical of a pregnancy.

TO MAKE THE DIAGNOSIS

In the history, ask:
- When did you start having urinary frequency?
- Do you have other urinary symptoms, like:
  - Pain on urination?
  - Difficult urination?
  - Blood in your urine?
- How old are you?
- Do you have pain in the lower abdomen? In the back? In the perineum?
- Have you ever had gonorrhea?
- Have you ever had an accident that caused blood in the urine?
- Have you ever had an operation on your bladder or penis?

In the physical exam, look for:
- Fever.
- A mass in the lower abdomen. Is it a pregnancy? Is it a full bladder?
- Tenderness in the lower abdomen.
- By rectal exam, a big or tender prostate.
- Fistulas or swelling in the perineum.

In the laboratory, do:
- A urine exam to look for:
  - White or red blood cells.
  - In a region where Schistosoma hematobium is frequent, the eggs of S. hematobium.

FREQUENT URINATION

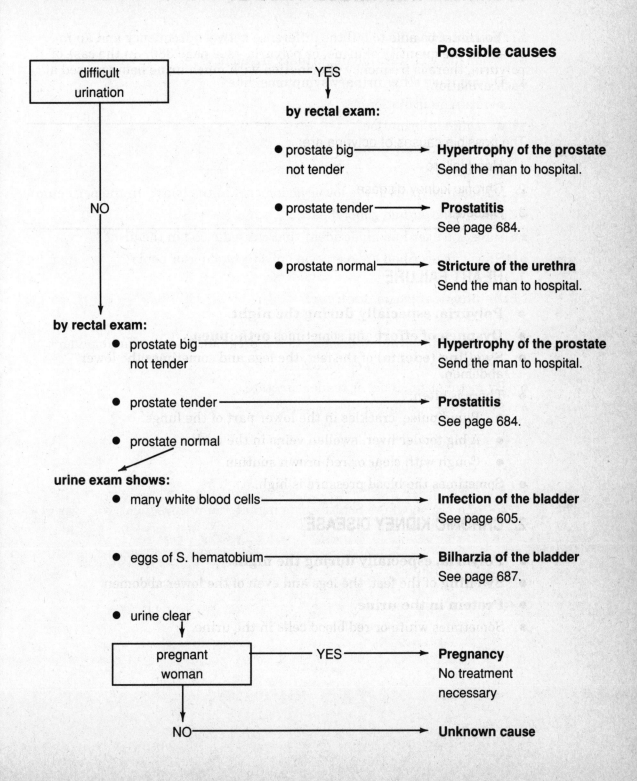

Possible causes

difficult urination ———— YES

by rectal exam:

- prostate big ———→ **Hypertrophy of the prostate**
  not tender   Send the man to hospital.

- prostate tender ———→ **Prostatitis**
           See page 684.

- prostate normal ———→ **Stricture of the urethra**
           Send the man to hospital.

NO

by rectal exam:

- prostate big ———————————→ **Hypertrophy of the prostate**
  not tender   Send the man to hospital.

- prostate tender ———————————→ **Prostatitis**
           See page 684.

- prostate normal

urine exam shows:

- many white blood cells ———————→ **Infection of the bladder**
           See page 605.

- eggs of S. hematobium ———————→ **Bilharzia of the bladder**
           See page 687.

- urine clear

  pregnant woman ———— YES ———→ **Pregnancy**
           No treatment
           necessary

  NO ———————————————→ **Unknown cause**

INCREASE IN THE QUANTITY OF URINE - POLYURIA

You must be able to tell the difference between frequency and an increase in the quantity of urine, or polyuria - see page 380. In the case of polyuria, there is frequency of urination with much urine being passed at each urination.

The possible causes of polyuria are:

1. Heart failure
2. Chronic kidney disease
3. Diabetes

1. HEART FAILURE

- **Polyuria, especially during the night**.
- **Dyspnea of effort** and sometimes **orthopnea**.
- **Swelling (edema)** of the feet, the legs and sometimes the lower abdomen.
- There is often:
  - Rapid pulse, crackles in the lower part of the lungs.
  - A big tender liver, swollen veins in the neck.
  - Cough with clear or red-brown sputum.
- Sometimes the blood pressure is high.

2. CHRONIC KIDNEY DISEASE

- **Polyuria, especially during the night**.
- **Swelling** of the feet, the legs and even of the lower abdomen.
- **Protein in the urine**.
- Sometimes white or red blood cells in the urine.

3. DIABETES

- **Polyuria both day and night**.
- Much thirst: the patient drinks much water.
- Increase of appetite: the patient eats very much.
- Loss of weight.
- **Sugar in the urine**.

TO MAKE THE DIAGNOSIS

In the history, ask:

- When did you start passing much urine?
- How much urine do you pass each time? Very much? Only a little?
- How many times do you pass urine during the night?
- How many times do you pass urine during the day?
- Do you have other symptoms, like swelling of the feet or legs, trouble breathing while working or while sleeping, cough, sputum?
- Are you always very thirsty or very hungry?
- Have you lost weight?

In the physical exam, look for:

- High blood pressure.
- Swelling of the feet or legs.
- Other signs of heart failure: rapid pulse, fast breathing, crackles in the bottom part of the lungs, a big tender liver, big veins in the neck.

In the laboratory, do:

- A urine exam to look for sugar, protein, white or red blood cells, or casts.

INCREASE IN THE QUANTITY OF URINE - POLYURIA

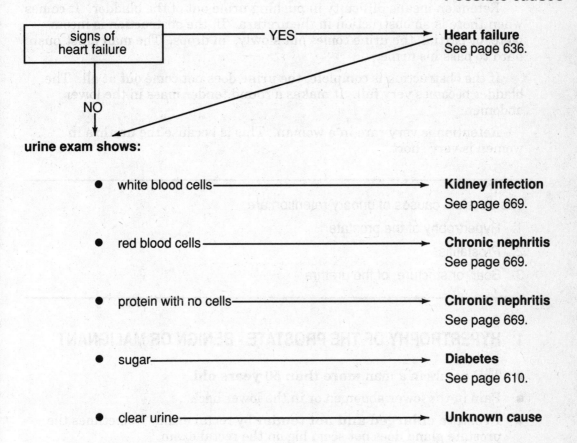

Possible causes

signs of heart failure —————YES—————→ **Heart failure**
See page 636.

NO

urine exam shows:

- white blood cells —————————————→ **Kidney infection**
  See page 669.

- red blood cells —————————————→ **Chronic nephritis**
  See page 669.

- protein with no cells ————————————→ **Chronic nephritis**
  See page 669.

- sugar ——————————————————→ **Diabetes**
  See page 610.

- clear urine ———————————————→ **Unknown cause**

If the cause is unknown and the patient seems ill, send him to hospital.

DIFFICULTY IN PASSING URINE IN A MAN-RETENTION

Retention means difficulty in pushing urine out of the bladder. It comes when there is an obstruction in the urethra. If the obstruction is incomplete, or partial, the urine comes out slowly, in drops. The man must push hard to pass his urine.

If the obstruction is complete, the urine does not come out at all. The bladder becomes very full. It makes a round tender mass in the lower abdomen.

Retention is very rare in a woman. This is because the urethra in women is very short.

The possible causes of urinary retention are:

1. Hypertrophy of the prostate
2. Prostatitis
3. Scar, or stricture, of the urethra

1. HYPERTROPHY OF THE PROSTATE - BENIGN OR MALIGNANT

- This occurs in a man **more than 50 years old**.
- Pain in the lower abdomen or in the lower back.
- **Prostate enlarged and not tender** by rectal exam. Sometimes the prostate gland does not seem big on the rectal exam.
- Often a round tender mass in the middle of the lower abdomen. This is a full bladder.
- Sometimes blood in the urine.
- The man needs an operation. Send him to hospital.

2. PROSTATITIS

- A disease that can come in a man **at any adult age**.
- Pain in the lower abdomen, in the lower back, or in the perineum.

- **Prostate very tender** on rectal exam. Often it is big.
- Sometimes fever, sometimes difficult urination.
- Sometimes pain on urination, or blood in the urine.

3. STRICTURE OF THE URETHRA

- This is scar tissue in the urethra. It makes the urethra very narrow.
- It can come in a man **at any age**.
- Often a history of gonorrhea or of an injury to the urethra.
- Prostate not tender, not big.
- Sometimes there is a complete obstruction of the urine. In this case, there will be a tender round mass in the lower abdomen. This is a very full bladder.
- A catheter will not pass into the bladder.
- Sometimes there are one or several urinary fistulas in the perineum, or signs of infection in the perineum: swelling, tenderness.
- The man needs an operation. Send him to hospital.

SYMPTOMATIC TREATMENT OF URINARY RETENTION

1. Start immediately the treatment for prostatitis - see page 684.
2. If the bladder is full and the patient cannot pass urine, send him immediately to hospital.
3. If the bladder is full but the hospital is far away, you must then take out the urine yourself.
   - First give meperidine, 75 mg or morphine, 10 mg.
   - If the cause of the retention is a big prostate, pass a catheter into the bladder. Sterilize the catheter first by boiling, or by an antiseptic solution. Pass the catheter into the bladder using sterile technique.
   - If the cause of the retention is a stricture of the urethra, or if you are unable to pass a catheter into the bladder in a man with a big prostate, take out the urine by aspiration. Use a big syringe and a big needle. Be sure they are sterile. Clean the lower abdomen of the man with an antiseptic solution. Make a puncture into the bladder in the middle line of the lower abdomen. Take out all of the urine by using the big syringe. Then send the man to hospital.

TO MAKE THE DIAGNOSIS

In the history, ask:

- How old are you?
- When did you first start having difficulty passing urine?
- Do you have pain when passing urine?
- Must you pass urine very often? When? Only at night? All of the time?
- Do you have blood in your urine?
- Do you have pain in the lower abdomen, in the back, or in the perineum?
- Have you ever had gonorrhea, or pus coming from the urethra?
- Have you ever had an accident followed by passing blood in the urine?
- Have you ever had an operation on your bladder, or on the urethra?

In the physical exam, look for:

- Fever.
- A round tender mass in the lower abdomen.
- Urinary fistulas, or signs of infection in the perineum.
- Do a rectal exam. See if the prostate is big or tender.

In the laboratory, do:

- A urine exam. Look for white or red blood cells.

DIFFICULTY IN PASSING URINE IN A MAN - RETENTION

Possible causes

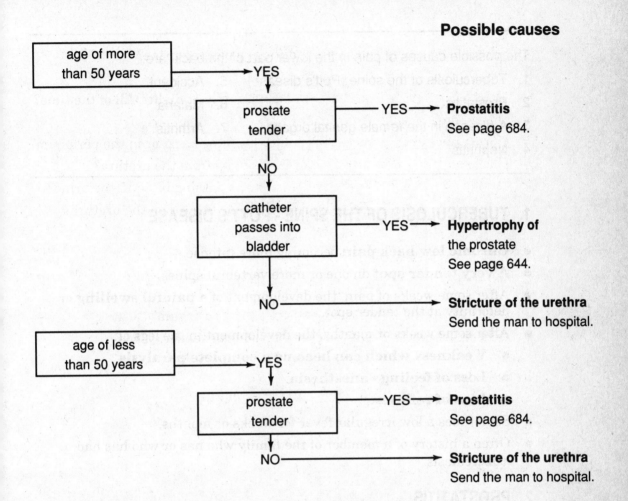

age of more than 50 years → YES

prostate tender → YES → **Prostatitis** See page 684.

NO ↓

catheter passes into bladder → YES → **Hypertrophy of** the prostate See page 644.

NO → **Stricture of the urethra** Send the man to hospital.

age of less than 50 years → YES

prostate tender → YES → **Prostatitis** See page 684.

NO → **Stricture of the urethra** Send the man to hospital.

LOW BACK PAIN

The possible causes of pain in the lower part of the back are:

1. Tuberculosis of the spine (Pott's disease)
2. Prostatitis
3. A disease in the female genital organs
4. Nephritis
5. Accident
6. Malaria
7. Arthritis

1. TUBERCULOSIS OF THE SPINE - POTT'S DISEASE

- **Chronic low back pain** becoming more intense.
- **A very tender spot** on one or more vertebral spines.
- After some weeks of pain, the development of a **painful swelling** or deformity at the tender spot.
- After some weeks or months, the development in the legs of:
  - **Weakness which can become a complete paralysis**.
  - **Loss of feeling - anesthesia**.
  - **Loss of reflexes**.
- Sometimes a low irregular fever for weeks or months.
- Often a history of a member of the family who has or who has had tuberculosis.

2. PROSTATITIS

- Acute or chronic pain in the lower back, the perineum, or the lower abdomen.
- By rectal exam, the prostate is **very tender**.
- No tenderness or swelling in the back.

3. DISEASE IN THE FEMALE GENITAL ORGANS

- **Low back pain related to the menstrual periods**.
- Sometimes a mass in the lower abdomen.
- Sometimes a mass coming down or out of the vagina.

4. NEPHRITIS - ACUTE OR CHRONIC

- Pain or tenderness in one or both flanks.
- **Protein** and often **white or red blood cells in the urine**.
- Swelling of the feet, the legs, and sometimes of the abdomen and the face.
- Sometimes high blood pressure.

5. ACCIDENT

- **History of a fall, a blow, or lifting a heavy load**.
- Start of the pain at the time of the accident.
- **Pain on movements of the lower back**.
- Sometimes a tender spot in the back, but no swelling.
- Sometimes a deformity of the back if the patient has had a fracture of the spine.

6. MALARIA

- Frequent attacks of fever.
- Low back pain coming with the fever.
- Positive thick smear during the attacks of fever.

7. ARTHRITIS

- **Pain on movements of the back**.
- **Pain during work, or when lifting a heavy load**.
- Sometimes the pain goes down one or both legs.
- Sometimes a change in the normal curve of the back, but no tender swelling.
- Sometimes tenderness of the spine, or of the muscles of the lower back.

TO MAKE THE DIAGNOSIS

In the history, ask:
- When did the pain begin?
- How did the pain start?
- Have you had a fall or a blow to the back?
- Did you lift something very heavy?
- Does the pain come with:
  - Menstrual periods?
  - Movements of the back?
  - Bending forward?
  - Work, or carrying heavy loads?
- Does anyone in your family have tuberculosis? Or has had it in the past?

In the physical exam, look for:
- Pain on movements of the back.
- Tender spot on the spine or in the muscles.
- A tender swelling of the spine.
- Weakness or paralysis of the legs.
- Anesthesia, or loss of reflexes in the legs.
- Tenderness of the prostate by rectal exam.
- Tenderness of the flanks.
- A deformity of the spine.
- Fever.
- High blood pressure.
- Swelling of the feet, the legs, the abdomen, or the face.
- In a woman, a mass in the lower abdomen or in the vagina.

In the laboratory, do:
- A urine exam to look for protein and blood cells.
- A thick blood smear to look for plasmodium.

LOW BACK PAIN

Possible causes

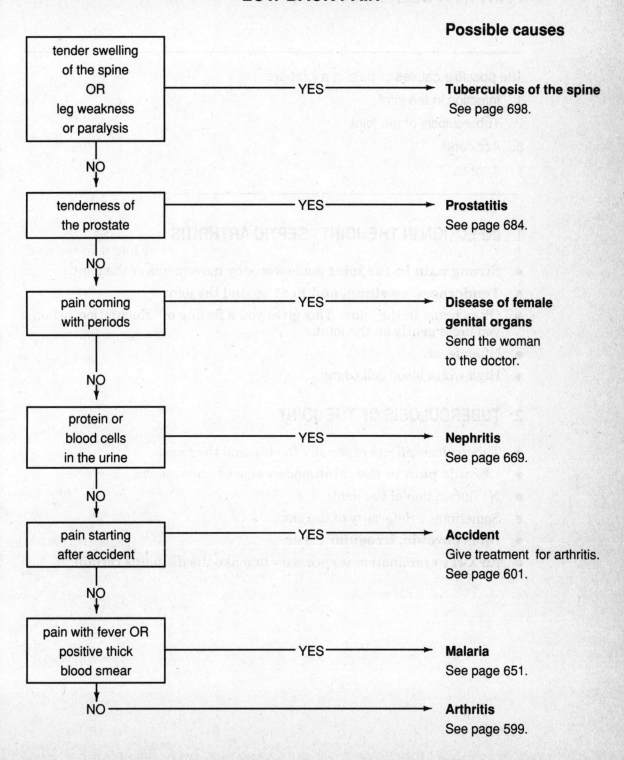

tender swelling of the spine OR leg weakness or paralysis	— YES →	**Tuberculosis of the spine** See page 698.
NO		
tenderness of the prostate	— YES →	**Prostatitis** See page 684.
NO		
pain coming with periods	— YES →	**Disease of female genital organs** Send the woman to the doctor.
NO		
protein or blood cells in the urine	— YES →	**Nephritis** See page 669.
NO		
pain starting after accident	— YES →	**Accident** Give treatment for arthritis. See page 601.
NO		
pain with fever OR positive thick blood smear	— YES →	**Malaria** See page 651.
NO		**Arthritis** See page 599.

PAIN IN A JOINT

The possible causes of pain in a joint are:
1. Infection in the joint
2. Tuberculosis of the joint
3. Accident
4. Arthritis

1. INFECTION IN THE JOINT - SEPTIC ARTHRITIS

- **Strong pain in the joint** made worse by movements of the joint.
- **Tenderness, swelling, and heat** around the joint.
- Often liquid in the joint. This gives you a feeling of "fluctuation" when you press gently on the joint.
- Often fever.
- High white blood cell count.

2. TUBERCULOSIS OF THE JOINT

- Tuberculosis affects especially the hip and the knee.
- **Chronic pain in the joint** made worse by movements.
- No fluctuation of the joint.
- Sometimes a deformity of the joint.
- Often **chronic, irregular fever**.
- An X-ray examination is necessary to make the diagnosis certain.

3. ACCIDENT - TRAUMATIC ARTHRITIS

- **History of a fall or of an injury to the joint**.
- Pain on movements of the joint.
- Often a tender swelling of the joint right after the accident.
- Often liquid in the joint right after the accident.
- No fever.

4. ARTHRITIS

- Acute or chronic pain made worse by movements of the joint.
- Sometimes stiffness of the joint, or a deformity of the joint.
- Sometimes liquid in the joint.
- Little or no tenderness in the joint.
- No fever.

TO MAKE THE DIAGNOSIS

In the history, ask:
- When did the pain start?
- Did you fall, or have an injury to the joint at the start of the pain?
- Have you had fever?
- Have you had tuberculosis? Has anyone in your family ever had it?

In the physical exam, look for:
- Fever.
- Tender swelling of the joint.
- Fluctuation in the joint.

In the laboratory, do:
- A white blood cell count.
- Sometimes the diagnosis is not certain. If there is liquid in the joint, make a puncture of the joint. Be sure that the syringe and needle are sterile. Clean the skin over the joint very carefully with an antiseptic solution. Look at the liquid under the microscope. Look for:
  - Many white blood cells: a sign of infection in the joint.
  - Few white blood cells: possibly tuberculosis of the joint.
  - Blood, or red blood cells: a sign of injury to the joint.
  - Clear liquid (no cells): a sign of simple arthritis.

PAIN IN A JOINT

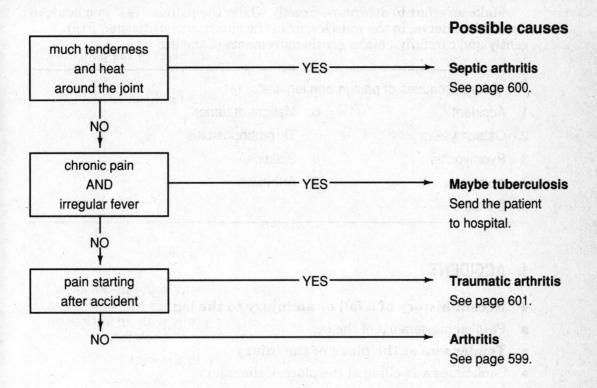

Possible causes

| much tenderness and heat around the joint | —YES→ | **Septic arthritis** See page 600. |

NO ↓

| chronic pain AND irregular fever | —YES→ | **Maybe tuberculosis** Send the patient to hospital. |

NO ↓

| pain starting after accident | —YES→ | **Traumatic arthritis** See page 601. |

NO→ **Arthritis** See page 599.

PAIN IN ONE LEG

Make an effort to determine exactly where the pain is. Is it in a bone, in a joint, in a nerve, in the muscles, or in the subcutaneous tissue? Feel gently and carefully. Make gentle movements of the leg.

The possible causes of pain in one leg are:

1. Accident
2. Osteomyelitis
3. Pyomyositis
4. Abscess
5. Cellulitis
6. Malignant tumor
7. Thrombophlebitis
8. Sciatica
9. Arthritis

1. ACCIDENT

- **Recent history of a fall or an injury to the leg**.
- Pain on movements of the leg.
- **Tenderness at the place of the injury**.
- Sometimes a swelling at the place of the injury.
- Look for signs of a fracture: see page 137.
  - Very tender spot in the bone at the place of the injury.
  - Abnormal movements in the middle of the injured bone.
  - Change in the line, the shape, and sometimes of the length of the bone and the leg.
  - "Crepitation" of bone fragments at the place of the injury.
- Look for signs of a sprain: see page 135.
  - Tenderness and swelling around a joint.
  - No signs of a fracture.
- Look for signs of a contusion: see page 137.
  - Tenderness and swelling at the place of the injury.
  - No signs of a fracture or of a sprain.

2. OSTEOMYELITIS

- **Strong deep pain in a bone** for one or more weeks.
- Pain made worse by using the leg, **but not by gentle movements of the leg**.
- Tenderness on deep pressure at the place of the pain.
- No swelling or thickening of the muscles or of the subcutaneous tissue.
- Often fever, especially in the evening.
- In the case of chronic osteomyelitis, there is often a fistula with pus at or near the place of the pain.
- An X-ray examination is necessary to make the diagnosis of osteomyelitis. It takes 2 weeks for X-ray signs of osteomyelitis to appear. So wait 2 weeks from the start of the pain before sending the patient for the X-ray examination.

3. PYOMYOSITIS - SEE PAGE 137

- Pain for some days in the muscles of the leg.
- **Pain made worse by every movement of these leg muscles**.
  - Pain when the patient uses these muscles.
  - Pain when you move the patient's leg.
- **Thickening of the painful muscles**.
- Tenderness at the place of the pain.
- No signs of pus: fluctuation, or changes of the skin. This is because the pus is deep inside the muscles. You cannot find it by palpation.
- Often fever, especially during the evening.

4. ABSCESS

- **Strong pain in one spot for one or more days**. The pain is not made worse by gentle movements.
- Tenderness at the place of the pain.
- **Heat, swelling and often fluctuation at the tender place**.
- The skin over the swelling becomes smooth and thin.

- Fever: often present, sometimes absent.
- Often tender lymph glands in the inguinal or femoral regions.
- Pus in the swelling found by sterile puncture and aspiration.
- High white blood cell count.

5. CELLULITIS

- **Pain in the skin and in the subcutaneous tissue**.
- **Heat and swelling of the skin and the subcutaneous tissue**.
- Tenderness of the affected region.
- Often a small wound or ulcer at the lower end of the infected region.
- Often fever; often a rapid pulse.
- Often tender lymph glands in the inguinal or femoral regions.
- High white blood cell count.

6. MALIGNANT TUMOR - OF THE BONE OR OF THE MUSCLES

- **Strong deep pain** for one or more weeks. Movements do not make the pain worse.
- Often **deep tender swelling**, and sometimes heat in the region.
- **No fever**, no tender lymph glands.
- A malignant bone tumor can look like osteomyelitis. It is necessary to do an X-ray examination to make the diagnosis clear.

7. THROMBOPHLEBITIS

- **Pain and tenderness in back of the lower leg made worse by walking**.
- **Pain made worse by bending the foot up**, in "dorsi-flexion."
- **Swelling of the ankle and of the lower leg**.
- Often fever.

8. SCIATICA

- **Pain in back of the leg, from the hip to the foot**, made worse by:
  - Bending forward while standing.
  - Extension of the straight leg.
  - Dorsi-flexion of the foot.

9. ARTHRITIS

- **Pain on movements of a joint**.
- Sometimes tenderness and sometimes swelling of the joint.
- No swelling or tenderness of the muscles or subcutaneous tissue.
- Sometimes liquid in the joint, with fluctuation of the joint.
- No fever.

SYMPTOMATIC TREATMENT OF PAIN IN ONE LEG

1. Give aspirin for the pain.
2. If there is much pain, put the patient in bed.
3. Send the patient to hospital if:
   - There is much pain and you cannot find the cause.
   - The general condition of the patient seems to be affected.
   - The pain continues for some days in spite of symptomatic treatment.

TO MAKE THE DIAGNOSIS

In the history, ask:

- When did the pain begin?
- Where do you feel the pain?
- Did the pain start right after a fall, or an injury?
- Does it hurt to use your leg?
- Do you have fever?

In the physical exam, look for:

- A tender place. Is it in the bone? In a joint? In a nerve? In the muscles? In the subcutaneous tissue? In the back of the lower leg?
- Pain when doing these things:
    - Bending forward.
    - Movements of a joint.
    - Movements of the muscles.
    - Dorsi-flexion of the foot.
    - Raising the leg in extension.
- Heat or swelling in a bone, in a joint, in some muscles, or in the subcutaneous tissue.
- Tenderness or abnormal movements in the middle of a bone.
- Changes in the line, the shape or the length of the leg.
- Crepitations in the bone.
- Tender thickening in the muscles.
- Fluctuation in the subcutaneous tissue.
- Fever.
- Tender lymph glands in the inguinal or femoral regions.
- Swelling of the ankle or of the lower leg.
- Wound, ulcer, or fistula.

In the laboratory, do:

- A white blood cell count.

PAIN IN ONE LEG

Possible causes

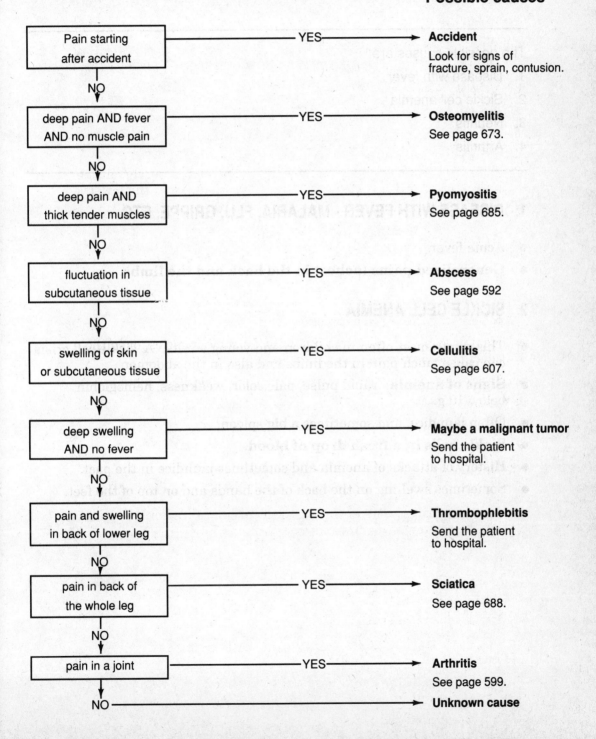

Pain starting after accident	—YES→	**Accident**
		Look for signs of fracture, sprain, contusion.
deep pain AND fever AND no muscle pain	—YES→	**Osteomyelitis**
		See page 673.
deep pain AND thick tender muscles	—YES→	**Pyomyositis**
		See page 685.
fluctuation in subcutaneous tissue	—YES→	**Abscess**
		See page 592
swelling of skin or subcutaneous tissue	—YES→	**Cellulitis**
		See page 607.
deep swelling AND no fever	—YES→	**Maybe a malignant tumor**
		Send the patient to hospital.
pain and swelling in back of lower leg	—YES→	**Thrombophlebitis**
		Send the patient to hospital.
pain in back of the whole leg	—YES→	**Sciatica**
		See page 688.
pain in a joint	—YES→	**Arthritis**
		See page 599.
NO ————————→		**Unknown cause**

PAIN IN MORE THAN ONE LIMB

The possible causes are:
1. Disease with fever
2. Sickle cell anemia
3. Neuritis
4. Arthritis

1. DISEASE WITH FEVER - MALARIA, FLU, GRIPPE, ETC.

- Acute fever.
- **Generalized pains (aches) in the back and the limbs.**

2. SICKLE CELL ANEMIA

- This comes most often in children and young adults. A sickle cell crisis can cause much pain in the limbs and also in the abdomen.
- **Signs of anemia**: rapid pulse, pale color, weakness, hemoglobin below 10 g.
- Often jaundice, and sometimes a big spleen.
- **Sickle cells in a fresh drop of blood.**
- History of attacks of anemia and sometimes jaundice in the past.
- Sometimes swelling on the back of the hands and on top of the feet.

3. NEURITIS

- **Chronic pain in the muscles or the bones**.
- Feelings of prickling or heat in the hands or feet.
- No pain on movements of the limbs.
- No pain in the joints.
- Sometimes a history of diabetes or arteriosclerosis.
- Sometimes a history of taking certain medicines, like INH for tuberculosis.

4. ARTHRITIS

- **Pain in several joints, made worse by movements**.
- Sometimes swelling or deformity of one or more joints.

TO MAKE THE DIAGNOSIS

In the history, ask:
- When did the pain begin?
- Exactly where do you feel the pain?
- Does moving your arms or legs make the pain worse?
- Do you have fever?
- Have you ever had anemia or jaundice in the past?
- Do you have diabetes, or some other chronic disease?
- Do you take any medicines regularly? If so, what medicine?

In the physical exam, look for:
- Fever.
- Swelling of one or more joints, or of the back of the hands or the top of the feet.
- Deformity of one or more joints.
- Signs of anemia: rapid pulse, pale color.
- Jaundice, a big spleen.

In the laboratory, do:
- In a child or a young adult, a fresh blood drop to look for sickle cells.
- A hemoglobin exam.
- If there is fever, a thick blood smear to look for plasmodium.

PAIN IN MORE THAN ONE LIMB

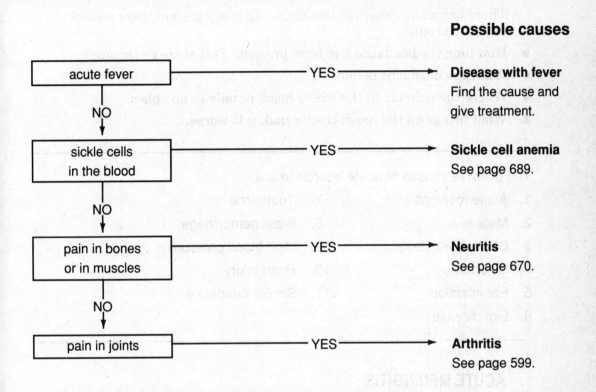

Possible causes

acute fever — YES → **Disease with fever**
Find the cause and give treatment.

NO

sickle cells in the blood — YES → **Sickle cell anemia**
See page 689.

NO

pain in bones or in muscles — YES → **Neuritis**
See page 670.

NO

pain in joints — YES → **Arthritis**
See page 599.

SYMPTOMATIC TREATMENT OF PAIN IN LIMBS

1. Give aspirin for the pain.
2. If there is much pain, put the patient in bed.
3. Send the patient to hospital if:
   - There is much pain and you cannot find the cause.
   - The general condition of the patient seems to be affected.
   - The pain continues for some days in spite of symptomatic treatment.

ACUTE HEADACHE

There are many causes of headache. In every patient, take a good history to find out:
- How long the headache has been present. Is it acute or chronic?
- What the headache is like.
- Where the pain is: in the whole head, or only in one place.
- What brings on the headache, or makes it worse.

The possible causes of acute headache are:

1. Acute meningitis
2. Malaria
3. Disease with fever
4. Sinusitis
5. Ear infection
6. Eye disease
7. Toothache
8. Brain hemorrhage
9. High blood pressure
10. Head injury
11. Simple headache

---

1. ACUTE MENINGITIS

- Strong pain in the whole head.
- **High fever**.
- **Stiffness of the neck**.
- **CSF cloudy**, containing many white blood cells.
- Sometimes convulsions, sometimes coma.

2. MALARIA

- Pain in the whole head.
- **Fever**.
- **Thick blood film positive for plasmodium**.
- Rapid improvement after treatment for malaria.

3. DISEASE WITH FEVER - PNEUMONIA, GRIPPE, FLU, HEPATITIS, TYPHOID FEVER

- Pain in the whole head.
- **Fever**.
- **Signs of the specific disease**.

4. SINUSITIS

- **Pain in the forehead or on one side of the face**.
- **Tenderness of the bones in the place of the pain**.
- Often fever, but not always.
- Often symptoms of a cold, with runny nose and blockage of the nose.

5. EAR INFECTION - OTITIS

- **Pain in an ear** and on the same side of the head.
- Often **pus coming from the ear canal**.
- Sometimes fever.

6. EYE DISEASE

- **Pain in one or both eyes**.
- Often **redness** of one or both eyes.
- Often diminished vision in one or both eyes. This is **very serious**.

7. TOOTHACHE

- Pain on one side of the face and head.
- **Pain and tenderness of one or more teeth**.
- Pain during chewing of food.

8. BRAIN HEMORRHAGE

- Very strong pain in the whole head, or on one side of the head.
- **High blood pressure**, often more than 160/110.

- **CSF pink or yellow**, with many red blood cells.
- Stiffness of the neck.
- Sometimes paralysis of one side of the body.
- Sometimes convulsions or coma.
- No fever.

9. HIGH BLOOD PRESSURE

- Pain in the whole head.
- **High blood pressure**, more than 160/100.

10. HEAD INJURY

- **History of a recent blow to the head**.
- Pain in the whole head, or at the place of the blow.
- Often a short period of coma right after the injury.
- Sometimes a wound or other signs of the injury.

11. SIMPLE HEADACHE

- **Vague pain** in the forehead, or in the whole head.
- Often a history of overwork, worries, nervousness.

SYMPTOMATIC TREATMENT OF ACUTE HEADACHE

1. Give aspirin, 0.5 g every 4 hours to calm the headache.
2. If you find no specific cause, look for other possible causes, such as over-work, worries, problems in the family or clan, fear or other strong emotions. Help the patient see how to overcome these problems.

TO MAKE THE DIAGNOSIS

In the history, ask:

- How long have you had the headache?
- Where does your head hurt?
  - Everywhere?
  - In the forehead?
  - In an ear?
  - In one or both eyes?
  - In a tooth?
- Do you have a runny nose? Or pus coming from an ear?
- How did the headache start?
- Have you had a fever?
- Do you have other symptoms, like a cough, pain in the throat, vomiting, diarrhea, pain in the abdomen?
- Do you have high blood pressure?
- Have you recently had an accident with a blow to the head? If so, did you lose consciousness right after the accident? For how long?
- Are you overworked? Do you have many worries or problems?

In the physical exam, look for:

- Fever.
- Stiffness of the neck.
- Signs of a disease with fever.
- Tenderness in the forehead, bones of the face, or one or more teeth.
- A runny nose or pus coming from the ear.
- Soreness or redness of one eye or both eyes.
- Diminished vision in one or both eyes.
- High blood pressure: more than 160/100.
- Paralysis of a part of the body.
- Signs of a head injury: wound, swelling, deformity.

In the laboratory, do:

- A thick blood film to look for plasmodium.
- A lumbar puncture in case of:
  - Fever and stiffness of the neck.
  - High blood pressure and stiffness of the neck.

ACUTE HEADACHE

Possible causes

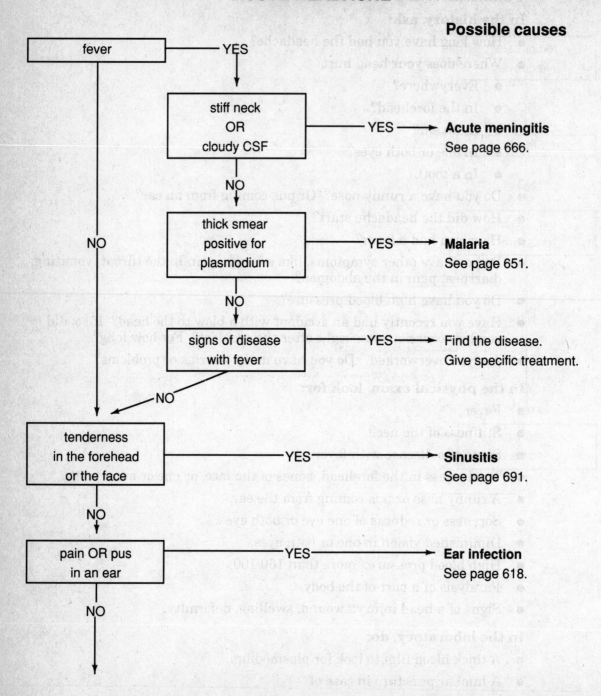

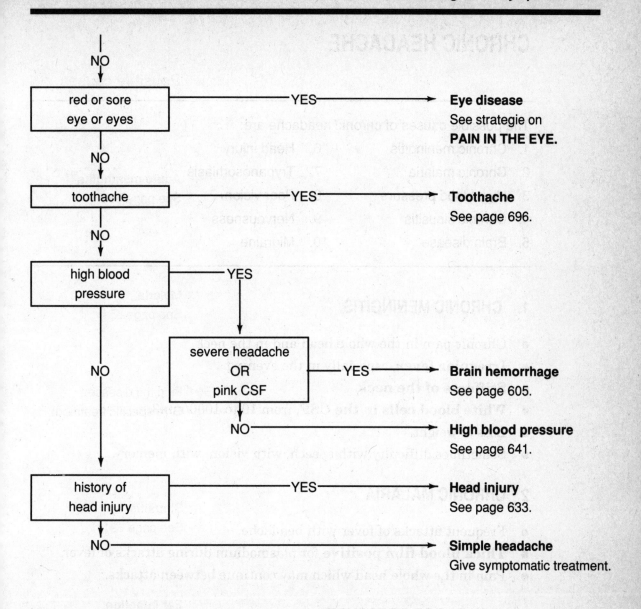

NO

| red or sore eye or eyes | ──YES──→ | **Eye disease** |
See strategie on
PAIN IN THE EYE.

NO

| toothache | ──YES──→ | **Toothache** |
See page 696.

NO

high blood pressure ──YES──

severe headache OR pink CSF ──YES──→ **Brain hemorrhage**
See page 605.

NO──→ **High blood pressure**
See page 641.

NO

| history of head injury | ──YES──→ | **Head injury** |
See page 633.

NO──→ **Simple headache**
Give symptomatic treatment.

CHRONIC HEADACHE

The possible causes of chronic headache are:

1. Chronic meningitis
2. Chronic malaria
3. High blood pressure
4. Chronic sinusitis
5. Brain disease
6. Head injury
7. Trypanosomiasis
8. Poor vision
9. Nervousness
10. Migraine

1. CHRONIC MENINGITIS

- Chronic pain in the whole head and in the neck.
- **Irregular fever**, especially in the evening.
- **Stiffness of the neck**.
- **White blood cells in the CSF**, from 10 to 1000/mm3.
- Loss of weight.
- Sometimes difficulty with speech, with vision, with memory.

2. CHRONIC MALARIA

- Frequent attacks of fever with headache.
- **Thick blood film positive** for plasmodium during attacks of fever.
- Pain in the whole head which may continue between attacks.

3. HIGH BLOOD PRESSURE

- Pain in the whole head or at the top of the head, especially in the morning.
- **High blood pressure**: more than 160/100.

4. CHRONIC SINUSITIS

- **Pain and tenderness in the forehead or on one side of the face.**
- Sometimes an irregular chronic fever.
- Often a purulent discharge from the nose.

5. BRAIN DISEASE - TUMOR, ABSCESS OF THE BRAIN

- **Paralysis** of one or more limbs, of one side of the face, or of an eye.
- **Difficulty with speech or of memory**.
- Sometimes convulsions; sometimes chronic vomiting.

6. HEAD INJURY

- **History of a blow to the head**, often followed by loss of consciousness for some minutes or hours.
- Headache beginning right after the injury.
- Pain in the whole head, or at the place of the injury.

7. TRYPANOSOMIASIS - AFRICAN SLEEPING SICKNESS

- This disease exists only in Central Africa.
- Chronic pain in the whole head.
- Often a **chronic irregular fever, with loss of weight**.
- Often difficulty with speech, memory, or behavior.
- **CSF with trypanosomes** and some white blood cells: from 4 to 1000/mm3.
- Sometimes trypanosomes in the lymph glands of the neck, or in a thick blood film.

8. POOR VISION

- Pain in the forehead, or in the back of the head and neck.
- **Headache made worse by reading, studying, or bright sunlight**.
- **Difficulty in seeing objects clearly**.

9. NERVOUSNESS

- Pain, or feeling of heat, usually at the top of the head.
- **Headache associated with overwork, worries**, bad dreams, problems in the family or clan, strong emotions.

10. MIGRAINE

- Repeated attacks of strong headache.
- **Pain often on only one side of the head**.
- Often **nausea, vomiting, and trouble seeing** at the beginning of the attack.
- Attacks of headache usually come with overwork, worries, menstrual periods, or problems with family, clan, or emotions.

TO MAKE THE DIAGNOSIS

In the history, ask:
- When did the headache start?
- Where do you feel the pain?
- At what time does the pain come?
- Do you have nausea, vomiting, or trouble seeing when the headache comes?
- Do you often have fever?
- Does the headache come only during attacks of fever?
- Have you lost weight?
- Do you have a thick discharge from the nose?
- Did you have a blow to the head at the beginning of the headache? If so, did you lose consciousness right after the blow? For how long?
- Do using your eyes or bright sunlight make the headache come or get worse?
- Do you have trouble seeing clearly?
- Do you often have bad dreams, or problems at home, in the family, or at work? Do these problems or bad dreams make the headache worse?

In the physical exam, look for:
- Fever.
- Signs of weight loss.
- Stiffness of the neck.
- High blood pressure.
- Tenderness of the forehead or of bones in the face.
- Paralysis of a part of the body, or of the face, or of an eye.
- Difficulty with speech or with memory.
- Signs of an old injury to the head.

In the laboratory, do:
- A thick blood film to look for plasmodium or trypanosomes.
- If there are lymph nodes in the neck, do a node puncture to look for trypanosomes.
- A lumbar puncture in case of fever with stiff neck or with convulsions, with difficulties of speech or memory, or with paralysis. Look for white blood cells (count them) and trypanosomes.

CHRONIC HEADACHE

Possible causes

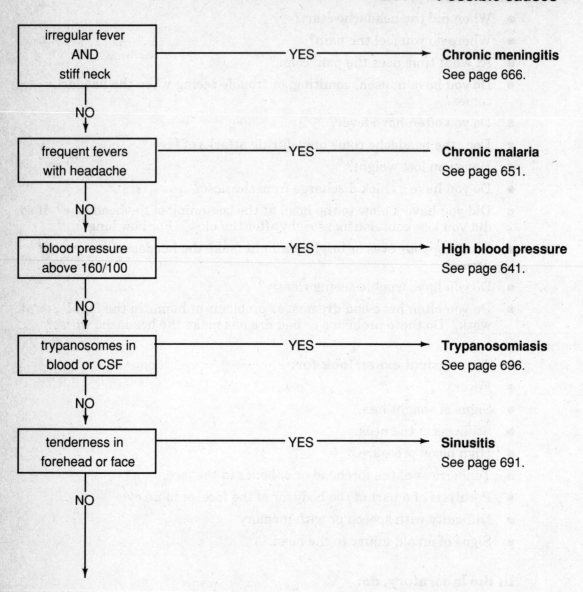

irregular fever
AND
stiff neck — YES — **Chronic meningitis**
See page 666.

NO

frequent fevers
with headache — YES — **Chronic malaria**
See page 651.

NO

blood pressure
above 160/100 — YES → **High blood pressure**
See page 641.

NO

trypanosomes in
blood or CSF — YES → **Trypanosomiasis**
See page 696.

NO

tenderness in
forehead or face — YES → **Sinusitis**
See page 691.

NO

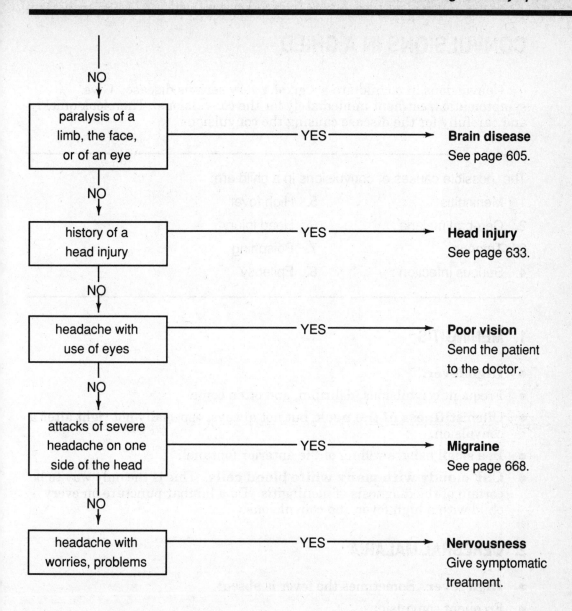

NO

| paralysis of a limb, the face, or of an eye | —— YES ——▶ | **Brain disease** See page 605. |

NO

| history of a head injury | —— YES ——▶ | **Head injury** See page 633. |

NO

| headache with use of eyes | —— YES ——▶ | **Poor vision** Send the patient to the doctor. |

NO

| attacks of severe headache on one side of the head | —— YES ——▶ | **Migraine** See page 668. |

NO

| headache with worries, problems | —— YES ——▶ | **Nervousness** Give symptomatic treatment. |

CONVULSIONS IN A CHILD

Convulsions in a child are a sign of a very serious disease. Give symptomatic treatment immediately for the convulsions. Then look quickly and carefully for the disease causing the convulsions.

The possible causes of convulsions in a child are:

1. Meningitis
2. Cerebral malaria
3. Tetanus
4. Serious infection
5. High fever
6. Head injury
7. Poisoning
8. Epilepsy

---

1. MENINGITIS

- **High fever.**
- Frequent convulsions, delirium, and often coma.
- Often **stiffness of the neck**, but not always, especially not right after a convulsion.
- In a small baby, swelling of the anterior fontanel.
- **CSF cloudy with many white blood cells**. This is the only way to be certain of the diagnosis of meningitis. Do a lumbar puncture on every child with a high fever and convulsions.

2. CEREBRAL MALARIA

- **High fever**. Sometimes the fever is absent.
- Frequent convulsions.
- **Delirium or coma between the convulsions**.
- No stiffness of the neck or swelling of the fontanel.
- **Thick blood film positive for plasmodium**.
- CSF clear, with no white blood cells.
- Sometimes a big spleen, but not always.

3. TETANUS

- Tetanus causes muscle spasms rather than true convulsions.
- **Frequent muscle spasms** caused by noise or by movements.
- **Inability to open the mouth**. The teeth are shut tightly together. We call this "trismus."
- **Stiffness of the neck and the whole back**.
- Fever. The fever is sometimes absent.
- No delirium or coma. **The consciousness is clear**.
- There is often a wound, a sore, a burn, chiggers, or an open fracture.
- Tetanus can affect a newborn baby.

4. SERIOUS INFECTION - PNEUMONIA, SEPTICEMIA, ABSCESS, GASTRO-ENTERITIS

- **High fever**.
- Rapid breathing, rapid pulse.
- **Signs of the specific infection**.

5. HIGH FEVER - FEBRILE CONVULSIONS

- A high fever alone can cause convulsions in small children.
- The consciousness is clear between the convulsions.
- No stiffness of the neck.

6. HEAD INJURY

- **History of a recent fall or blow to the head**.
- Often a loss of consciousness right after the accident.
- Delirium or coma.
- Often vomiting.
- No fever or stiffness of the neck.

7. POISONING

- **History of the child having eaten or drunk something poisonous, like too much medicine, or a poisonous substance**.
- Often delirium or coma.
- No fever or stiffness of the neck.

8. EPILEPSY

- **History of frequent convulsions during the past months or years**.
- The convulsions come without fever.
- The child appears normal between the convulsions.

SYMPTOMATIC TREATMENT OF CONVULSIONS IN A CHILD

1. Protect the child from injury during the convulsion.
2. Turn the child on one side with the head back.
3. Take out all the secretions and vomit from the mouth.
4. Put a sponge or other cloth into the mouth between the teeth to keep the child from biting the tongue.
5. In case of fever:
   - Give the child aspirin, 10 mg/kilo of weight every 4 hours.
   - After the convulsion, give him a cool bath to bring down the fever.
6. Give him an anticonvulsive medicine:
   - Diazepam (*Valium) 0.2 mg/kilo, or
   - Phenobarbital 5 mg/kilo.
   - Repeat the dose after one hour if the convulsions continue.
7. If the convulsions continue for more than 6 hours after you begin the treatment, send the child to hospital.

TO MAKE THE DIAGNOSIS

In the history, ask the parents:
- When did the convulsions first begin?
- Was there a fever? Or difficulty breathing? Or a strong cough?
- Has the child often had convulsions in the past?
- If so, do the convulsions come only when the child has a fever?
- Can the child open the mouth? Can he eat? Can he drink?
- Has the child recently had a fall, or a blow to the head?
- Has the child just swallowed some medicine, or another substance which could be poisonous?

In the physical exam, look for:
- Fever.
- A stiff neck or back.
- A swollen fontanel.
- Delirium or coma between the convulsions.
- Muscle spasms caused by noise or movements.
- Trismus. See how wide the mouth will open. Try to open it gently yourself.
- A wound, sore, burn, or chiggers.
- Signs of dyspnea; crackles in the lungs.
- An abscess or other infection somewhere.

In the laboratory, do:
- A lumbar puncture on every child with fever and convulsions. Look at the CSF. Is it cloudy? Look at it under the microscope to look for white blood cells.
- A thick blood film to look for plasmodium.

CONVULSIONS IN A CHILD

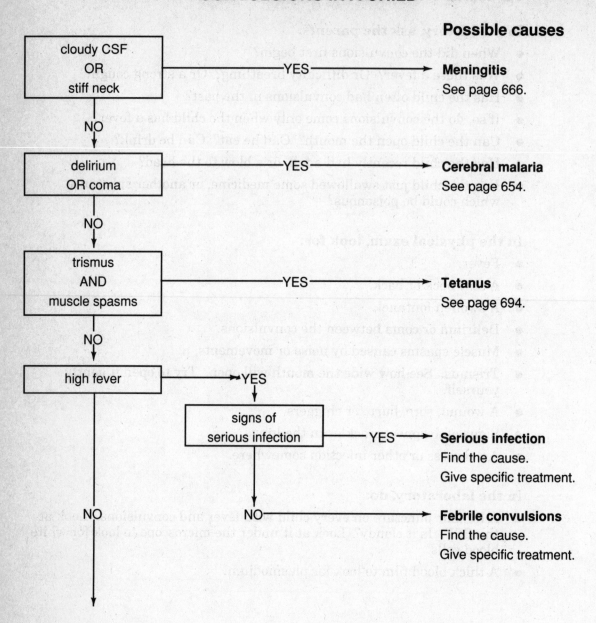

Possible causes

cloudy CSF OR stiff neck → YES → **Meningitis**
See page 666.

NO ↓

delirium OR coma → YES → **Cerebral malaria**
See page 654.

NO ↓

trismus AND muscle spasms → YES → **Tetanus**
See page 694.

NO ↓

high fever → YES →

signs of serious infection → YES → **Serious infection**
Find the cause.
Give specific treatment.

NO → **Febrile convulsions**
Find the cause.
Give specific treatment.

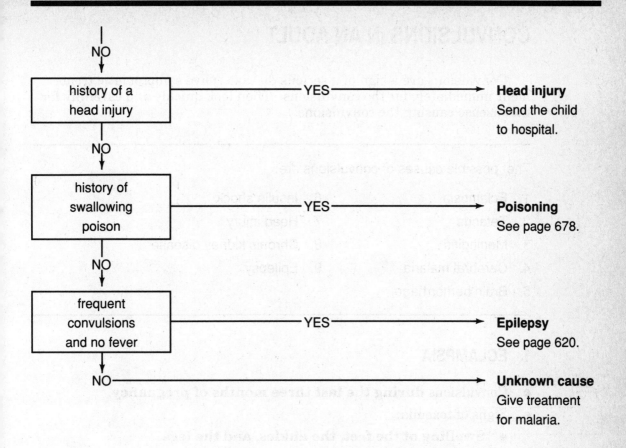

NO

| history of a head injury | —YES——→ | **Head injury** Send the child to hospital. |

NO

| history of swallowing poison | —YES——→ | **Poisoning** See page 678. |

NO

| frequent convulsions and no fever | —YES——→ | **Epilepsy** See page 620. |

NO————————————————→ **Unknown cause** Give treatment for malaria.

CONVULSIONS IN AN ADULT

Convulsions are a sign of a serious disease. Give symptomatic treatment immediately for the convulsions. Then look quickly and carefully for the disease causing the convulsions.

The possible causes of convulsions are:

1. Eclampsia
2. Tetanus
3. Meningitis
4. Cerebral malaria
5. Brain hemorrhage
6. Insulin shock
7. Head injury
8. Chronic kidney disease
9. Epilepsy

---

1. ECLAMPSIA

- Convulsions **during the last three months of pregnancy**.
- Signs of toxemia:
  - **Swelling of the feet, the ankles, and the legs**.
  - **Protein in the urine**.
  - **High blood pressure**, more than 130/90.

2. TETANUS

- Tetanus causes muscle spasms rather than true convulsions.
- **Frequent muscle spasms** caused by noise or by movements.
- **Inability to open the mouth**. The teeth are tightly shut together. We call this "trismus."
- **Stiffness of the neck and the whole back**.
- Fever. The fever is sometimes absent.
- No delirium or coma. **The consciousness is clear**.
- There is often a wound, a sore, a burn, chiggers, or an open fracture.

3. MENINGITIS

- **High fever**.
- Frequent convulsions, delirium and often coma.
- **Stiffness of the neck**.
- **CSF cloudy with many white blood cells**.

4. CEREBRAL MALARIA

- High fever. Sometimes the fever is absent.
- Delirium or coma between the convulsions.
- No stiffness of the neck.
- **Thick blood film positive for plasmodium**.
- CSF clear, with no white blood cells.
- Sometimes a big spleen, but not always.

5. BRAIN HEMORRHAGE

- **High blood pressure**, more than 160/100.
- Coma.
- Often **paralysis** of a leg, an arm, one side of the face, or an eye.
- Sometimes stiffness of the neck.
- **CSF pink or yellow**, with many red blood cells.

6. INSULIN SHOCK

- **History of diabetes**.
- **An injection of insulin a few hours before**. The patient has eaten little or no food since the injection.
- Slow pulse, moist skin, dilated pupils.
- There is usually no sugar in the urine.

7. HEAD INJURY

- **History of a recent accident with a blow to the head**.
- Often a loss of consciousness for a short time right after the accident.
- The convulsions may start some weeks after the accident. This is a sign of a hemorrhage inside the skull. It is very serious.
- Often vomiting.
- No fever or stiffness of the neck.

8. CHRONIC KIDNEY DISEASE

- **Protein and often white or red blood cells in the urine**.
- **Swelling of the feet, the legs, the abdomen, or the face**.
- Sometimes delirium, even coma.
- Breathing which is very deep and rapid.

9. EPILEPSY

- **History of repeated convulsions for months or years with no fever**.
- The patient appears normal between the periods of convulsion.

SYMPTOMATIC TREATMENT OF CONVULSIONS IN AN ADULT

1. Protect the patient from injury during the convulsion.
2. Lay the patient on one side with his head back.
3. Take out all secretions and vomit from his mouth.
4. Put a sponge or other cloth into the patient's mouth between his teeth to prevent him from biting his tongue.
5. Give an anticonvulsive medicine:
   - Diazepam (*Valium) 10mg, or phenobarbital 100 mg.
   - Repeat the dose in one hour if the convulsions continue.
6. If the convulsions continue for more than 12 hours after you begin the treatment, send the patient to hospital.

TO MAKE THE DIAGNOSIS

In the history, ask:

- When did the convulsions start?
- How often do the convulsions come?
- In the case of a woman, are you pregnant? If so, how many months?
- Can you open your mouth wide?
- Do you have muscle spasms?
- Have you had a fever? Or vomiting?
- Do you have diabetes? If so, have you had an insulin shot today?
- Have you recently had an accident with a blow to the head?
- Did you lose consciousness right after the accident? For how long?

In the physical exam, look for:

- A pregnancy in the last trimester, with swelling and high blood pressure.
- Muscle spasms caused by noise or movements.
- Trismus. Ask the patient to open the mouth wide.
- Fever.
- Stiffness of the neck or of the back.
- Delirium or coma.
- High blood pressure.
- Paralysis of a leg, an arm, one side of the face, or an eye.
- Signs of a recent head injury.
- Swelling of the feet, the legs, the abdomen, or the face.
- Deep and rapid breathing.

In the laboratory, do:

- A thick blood film to look for plasmodium.
- A urine exam to look for protein and white or red blood cells.
- A lumbar puncture to look for white or red blood cells.

CONVULSIONS IN AN ADULT

Possible causes

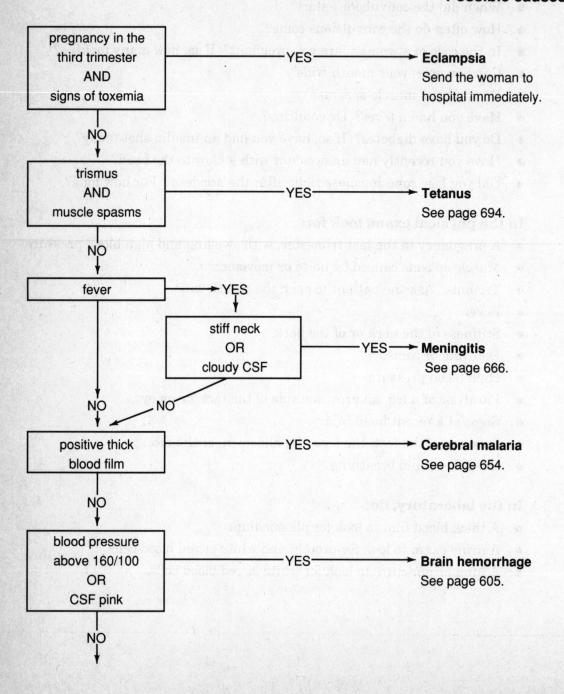

pregnancy in the third trimester AND signs of toxemia ——YES——→ **Eclampsia**
Send the woman to hospital immediately.

NO

trismus AND muscle spasms ——YES——→ **Tetanus**
See page 694.

NO

fever ——→YES

stiff neck OR cloudy CSF ——YES——→ **Meningitis**
See page 666.

NO   NO

positive thick blood film ——YES——→ **Cerebral malaria**
See page 654.

NO

blood pressure above 160/100 OR CSF pink ——YES——→ **Brain hemorrhage**
See page 605.

NO

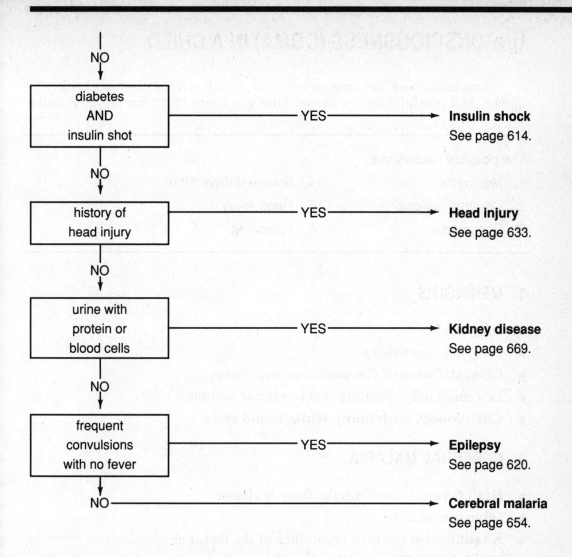

NO
↓

| diabetes AND insulin shot | —YES→ | **Insulin shock** See page 614. |

NO
↓

| history of head injury | —YES→ | **Head injury** See page 633. |

NO
↓

| urine with protein or blood cells | —YES→ | **Kidney disease** See page 669. |

NO
↓

| frequent convulsions with no fever | —YES→ | **Epilepsy** See page 620. |

NO———————————————→ **Cerebral malaria** See page 654.

UNCONSCIOUSNESS (COMA) IN A CHILD

Unconsciousness, or coma, comes from a very serious disease. Look quickly and carefully for the cause. Give good care to the unconscious child.

The possible causes are:

1. Meningitis
2. Cerebral malaria
3. Pneumonia
4. Severe dehydration
5. Head injury
6. Poisoning

1. MENINGITIS

- **High fever**.
- Frequent convulsions.
- Often **stiffness of the neck**, but not always.
- In a small baby, swelling of the anterior fontanel.
- **CSF cloudy, with many white blood cells**.

2. CEREBRAL MALARIA

- **High fever**. Sometimes the fever is absent.
- Often convulsions.
- No stiffness of the neck or swelling of the fontanel.
- **Thick blood film positive for plasmodium**.
- CSF clear, with no white blood cells.
- Sometimes a big spleen, but not always.

3. PNEUMONIA

- **Signs of dyspnea**:
  - Rapid breathing, 40 times per minute or more.
  - Retraction of the lower ribs and between the ribs during inspiration.
  - Dilating of the openings of the nose during inspiration.
- **High fever**. The fever is sometimes absent.

- The coma comes because little air goes from the lungs into the blood and then into the brain. Coma in pneumonia is a very serious sign.

4. SEVERE DEHYDRATION - SEE PAGE 171

- From severe diarrhea or vomiting, or from a burn.
- **Mouth dry**.
- **Skin dry**, with many folds. The skin is no longer elastic.
- **Eyes dry**, sunken deep in the eye sockets, with no tears.
- Little or no urine for many hours.

5. HEAD INJURY

- **History of a recent fall or blow to the head**.
- Often a loss of consciousness for a short time right after the fall or blow.
- Sometimes signs of injury, or a wound.
- No fever or stiff neck.
- Often vomiting; sometimes convulsions.

6. POISONING

- **History of the child having eaten or drunk too much medicine or a poisonous substance**.
- Sometimes convulsions.
- No fever or stiffness of the neck.

SYMPTOMATIC TREATMENT OF COMA IN A CHILD

1. Keep the child in bed and very quiet. Put a good mattress on the bed.
2. Keep the bed and the bedding clean. Give regular baths to the child.
3. Turn him from one side to the other every 3 hours. This will keep him from getting bed sores.
4. Give him much liquid by vein, rectal infusion, or stomach tube.
5. If he has convulsions, give him treatment for convulsions: page 424.
6. If he stays in coma for more than 12 hours, send him to hospital.

TO MAKE THE DIAGNOSIS

In the history, ask the parents:

- When did the child lose consciousness?
- Was there a fever?
- Were there convulsions? Vomiting? Diarrhea?
- Has he had a strong cough? Or trouble breathing?
- Did he fall? Was there a blow to his head? If so, did he lose consciousness right after the fall or the blow?
- Did he swallow too much medicine? Or another poisonous substance?

In the physical exam, look for:

- Fever.
- Stiffness of the neck.
- Swelling of the anterior fontanel.
- A big spleen.
- Signs of dyspnea:
  - Rapid breathing.
  - Retraction of the lower ribs or between the ribs during inspiration.
  - Dilating of the openings of the nose during inspiration.
- Signs of dehydration:
  - Dry mouth.
  - Dry skin with many folds and loss of elasticity.
  - Dry sunken eyes, with no tears.
- Signs of a head injury.

In the laboratory, do:

- A thick blood film to look for plasmodium.
- A lumbar puncture to look for white blood cells .

UNCONSCIOUSNESS (COMA) IN A CHILD

Possible causes

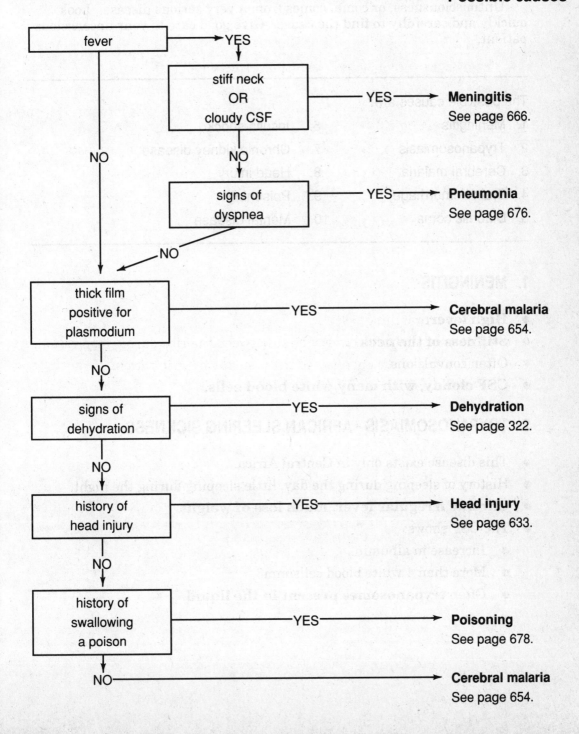

fever → **YES** → stiff neck OR cloudy CSF → **YES** → **Meningitis** See page 666.

stiff neck OR cloudy CSF → **NO** → signs of dyspnea → **YES** → **Pneumonia** See page 676.

fever → **NO**

signs of dyspnea → **NO**

thick film positive for plasmodium → **YES** → **Cerebral malaria** See page 654.

thick film positive for plasmodium → **NO**

signs of dehydration → **YES** → **Dehydration** See page 322.

signs of dehydration → **NO**

history of head injury → **YES** → **Head injury** See page 633.

history of head injury → **NO**

history of swallowing a poison → **YES** → **Poisoning** See page 678.

history of swallowing a poison → **NO** → **Cerebral malaria** See page 654.

UNCONSCIOUSNESS (COMA) IN AN ADULT

Unconsciousness, or coma, comes from a very serious disease. Look quickly and carefully to find the cause. Give good care to your unconscious patient.

The possible causes are:

1.	Meningitis	6.	Insulin shock
2.	Trypanosomiasis	7.	Chronic kidney disease
3.	Cerebral malaria	8.	Head injury
4.	Brain hemorrhage	9.	Poisoning
5.	Diabetic coma	10.	Mental disease

---

1. MENINGITIS

- **High fever**.
- **Stiffness of the neck**.
- Often convulsions.
- **CSF cloudy, with many white blood cells**.

2. TRYPANOSOMIASIS - AFRICAN SLEEPING SICKNESS

- This disease exists only in Central Africa.
- History of sleeping during the day, little sleeping during the night.
- **Chronic irregular fever, much loss of weight**.
- The CSF shows:
  - Increase in albumin.
  - More than 4 white blood cells/mm3.
  - Often **trypanosomes present in the liquid**.

3. CEREBRAL MALARIA

- Sudden loss of consciousness.
- **High fever**. Sometimes the fever is absent.
- No stiffness of the neck.
- **Thick blood film positive for plasmodium**.
- CSF clear, with no white blood cells.

4. BRAIN HEMORRHAGE

- **High blood pressure**, above 160/100.
- Often paralysis of a leg, an arm, one side of the face, or an eye.
- Sometimes stiffness of the neck.
- **CSF pink or yellow, with many red blood cells**.

5. DIABETIC COMA

- **History of diabetes**, or of passing very much urine.
- Breathing very deep and rapid.
- Dehydration.
- **Sugar in the urine**.

6. INSULIN SHOCK

- **History of diabetes**.
- **An injection of insulin a few hours before**. The patient has eaten little or no food since the injection.
- Slow pulse, moist skin, pupils dilated.
- Often convulsions.
- There is usually no sugar in the urine.

7. CHRONIC KIDNEY DISEASE

- Breathing very deep and rapid.
- **Protein, and often white or red blood cells in the urine**.
- **Swelling** of the feet, the legs, the abdomen, or the face.
- Often high blood pressure of more than 150/100.

8. HEAD INJURY

- **History of a recent accident with a blow to the head**.
- Often a loss of consciousness for a short time right after the blow.
- Sometimes convulsions and sometimes a paralysis.
- No fever or stiffness of the neck.

9. POISONING

- **History of having swallowed too much medicine or another poisonous substance**, or of having an injection just before the start of the coma.
- Sometimes a history of having drunk a large amount of alcoholic drink.
- No fever and no stiff neck.

10. MENTAL DISEASE

- History of many problems or much worry.
- Or a history of a **sudden severe psychological difficulty**.
- No fever or stiff neck.
- No signs of severe or chronic disease.

SYMPTOMATIC TREATMENT OF COMA IN AN ADULT

1. Keep the patient in bed and very quiet. Put a good mattress on the bed.
2. Keep the bed and the bedding clean. Give him regular baths.
3. Turn him from one side to the other every 3 hours. This will keep him from getting bed sores.
4. Give him much liquid, either by vein, by rectal infusion, or by stomach tube.
5. If he has convulsions, give him treatment for convulsions. See page 430.
6. If he stays in coma for more than 12 hours, send him to hospital.

TO MAKE THE DIAGNOSIS

In the history, ask the relatives of the patient:
- When did the patient lose consciousness?
- Did it happen quickly, or slowly over some days?
- Did something happen that could have caused this coma?
- Has he had convulsions?
- Does he sleep much during the day and only a little at night?
- Does he receive treatment for a chronic disease, like high blood pressure, kidney disease, diabetes, sleeping sickness?
- Has he recently had an accident or a blow to the head?
- Has he just taken some medicine, or just had an injection?
- Has he swallowed much medicine, or another substance that could be poisonous?
- Has he just drunk much alcoholic drink?
- Does he seem to have many serious problems, or worries?
- Has he just had a very severe difficulty in his life? Or in his family? Or at work? Or in the home?

In the physical exam, look for:
- Fever.
- High blood pressure.
- Stiff neck.
- Deep rapid respirations.
- Signs of dehydration.
- Signs of weight loss.
- Swelling of the feet, the legs, the abdomen, or the face.
- Signs of head injury.
- Paralysis of a leg, an arm, one side of the face, or an eye.

In the laboratory, do:
- A thick blood film to look for plasmodium.
- A urine exam to look for sugar, protein, white or red blood cells.
- A lumbar puncture to look for white or red blood cells and trypanosomes.

UNCONSCIOUSNESS (COMA) IN AN ADULT

Possible causes

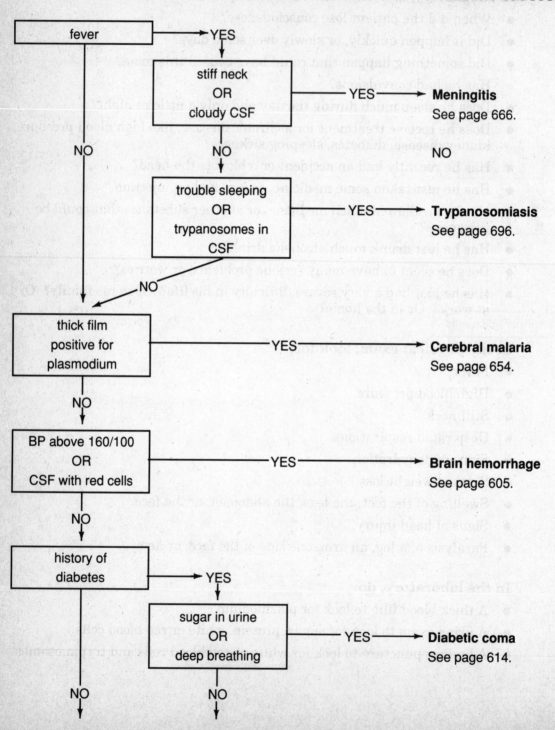

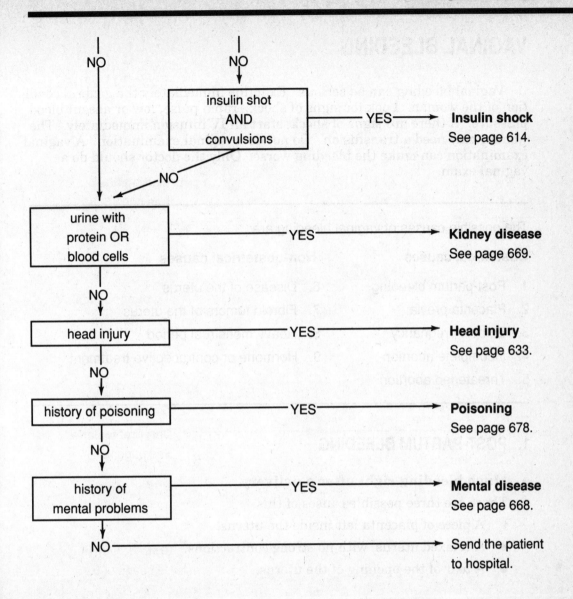

NO   NO

insulin shot
AND
convulsions ──── YES ──→ **Insulin shock**
                          See page 614.

        NO

urine with
protein OR   ──────── YES ──────→ **Kidney disease**
blood cells   See page 669.

   NO

head injury ──────── YES ──────→ **Head injury**
                                  See page 633.

   NO

history of poisoning ──── YES ──→ **Poisoning**
                                  See page 678.

   NO

history of
mental problems ──── YES ──→ **Mental disease**
                             See page 668.

   NO ──────────────────────→ Send the patient
                              to hospital.

VAGINAL BLEEDING

Vaginal bleeding can be serious. Examine immediately the general condition of the woman. Look for signs of shock: rapid pulse, low or absent blood pressure. If there are signs of shock, start an IV infusion immediately. The woman may need a transfusion. Do not do a vaginal examination. A vaginal examination can make the bleeding worse. Only the doctor should do a vaginal exam.

The possible causes of vaginal bleeding are:

Obstetrical causes

1. Post-partum bleeding
2. Placenta previa
3. Ectopic pregnancy
4. Incomplete abortion
5. Threatened abortion

Non-obstetrical causes

6. Disease of the uterus
7. Fibroid tumors of the uterus
8. Heavy menstrual period
9. Hormone or contraceptive treatment

---

1. POST-PARTUM BLEEDING

- **Much bleeding right after a delivery**.
- There are three possible causes of this:
  - A piece of placenta left inside the uterus.
  - A relaxed uterus, with no strong contractions.
  - A tear of the opening of the uterus.

2. PLACENTA PREVIA

- This occurs during **the last three months of the pregnancy**. We call this period the last trimester.
- There may be much vaginal bleeding, or only a little.
- Send to hospital **immediately** any woman in the last trimester of pregnancy who has vaginal bleeding. Do this even if there is only a little bleeding. DO NOT DO A VAGINAL EXAMINATION.

3. ECTOPIC PREGNANCY

- The pregnancy develops outside of the uterus, in the tube or in the abdominal cavity. During the first trimester, the pregnancy ruptures. There is bleeding inside the abdomen. This causes signs of peritonitis, with no signs of infection. Sometimes there is also vaginal bleeding.

- **History of no periods for one or more months**. But the history of menstrual periods is often not correct. So think about the possibility of a ruptured ectopic pregnancy in any woman who has vaginal bleeding during her reproductive years.

- **Abdomen very tender, with rebound pain**.

- **Signs of anemia**: pale color, rapid pulse, low or absent blood pressure, low hemoglobin.

- Swelling of the abdomen.

- No fever.

4. INCOMPLETE ABORTION

- **History of no periods for one month or more**.

- **Severe pain in the lower abdomen**, no tenderness or rebound pain.

- Much vaginal bleeding.

5. THREATENED ABORTION

- **History of no periods for one month or more**.

- **Some pain in the lower abdomen**, with no tenderness.

- Only a little vaginal bleeding.

6. DISEASE OF THE UTERUS

- **Vaginal bleeding coming when there is no menstrual period**.

- Any woman after her menopause who has vaginal bleeding must go **immediately** to the doctor. She may have cancer.

7. FIBROID TUMORS OF THE UTERUS

- Often an increase in the bleeding during menstrual periods.

- **An irregular hard mass in the lower abdomen**.

- Often the woman has no children, or only one or two.

8. HEAVY MENSTRUAL PERIOD

- **Much bleeding during one or more menstrual periods**.
- There are many possible causes of this. Send the woman to the doctor.

9. HORMONE OR CONTRACEPTIVE TREATMENT

- These products can change the working of the ovaries and of the uterus. They can increase or decrease menstrual bleeding. They can even cause vaginal bleeding when there is no period. So ask the woman with vaginal bleeding if she is taking hormone or contraceptive treatment. If so, and if there is much bleeding, send her to the doctor.

TO MAKE THE DIAGNOSIS

In the history, ask:
- How long have you been bleeding?
- Have you just had a baby?
- Are you pregnant? If so, how many months is the pregnancy?
- Do you have pain in the abdomen? If so, where is it? When did it start?
- Do you have periods every month? If so, are they normal?
- Does your vaginal bleeding come just during your periods?
- Or does it come when you do not have a period?
- Have you missed any periods? If so, how many?
- How many children do you have?
- Do you take any medicines regularly? If so, which ones? What for? Since when? Who prescribed them for you?
- Do you take contraceptive medicines to keep from becoming pregnant?

In the physical exam, look for:
- Signs of anemia: pale color, rapid pulse, low or absent blood pressure.
- Tenderness in the abdomen.
- Rebound pain in the abdomen.
- A pregnancy: how many months?
- Another mass in the abdomen.

In the laboratory, do:
- A hemoglobin exam.

VAGINAL BLEEDING

Possible causes

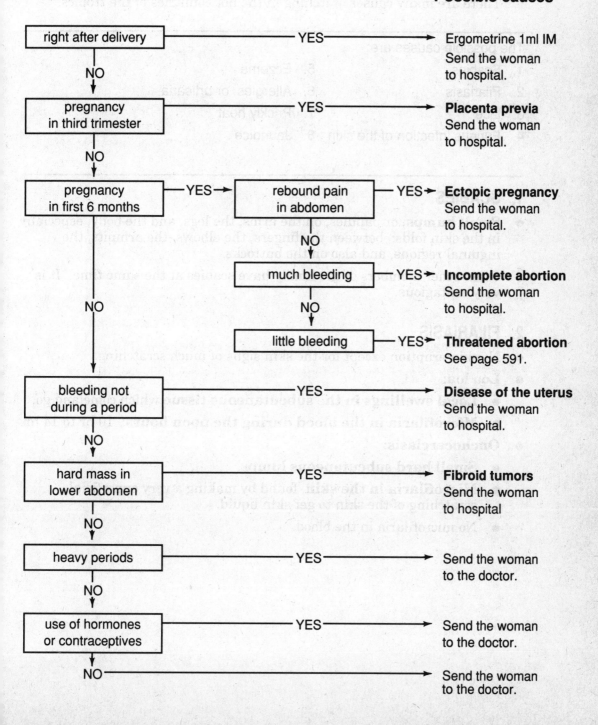

ITCHING

There are many causes of itching in the hot countries of the tropics.

The possible causes are:

1. Scabies
2. Filariasis
3. Lice
4. Fungus infection of the skin

5. Eczema
6. Allergies, or urticaria
7. Prickly heat
8. Jaundice

---

1. SCABIES

- **Small bumps,** or papules, on the arms, the legs, and the body, especially in the skin folds: between the fingers, the elbows, the armpits, the inguinal regions, and also on the buttocks.

- Often other members of the family have scabies at the same time. It is very contagious.

2. FILARIASIS

- No skin eruption except for the skin signs of much scratching.

- **Loa loa:**
  - **Local swellings in the subcutaneous tissue** which come and go.
  - **Microfilaria in the blood during the noon hours:** 10 hr to 14 hr.

- **Onchocerciasis:**
  - **Small hard subcutaneous lumps.**
  - **Microfilaria in the skin,** found by making a very superficial scratching of the skin to get skin liquid.
  - No microfilaria in the blood.

3. LICE

- **Small insects living in the hairy regions of the body**: the head, the armpits, the pubic region.
- Small bumps, or papules, in the regions that itch.

4. FUNGUS INFECTION OF THE SKIN

- **Large chronic plaques, dry, with a definite edge or border** - see figure on page 118.
- Much itching in these plaques.
- The infection is often on the buttocks, in the inguinal, pubic, or femoral regions, or under the armpits or the breasts.

5. ECZEMA

- A bacterial infection of the skin.
- **A large acute plaque, with liquid secretions and often pustules**.
- Pain in the plaque.
- Often **fever**.
- Often tender lymph nodes in the area.

6. ALLERGY - URTICARIA

- **Big irregular bumps in the skin**, with much itching.
- They come quickly and go away after a few hours.

7. PRICKLY HEAT

- **Very small bumps in areas where there is much sweating**: under the armpits or breasts, the neck, around the waist.
- Much itching, made worse by sweating.
- The bumps are swellings of the sweat glands.

8. JAUNDICE

- Deep jaundice can cause general itching over the whole body.
- There is no skin eruption.
- Yellow color of the eyes, the mucus membranes, and even of the skin.
- Often a big tender liver.

SYMPTOMATIC TREATMENT OF ITCHING

1. It is important to keep the skin clean, especially when there is an eruption. A daily bath with soap and water is necessary.
2. The patient must dry the skin well after each bath.
3. Talcum powder on the dry skin will help keep the skin from itching.
4. The best treatment for the itching is the specific treatment for the disease causing the itching.
5. There are other lotions and ointments which can help stop the itching, such as those with menthol or an antihistamine like promethazine.
6. The patient must keep his finger nails short and clean. He must try not to scratch the itching places.

TO MAKE THE DIAGNOSIS

In the history, ask:

- When did the itching start?
- Where do you itch?
- Are there others in your family who itch also?
- Do you have swellings that come and go? If so, where? On the skin? Or under the skin? How long do they stay?
- Have you had fever? Or jaundice?

In the physical exam, look for:

- Small bumps or papules on the skin: Where are they?
- Small hard lumps in the subcutaneous tissues.
- Small crawling insects (lice) in the hairy regions of the body.
- One or more large plaques in the skin, with much itching.
  - Are they acute or chronic?
  - Are they dry with a definite border?
  - Are there secretions from the plaques?
  - Is there pain in the plaques?
  - Are there tender lymph nodes in the region?
- Big irregular bumps in the skin coming quickly and going away soon.
- Fever.
- Jaundice.
- A big tender liver.

In the laboratory, do:

- A fresh blood drop exam during the noon hours to look for microfilaria.
- A skin scratch test to look for microfilaria. Do this near one of the lumps in the subcutaneous tissue.

ITCHING

Possible causes

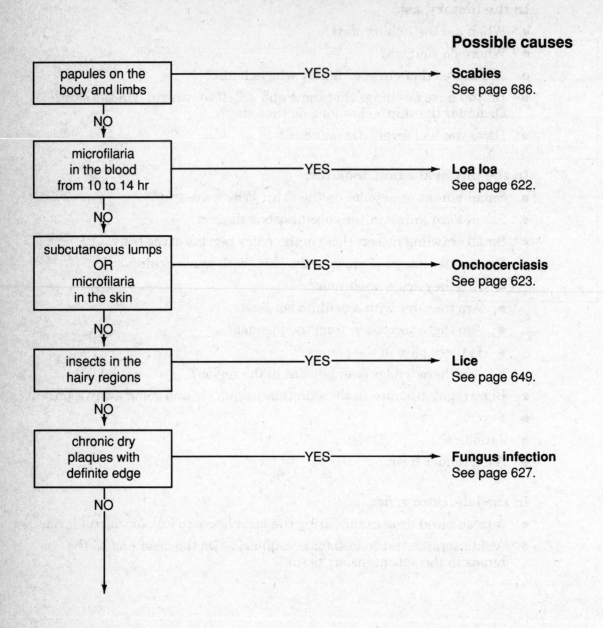

papules on the body and limbs —YES→ **Scabies** See page 686.

NO

microfilaria in the blood from 10 to 14 hr —YES→ **Loa loa** See page 622.

NO

subcutaneous lumps OR microfilaria in the skin —YES→ **Onchocerciasis** See page 623.

NO

insects in the hairy regions —YES→ **Lice** See page 649.

NO

chronic dry plaques with definite edge —YES→ **Fungus infection** See page 627.

NO

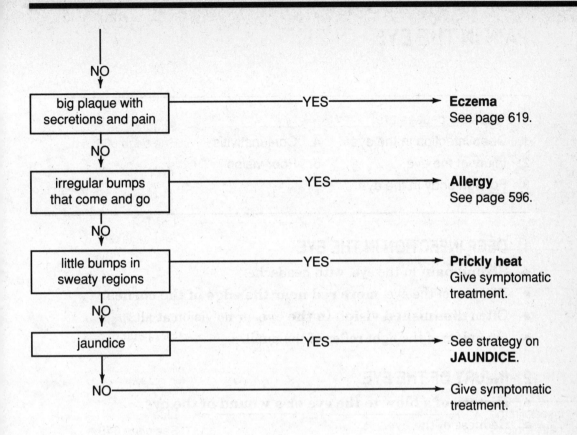

NO

big plaque with secretions and pain ──────YES──────→ **Eczema**
See page 619.

NO

irregular bumps that come and go ──────YES──────→ **Allergy**
See page 596.

NO

little bumps in sweaty regions ──────YES──────→ **Prickly heat**
Give symptomatic treatment.

NO

jaundice ──────YES──────→ See strategy on **JAUNDICE**.

NO──────────────────────────────→ Give symptomatic treatment.

PAIN IN THE EYE

The possible causes are:

1. Deep infection in the eye
2. Injury of the eye
3. Foreign body in the eye
4. Conjunctivitis
5. Poor vision

1. DEEP INFECTION IN THE EYE

- **Strong pain** in the eye, with headache.
- Redness of the eye, **more red near the edge of the cornea**.
- Often **diminished vision in the eye**, or no vision at all.
- Often loss of the light reflex of the pupil.

2. INJURY OF THE EYE

- **History of a blow to the eye or a wound of the eye**.
- Redness of the eye.
- Often a wound of the lid, of the conjunctiva, or of the cornea.

3. FOREIGN BODY IN THE EYE

- **History of something going into the eye**.
- Feeling of scratching in the eye.
- Sometimes redness of the eye.
- **A small piece of matter on the cornea, or in the conjunctival sack**.

4. CONJUNCTIVITIS

- Redness of one or both eyes, **more red away from the cornea**.

- Feeling of scratching in the eye.
- Sometimes trouble seeing.

5. POOR VISION

- Little or no redness of the eye.
- **Difficulty seeing objects clearly**.
- Pain worse after reading, studying.
- Often headache in the forehead, or in the back of the head.

TO MAKE THE DIAGNOSIS

In the history, ask:

- When did your eye, or eyes, start hurting?
- What treatment have you already had?
- Has something hit your eye?
- Has anything gone into your eye?
- Do you have trouble seeing with that eye?
- Do you have trouble reading, or seeing clearly things that are far away?
- Do you frequently have headaches?

In the physical exam, look for:

- Redness of the eye. Is there more redness near the cornea? Or is it more away from the cornea and in the conjunctival sack?
- The light reflex of the pupil. Is it present or absent? See page 70.
- A wound of the eye.
- Look very carefully at the cornea and in the conjunctival sack for a small piece of matter. Look inside both upper and lower eyelids. Use a good light to do this.
- Do a vision test on each eye. See page 71.

In the laboratory, do:

- In a region where there is onchocerciasis, do a skin scratch test near the clavicle or near the iliac crest. Look for microfilaria. Microfilaria of onchocerciasis can cause eye trouble.

PAIN IN THE EYE

Possible causes

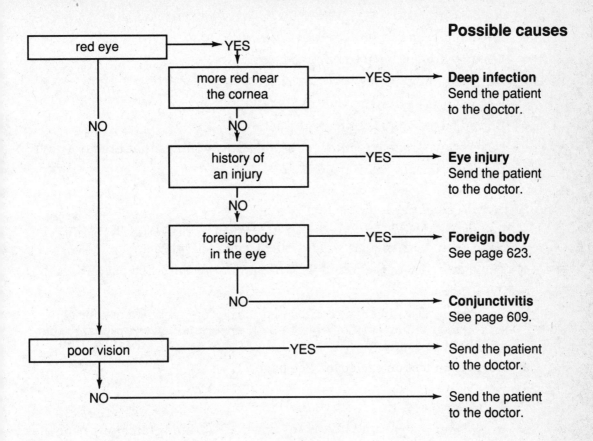

Deep infection
Send the patient
to the doctor.

Eye injury
Send the patient
to the doctor.

Foreign body
See page 623.

Conjunctivitis
See page 609.

Send the patient
to the doctor.

Send the patient
to the doctor.

Chapter 9
STRATEGIES FOR SIGNS

FEVER

Fever is a very frequent sign of disease. Very often the fever is a sign of an infection. Most often the patient will have other symptoms and signs of disease. Follow the strategies of the other symptoms and signs of the patient. In this way you will almost always find the disease causing the fever. So take a good history. Do a careful physical examination. Do any necessary laboratory exams to make the diagnosis certain.

TO MAKE THE DIAGNOSIS

In the history, ask:

- How long have you had a fever? For a few days? Or for some weeks or months?

- What is the fever like? Very high, or not high?

- How did the fever start? Suddenly? Or slowly over some days?

- Is it present all the time? Or does it come and go?

- Have you often had attacks of fever in the past?

- Have you had chills with the fever? Or much sweating at night?

- What treatment have you already taken for the fever or the disease?

- Have you had other symptoms, like:

  - Sore throat, earache?

  - Cough, trouble breathing, pain in the chest?

  - Pain in the abdomen, vomiting, diarrhea, jaundice?

  - Pain on urinating, frequent urination, difficulty in urinating, pus or blood in the urine?

  - Headache, convulsions, stiff neck, unconsciousness?

  - Pain elsewhere, loss of weight, swelling, secretions from the vagina?

- Do a good review of systems. Follow the strategy of each important symptom the patient has.

In the physical exam, look for:
- The seriousness of the fever. Is it high or low?
- Other signs of disease:
  - Stiffness of the neck or, in a small baby, a swollen fontanel.
  - Pus in the ear canal.
  - Redness of the throat, or white spots of pus in the throat or on the tonsils.
  - Painful swellings or tender lymph nodes.
  - Signs of dyspnea: rapid breathing and, in a small child, retraction of the ribs and dilating of the openings of the nose with breathing.
  - Crackles in the lungs.
  - Tenderness in the abdomen: where is it?
  - Rebound tenderness in the abdomen.
  - Big or tender liver, or jaundice.
  - Mass in the abdomen. Where is it? What is it like?
  - Swelling or tenderness in a limb or in a joint.
- Follow the strategy for each sign you find.

In the laboratory, do:
- A thick blood film to look for malaria.
- A urine exam to look for protein and white or red blood cells.
- A white blood cell count. A high white blood cell count, above 10,000/mm3, is a sign of a bacterial infection.
- A lumbar puncture if there are:
  - Fever and convulsions.
  - Fever and stiffness of the neck or a swollen fontanel.
  - Chronic fever with headache, convulsions, or coma.
- 3 sputum exams for tubercle bacilli if the patient has a cough with sputum.

SYMPTOMATIC TREATMENT OF FEVER

1. In a region where there is much malaria, there is a temptation to give malaria treatment to everyone who has fever. This is not good treatment. It will help the plasmodium become resistant to treatment. So always do a thick blood film first. Give malaria treatment only to patients who have plasmodium in the blood. Always give a complete cure. An incomplete cure is another cause for malaria to become resistant to treatment.

2. Be careful about giving treatment with antibiotics. Give antibiotics only when you find an infection which antibiotics will treat. Antibiotics do not take away fever. They do not act against infections from a virus like measles, hepatitis, polio, a cold, flu, or grippe.

3. Fever can be dangerous for a small child. It can cause convulsions. In a child with a fever of 39° or more, give him a cool bath for 15 minutes. This will help bring down the fever. It will help prevent convulsions. Give him aspirin, 10 mg/kg every 4 hours if necessary.

4. A patient with a high fever loses much water by sweating. He will soon become dehydrated. The dehydration will make the fever worse. So give him much liquid to drink: water, tea, or breast milk to a small baby. If necessary, give liquid by rectal infusion or by IV infusion.

Sometimes a patient has a disease that usually causes a fever. But he has no fever at the time of the consultation. There are 4 possible reasons for this:

1. A treatment already received at home or elsewhere that makes the fever go away: aspirin, chloroquine, an antibiotic.

2. Malnutrition, old age, a chronic disease. The patient's body is weak and does not develop a fever even when there is an infection.

3. The infection, such as a chronic abscess or chronic hepatitis, has been present a long time. The body of the patient is used to the infection and no longer develops a fever.

4. The fever is irregular, and you have examined the patient at a moment when the fever is not present. This can happen with tuberculosis, trypanosomiasis, kidney infection, a chronic abscess. In this case, it is important to take the temperature at least 3 times during the day, sometimes for several days. Write down the temperature each time. Then you can see what happens to the temperature during several days.

WEIGHT LOSS IN A CHILD

The possible causes are:

1. Malnutrition
2. Tuberculosis
3. Another infection
4. A chronic disease
5. Intestinal worms

1. MALNUTRITION

This is the most frequent cause of weight loss in small children. Loss of weight is the first sign of malnutrition. It comes before the other signs come.

1. **Protein-calorie malnutrition** - kwashiorkor.
   - Changes in the color of the skin and the hair.
   - Loss of interest in playing.
   - Swelling of the feet, the legs, and the face.
2. **Marasmus** - starvation.
   - History of famine or lack of all kinds of food.
   - Severe weight loss.
   - No swelling and no changes in the color of the skin or hair.

2. TUBERCULOSIS

This is a difficult diagnosis to make in a child. Only the doctor can make this diagnosis. Send to the doctor any child who has:

- A **chronic fever** that does not respond to other treatment.
- A respiratory infection that does not respond to penicillin or other antibiotics.
- Weight loss or malnutrition that does not improve with good food.
- **Another member of the family who has, or who has had, tuberculosis.**

3. ANOTHER INFECTION

● Measles, whooping cough, pneumonia, severe diarrhea, or another chronic infection can cause much loss of weight. The infection keeps the child from eating well. So he loses weight.

● **Symptoms and signs of the infection**.

4. A CHRONIC DISEASE - CIRRHOSIS, TUMOR

● Big liver, or big mass in the abdomen.

● Big lymph nodes.

5. INTESTINAL WORMS

● Especially ascaris, hookworm, and tapeworm.

● The weight loss comes because the child does not absorb the food he eats.

● **Worm eggs or larva in the stools**.

● Sometimes anemia.

TO MAKE THE DIAGNOSIS

In the history, ask:

- When did the child start to lose weight?

- Does he have a fever? A cough? Trouble breathing?

- Has he recently had measles, whooping cough, pneumonia, severe diarrhea, or another disease?

- If so, what was the treatment? What was the result of the treatment?

- Is there anyone in your family who has tuberculosis, or who has had it in the recent past?

In the physical exam, look for:

- Signs of malnutrition.

- Fever. It may be necessary to take the temperature of the child three times a day for several days. Write down the temperature each time. Then you can see if he has a fever and how much it is.

- Big lymph nodes.

- Signs of dyspnea, or crackles in the lungs.

- Skin eruption.

- Abscess, tender mass somewhere, mass in the abdomen.

- Big liver or spleen.

In the laboratory, do:

- A hemoglobin exam.

- A stool exam to look for worm eggs or larva.

- A urine exam to look for protein and white or red blood cells.

WEIGHT LOSS IN A CHILD

Possible causes

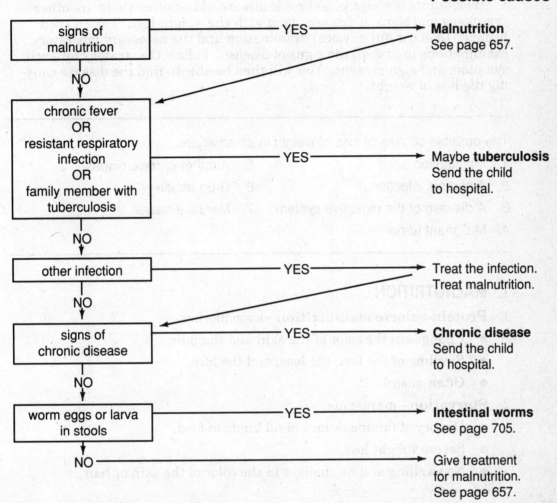

signs of
malnutrition
— YES → **Malnutrition**
See page 657.

NO ↓

chronic fever
OR
resistant respiratory
infection
OR
family member with
tuberculosis
— YES → Maybe **tuberculosis**
Send the child
to hospital.

NO ↓

other infection
— YES → Treat the infection.
Treat malnutrition.

NO ↓

signs of
chronic disease
— YES → **Chronic disease**
Send the child
to hospital.

NO ↓

worm eggs or larva
in stools
— YES → **Intestinal worms**
See page 705.

NO → Give treatment
for malnutrition.
See page 657.

WEIGHT LOSS IN AN ADULT

Weight loss is a sign of a chronic disease. Most often there are other symptoms and signs of disease along with the weight loss. Take a good history. Do a careful physical examination and the necessary laboratory examinations to find all the signs of disease. Follow the strategy for each symptom and sign present. You will then be able to find the disease causing the loss of weight.

The possible causes of loss of weight in an adult are:

1. Malnutrition
2. A chronic infection
3. A disease of the digestive system
4. Malignant tumor
5. Another chronic disease
6. Drug abuse
7. Mental disease

---

1. MALNUTRITION

1. **Protein-calorie malnutrition** - kwashiorkor.
   - Changes in the color of the skin and the hair.
   - Swelling of the feet, the legs, and the face.
   - Often anemia.

2. **Starvation** - marasmus.
   - History of famine or lack of all kinds of food.
   - Severe weight loss.
   - No swelling and no changes in the color of the skin or hair.

2. A CHRONIC INFECTION

- **Tuberculosis**: chronic cough, sputum often with blood, dyspnea, pain in the chest, chronic irregular fever.
- **Kidney infection**: protein and white blood cells in the urine.
- **Trypanosomiasis**: chronic fever, mental troubles, CSF with some white cells and often trypanosomes.
- **Intestinal worms**: pain or colic in the abdomen, worm eggs or larva in the stools.

- **Abscess or other chronic infection**.
- **AIDS**: chronic fever, chronic diarrhea, chronic big lymph nodes.

3. A DISEASE OF THE DIGESTIVE SYSTEM

- Chronic gastritis, peptic ulcer.
- Chronic diarrhea: amebiasis, tuberculosis, intestinal parasites.
- **Symptoms and signs of the digestive system**.

4. MALIGNANT TUMOR

- Liver, stomach, uterus, lymph nodes, or elsewhere.
- **Hard, irregular mass** in the abdomen, in the liver, in lymph nodes, in the neck, or elsewhere.
- Often pain associated with the mass.
- Sometimes chronic bleeding: from the vagina, from the stomach, in the stools.
- Sometimes chronic diarrhea.

5. ANOTHER CHRONIC DISEASE

- **Heart failure**: dyspnea, cough, rapid pulse, swelling of the feet and legs, crackles in the lungs.
- **Diabetes**: sugar in the urine, much urine.
- **Cirrhosis**: big hard liver, ascites, swelling of the feet and legs.
- **Hyperthyroidism**: rapid pulse, trembling of the hands, lack of sleep (insomnia), sometimes a goiter, sometimes bulging eyes.

6. DRUG ABUSE - ALCOHOLISM, USE OF DRUGS, USE OF HEMP

- No desire to eat, to work, or to keep clean.
- The weight loss comes because the patient prefers to drink or to use drugs rather than to eat.

7. MENTAL DISEASE

- Much stress, many worries, fear, sadness, or a real mental illness (psychosis).
- The patient does not want to eat. This is why the patient loses weight.

TO MAKE THE DIAGNOSIS

In the history, ask:
- How are you eating? Is it difficult to find enough to eat?
- What did you eat today? What did you eat yesterday?
- How many times each week do you eat meat? Fish? Corn? Groundnuts? Other sources of protein?
- Do you often have a fever?
- Do you have a cough?
- Do you have sputum? If so, what is it like?
- Do you have trouble breathing, pain in the chest, swelling of your feet or legs?
- Do you have heart burn, vomiting, diarrhea, pain in your abdomen, blood in your stools, jaundice?
- Do you have pain when urinating, much urine, blood or pus in the urine?
- Do you have pain elsewhere, a swelling or lump, headache, dizziness, convulsions, trembling of the hands, trouble sleeping?
- Have you had any bleeding from the nose, the mouth, the rectum, the vagina?
- Do you drink much alcoholic drinks? Do you use drugs? Hemp? To find out about this, you must often ask another member of the patient's family about this.
- Ask questions about stress, worries, bad dreams, other problems.

In the physical exam, look for:
- Fever, rapid pulse.
- Signs of malnutrition.
- Big lymph nodes.
- Dyspnea, crackles in the lungs.
- Big liver, big spleen.
- Mass in the abdomen.

- Swelling of the feet, the legs, the abdomen, the face.
- Other lumps or masses.
- A goiter, or fine trembling of the hands.

In the laboratory, do:
- A hemoglobin exam.
- A stool exam to look for worm eggs or larva, or other parasites.
- A urine exam to look for sugar, protein, or blood cells.
- 3 sputum exams to look for TB bacilli if there is a cough with sputum.
- A lumbar puncture if there are signs of trypanosomiasis or chronic meningitis.

WEIGHT LOSS IN AN ADULT

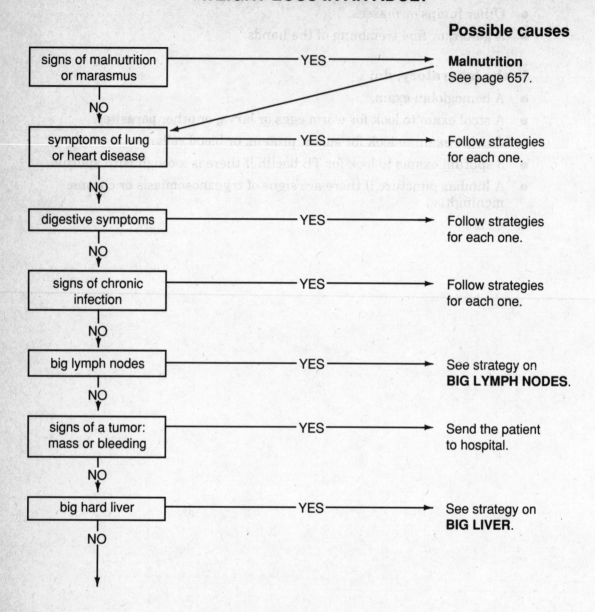

Possible causes

signs of malnutrition or marasmus — YES → **Malnutrition** See page 657.

NO

symptoms of lung or heart disease — YES → Follow strategies for each one.

NO

digestive symptoms — YES → Follow strategies for each one.

NO

signs of chronic infection — YES → Follow strategies for each one.

NO

big lymph nodes — YES → See strategy on **BIG LYMPH NODES**.

NO

signs of a tumor: mass or bleeding — YES → Send the patient to hospital.

NO

big hard liver — YES → See strategy on **BIG LIVER**.

NO

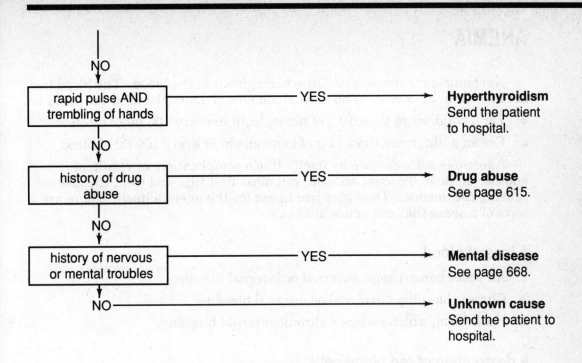

rapid pulse AND trembling of hands ——————YES—————→ **Hyperthyroidism**
Send the patient to hospital.

history of drug abuse ——————YES—————→ **Drug abuse**
See page 615.

history of nervous or mental troubles ——————YES—————→ **Mental disease**
See page 668.

NO ——————————————————————→ **Unknown cause**
Send the patient to hospital.

ANEMIA

Anemia means there is too little hemoglobin in the blood. The blood has become "thin" or "weak." The normal amount of hemoglobin in the blood is:

- For a child, more than 10 g of hemoglobin in every 100 ml of blood.
- For an adult, more than 12 g of hemoglobin in every 100 ml of blood.

Anemia is not a disease by itself. It is a complication, or result, of another disease. To treat anemia, you must first find and treat the disease causing the anemia. Then give treatment for the anemia itself. There are 4 sorts of disease that can cause anemia:

A loss of blood.

1. An acute hemorrhage: external or internal bleeding.
2. Chronic bleeding: external or internal bleeding.
3. Hookworm, which causes a chronic internal bleeding.

A destruction of red blood cells.

We call this a "hemolytic anemia."

1. Malaria. The plasmodium destroy the red blood cells.
2. Sickle cell anemia. The red blood cells are very fragile. They break down very easily inside the blood vessels and are destroyed.

Snake bite

- The snake venom destroys many red blood cells - a hemolytic anemia.
- The snake venom also causes much bleeding into the tissues.

Lack of protein or iron in the diet

These two elements are essential for the body to make hemoglobin. If there is only a little protein or iron in the food, the patient will develop anemia. We call this a "deficiency anemia." It comes in:

1. Malnutrition: a lack of protein.
2. Anemia of pregnancy: a lack of iron and folic acid.
3. A chronic disease.

1. ACUTE EXTERNAL BLEEDING

- **History of recent bleeding**:
  - Vomiting of blood.
  - Vaginal bleeding.
  - Bleeding from the intestine: stools red or black.
  - Hemoptysis: sputum with much blood.
  - A big wound, with much bleeding.
  - Severe nose bleed.
- **Signs of acute anemia**: weakness, rapid pulse, pale color of the mucus membranes, low or absent blood pressure.

2. ACUTE INTERNAL BLEEDING

- **In the abdomen or in the intestine**:
  - Much pain and tenderness in the abdomen.
  - Often rebound tenderness in the abdomen.
- **After an accident with internal injuries**:
  - Fracture of the spine or of the femur, a large burn, injury to the chest or abdomen with bleeding inside.
- Signs of the injury.
- Signs of acute anemia.

3. CHRONIC BLEEDING

- Heavy menstrual periods.
- Other vaginal bleeding.
- Blood in the stools.
- Sputum with blood.
- Frequent nose bleeds.
- A wound or sore that keeps bleeding.

4. HOOKWORM

- Abdominal pain or colic.
- **Hookworm eggs or larva in the stools.**

5. SNAKE BITE

- History of a snake bite in the last few hours.
- Signs of severe acute anemia.
- Often very much swelling near the region of the snake bite.
- Sometimes jaundice.

6. MALARIA

- History of **frequent attacks of fever**.
- **Thick blood film positive for plasmodium during an attack of fever**.
- **Often a big spleen**.

7. SICKLE CELL DISEASE

- This is a disease of children and young adults.
- **History of frequent attacks of anemia and jaundice**.
- Often a history of frequent attacks of pain in the limbs or in the abdomen.
- **Sickle cells in the blood seen in a fresh blood drop exam**.
- Sometimes jaundice.

8. MALNUTRITION

- Weight loss.
- Swelling of the feet, the legs, and often of the face.
- Changes in the color of the skin or the hair.

9. ANEMIA OF PREGNANCY

- Pregnancy between the 4th and the 9th months.
- Pale color of the mucus membranes.
- Sometimes swelling of the feet and legs.

10. CHRONIC DISEASE

- Tuberculosis, chronic infection, chronic kidney disease, malignant tumor, cirrhosis, diabetes.
- Signs of the disease.
- Weight loss, and sometimes a chronic fever.

TO MAKE THE DIAGNOSIS

For a child, in the history, ask the parents:

- Has he been bleeding from anywhere?
- Has he just had an accident? Or been bitten by a snake?
- Does he often have fever? Or jaundice?
- Does he often have pain in the arms or legs? Or in the abdomen?
- Does he have swelling of the feet or legs?
- Has he lost weight?
- Is he often sick?
- Does he have a cough, trouble breathing, diarrhea, vomiting?
- Is he taking treatment for another disease? If so, what? For what disease?

For an adult, ask:

- Have you been bleeding from anywhere? From the vagina? From the stomach? In your stools? In your sputum? From your nose? From a wound or sore?
- Have you just had an accident? Or a snake bite?
- Do you have pain in your abdomen? If so, where? What is it like?
- Do you often have fever? Or jaundice?
- In a woman: are you pregnant? If so, for how many months? Have you been bleeding from the vagina?
- Do you have heavy menstrual periods?
- Do you have fever, weakness, a cough, pain anywhere, diarrhea, trouble urinating, or weight loss?
- Do you have some other serious disease?
- Are you taking treatment for some other disease? If so, what?

In the physical exam, look for:

- Signs of shock: rapid pulse, low or absent blood pressure.
- Bleeding from some place.
- A wound, or a snake bite.
- Much tenderness, or rebound tenderness, in the abdomen.

- Fever, jaundice, a big spleen.
- Signs of malnutrition.
- A pregnancy.
- Signs of a chronic disease: loss of weight, mass in the abdomen, a big liver, swelling of the feet or legs.

In the laboratory, do:

- A hemoglobin exam to see how severe the anemia is.
- A thick blood film to look for plasmodium.
- A fresh blood drop exam to look for sickle cells.
- A stool exam to look for hookworm eggs or larva.
- A urine exam to look for sugar, protein, or blood cells.

REMEMBER:

A patient often has more than one cause of anemia. For example, a patient may have malnutrition and hookworm and even malaria. So with every patient with anemia, look for every possible cause. Give treatment for every cause as well as for the anemia itself.

ANEMIA IN AN ADULT

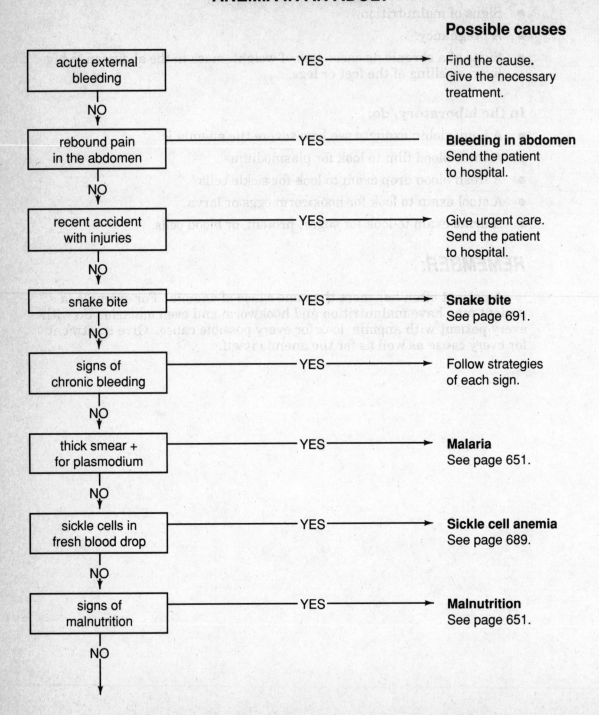

Possible causes

acute external bleeding —— YES ——→ Find the cause.
Give the necessary treatment.

NO

rebound pain in the abdomen —— YES ——→ **Bleeding in abdomen**
Send the patient to hospital.

NO

recent accident with injuries —— YES ——→ Give urgent care.
Send the patient to hospital.

NO

snake bite —— YES ——→ **Snake bite**
See page 691.

NO

signs of chronic bleeding —— YES ——→ Follow strategies of each sign.

NO

thick smear + for plasmodium —— YES ——→ **Malaria**
See page 651.

NO

sickle cells in fresh blood drop —— YES ——→ **Sickle cell anemia**
See page 689.

NO

signs of malnutrition —— YES ——→ **Malnutrition**
See page 651.

NO

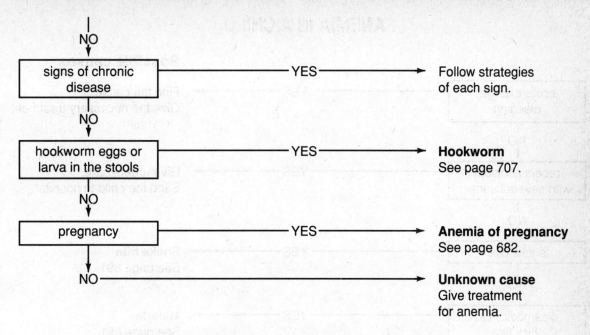

NO		
signs of chronic disease	——YES——→	Follow strategies of each sign.
NO		
hookworm eggs or larva in the stools	——YES——→	**Hookworm** See page 707.
NO		
pregnancy	——YES——→	**Anemia of pregnancy** See page 682.
NO ————————————————————→		**Unknown cause** Give treatment for anemia.

Look for all these causes in every adult patient with anemia.

ANEMIA IN A CHILD

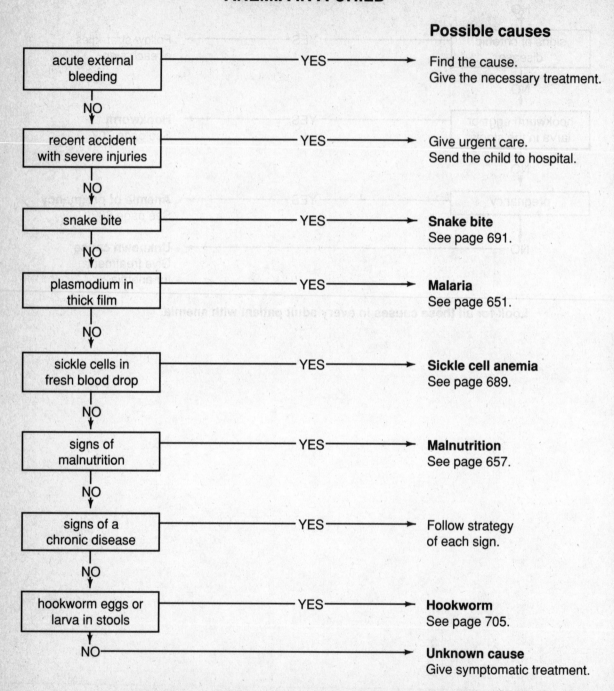

Possible causes

acute external bleeding —YES→ Find the cause.
Give the necessary treatment.

NO

recent accident with severe injuries —YES→ Give urgent care.
Send the child to hospital.

NO

snake bite —YES→ **Snake bite**
See page 691.

NO

plasmodium in thick film —YES→ **Malaria**
See page 651.

NO

sickle cells in fresh blood drop —YES→ **Sickle cell anemia**
See page 689.

NO

signs of malnutrition —YES→ **Malnutrition**
See page 657.

NO

signs of a chronic disease —YES→ Follow strategy
of each sign.

NO

hookworm eggs or larva in stools —YES→ **Hookworm**
See page 705.

NO→ **Unknown cause**
Give symptomatic treatment.

Look for all of these possible causes in every child with anemia.

SYMPTOMATIC TREATMENT OF ANEMIA

1. If the hemoglobin is below 6 g, the patient will probably need a transfusion. If you cannot give it, send him to hospital.

2. In severe anemia, the patient can develop heart failure. In this case, he will need treatment for heart failure. He may also need a transfusion given slowly.

3. The patient must eat food rich in protein and in iron. This will help him make hemoglobin and red blood cells.

4. Some patients will need iron, such as ferrous sulfate:

   - A child needs 10 mg/kg 3 times a day.

   - An adult needs 300 mg 3 times a day.

   If after 2 weeks of treatment the anemia is still serious, send the patient to hospital.

5. Patients with hemolytic anemia do not need iron. Do not give it to them. They have much iron in their body from the destroyed red blood cells.

6. For the anemia of pregnancy, give:

   - Ferrous sulfate, 300 mg 3 times a day.

   - Folic acid, 5 mg 2 times a day to the end of the pregnancy.

   - Instructions to eat food rich in protein every day.

SWELLING (EDEMA) IN A CHILD

The possible causes are:

1. Malnutrition
2. Anemia
3. Heart failure
4. Nephritis
5. Nephrosis
6. Cirrhosis

1. MALNUTRITION

- Malnutrition occurs most often in children from 1 to 6 years old.
- **Loss of weight**. The upper arms become very thin.
- **Changes in the color of the skin and the hair**.
- Swelling of the feet and legs and often of the face.
- Swelling of the abdomen.
- Weakness and loss of interest in playing.
- Sometimes anemia.

2. ANEMIA

- Swelling of the feet and legs and often of the face.
- The swelling in sickle cell anemia is often on the top of the feet and on the back of the hands.
- **Pale color of the mucous membranes**.
- **Hemoglobin below 8 g**.
- Jaundice if it is a hemolytic anemia.

3. HEART FAILURE - SEE CHAPTER 4, PAGE 189

- Swelling is a late sign of heart failure, especially in a baby.
- **Dyspnea**, with rapid respirations of more than 40/minute.
- **Rapid pulse**: more than 120/minute.
- **Big tender liver**.
- Sometimes crackles in the lungs.

4. NEPHRITIS

- **Swelling of the face and eyelids**, and also of the feet and legs.
- Often fever.
- Often high blood pressure: more than 100/60.
- Tenderness in one or both flanks.
- **Red blood cells and often protein in the urine**.

5. NEPHROSIS

- **Very much swelling** of the legs, the arms, the face and the abdomen.
- Often ascites.
- **Much protein in the urine, but no blood cells**.

6. CIRRHOSIS - SEE CHAPTER 4, PAGE 183

- Swelling of the feet and legs and sometimes of the abdomen.
- Liver big, hard, irregular and usually not tender.
- Sometimes ascites.

SYMPTOMATIC TREATMENT OF EDEMA IN A CHILD

1. The most important treatment is the treatment of the disease causing the swelling.
2. The child must eat foods rich in protein - see page 658.
3. Perhaps you will not find the cause. But the child seems very ill. In this case, send him to hospital. If he does not seem very ill, talk to the parents about the food he must eat, foods rich in protein. Do a stool exam to look for worm eggs or larva. Examine him again after one week.

TO MAKE THE DIAGNOSIS

In the history, ask the parents:
- When did the swelling start?
- Has the child lost weight?
- Has he had jaundice? Or pains in the arms and legs?
- Does he have trouble breathing?
- Has he had fever?

In the physical exam, look for:
- Where the swelling is, and how much there is.
- Signs of malnutrition:
  - Weight loss. Are the upper arms very thin?
  - Changes in the color of the skin and hair.
  - Swelling of the abdomen.
  - Ascites.
- Pale color of the mucus membranes, jaundice.
- Signs of heart failure:
  - Signs of dyspnea: rapid respirations, retraction of the ribs, dilating of the openings of the nose during breathing.
  - Rapid pulse.
  - Big tender liver.
  - Crackles in the lungs.
- Fever.
- High blood pressure: more than 100/60.
- Tenderness in the flanks.
- Liver that is big, hard, irregular and not tender.

In the laboratory, do:
- A hemoglobin exam.
- A fresh blood drop exam to look for sickle cells.
- A urine exam to look for protein and for blood cells.

SWELLING (EDEMA) IN A CHILD

Possible causes

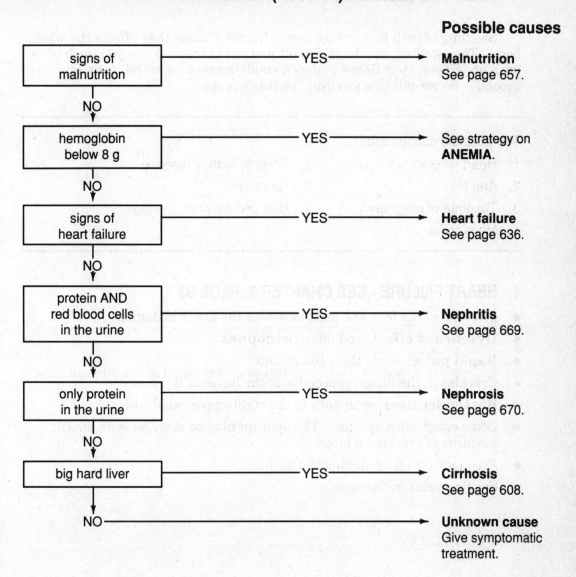

signs of malnutrition	—YES→ **Malnutrition** See page 657.
NO ↓	
hemoglobin below 8 g	—YES→ See strategy on **ANEMIA**.
NO ↓	
signs of heart failure	—YES→ **Heart failure** See page 636.
NO ↓	
protein AND red blood cells in the urine	—YES→ **Nephritis** See page 669.
NO ↓	
only protein in the urine	—YES→ **Nephrosis** See page 670.
NO ↓	
big hard liver	—YES→ **Cirrhosis** See page 608.
NO →	**Unknown cause** Give symptomatic treatment.

SWELLING (EDEMA) IN AN ADULT

Swelling of both feet or legs comes from a disease that affects the whole body. The swelling, or edema, is soft and not tender. When you push on it with one finger, your finger makes a small depression, or pit, for a few seconds. So we call this swelling "pitting edema."

The possible causes are:

1. Heart failure
2. Anemia
3. Toxemia of pregnancy
4. Malnutrition
5. Chronic kidney disease
6. Cirrhosis
7. Bad circulation in the legs

1. HEART FAILURE - SEE CHAPTER 3, PAGE 93

- Swelling of the feet, the legs, and even the lower abdomen.
- **Dyspnea of effort**, and often **orthopnea**.
- **Rapid pulse**: more than 100/minute.
- Crackles in the lungs, especially at the bases of the lungs.
- **Big tender liver**, with pain in the right upper quadrant.
- Often cough with sputum. The sputum may be clear, or with small amounts of red-brown blood.
- Frequent urination during the night.
- Swollen veins in the neck.

2. ANEMIA

- Swelling of the feet and legs and even of the face.
- **Pale color of the mucous membranes**.
- Weakness, dizziness.
- **Hemoglobin below 8 g**.
- If the anemia is severe, there may be signs of heart failure.

3. TOXEMIA OF PREGNANCY - SEE CHAPTER 3, PAGE 128

- Pregnancy in the last three months, the third trimester.
- **Protein in the urine**.
- **High blood pressure: more than 130/90**.
- In any pregnant woman with swelling of the legs, take her blood pressure and do a urine exam to look for protein.

4. MALNUTRITION

- Swelling of the feet, the legs, and often of the face.
- **Signs of weight loss**.
- **Changes in the color of the skin and the hair**.
- Weakness, loss of energy to work.
- Sometimes anemia.

5. CHRONIC KIDNEY DISEASE

- Such as nephritis, pyelonephritis, nephrosis.
- Swelling of the feet, the legs, and even of the face.
- Often high blood pressure.
- **Protein and often red or white blood cells in the urine**.

6. CIRRHOSIS - SEE CHAPTER 3, PAGE 106

- Swelling of the feet and legs and sometimes of the lower abdomen.
- **Liver big, hard, irregular**, and usually not tender.
- Signs of weight loss.
- Often ascites.
- Sometimes vomiting of blood.
- No jaundice except when the cirrhosis is very severe.

7. BAD CIRCULATION OF THE LEGS

- No signs of general disease.
- Sometimes big swollen veins of the legs.
- Sometimes shallow ulcers of the skin of the lower legs. These ulcers have no signs of infection.
- Pain in the legs made worse by walking or working.

SYMPTOMATIC TREATMENT OF EDEMA IN AN ADULT

1. The patient must not eat salt or any food containing much salt.

2. He must eat food with much protein - see page 658.

3. He may have pain in the legs because of the swelling. In this case, put elastic bandages around the legs. Start at the base of the toes. Be sure to cover the heel. Continue the bandage up to just below the knees.

4. Treat every ulcer or sore of the lower legs.
    - Daily dressings.
    - Elastic bandage.
    - Antibiotics in case of infection.

5. Do not give a diuretic medicine to every patient who has edema. Give it only if the patient has a specific disease that needs a diuretic.

6. The most effective diuretic is water to drink. Tell each patient with edema to drink much water: 3 to 5 liters a day. This will make him have much urine. The edema liquid and salt will go out in the urine.

TO MAKE THE DIAGNOSIS

In the history, ask:
- When did the swelling start?
- Do you have a cough?
- Do you have sputum? If so, what is the sputum like?
- Do you have trouble breathing? If so, when? While working? While sleeping?
- How many times do you urinate during the night?
- Have you lost weight?
- Are you often dizzy or weak?
- Have you vomited blood?
- Are you pregnant? If so, how many months?
- Do you have pains in your legs?

In the physical exam, look for:
- Where the swelling is and how much there is.
- Signs of heart failure:
  - Rapid pulse, rapid breathing, crackles in the bases of the lungs, big tender liver, swollen veins in the neck.
- Pale color of the mucous membranes.
- Signs of malnutrition:
  - Signs of weight loss.
  - Changes in the color of the skin or the hair.
- A pregnancy: how many months?
- High blood pressure.
- Liver big, hard, irregular.
- Ascites.
- Swollen veins in the legs.
- Shallow ulcers on the lower legs.

In the laboratory, do:
- A hemoglobin exam.
- A urine exam to look for protein and for blood cells.

SWELLING (EDEMA) IN AN ADULT

Possible causes

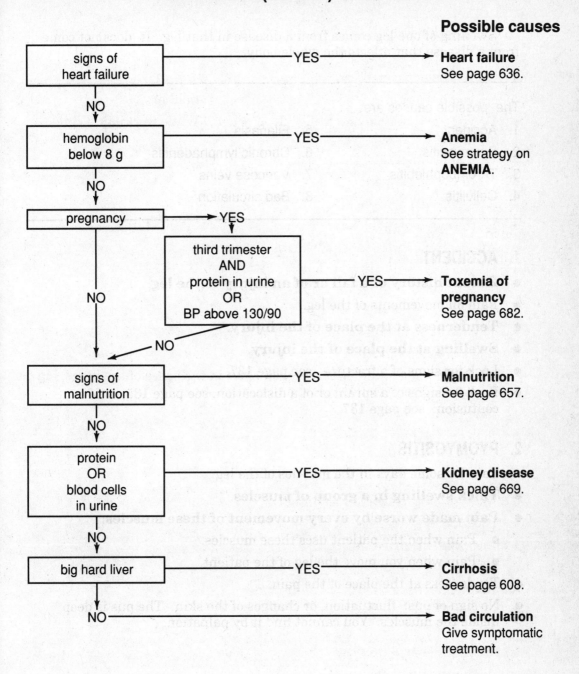

signs of
heart failure —————YES—————▶ **Heart failure**
See page 636.

NO

hemoglobin
below 8 g —————YES—————▶ **Anemia**
See strategy on
ANEMIA.

NO

pregnancy ——————▶ YES

NO

third trimester
AND
protein in urine
OR
BP above 130/90 —————YES—————▶ **Toxemia of
pregnancy**
See page 682.

NO

signs of
malnutrition —————YES—————▶ **Malnutrition**
See page 657.

NO

protein
OR
blood cells
in urine —————YES—————▶ **Kidney disease**
See page 669.

NO

big hard liver —————YES—————▶ **Cirrhosis**
See page 608.

NO—————————————————▶ **Bad circulation**
Give symptomatic
treatment.

SWELLING OF ONE LEG

Swelling of one leg comes from a disease in that leg. It does not come from a disease that affects the whole body.

The possible causes are:

1. Accident
2. Pyomyositis
3. Thrombophlebitis
4. Cellulitis
5. Filariasis
6. Chronic lymphadenitis
7. Varicose veins
8. Bad circulation

1. ACCIDENT

- **Recent history of a fall or of an injury to the leg**.
- Pain on movements of the leg.
- **Tenderness at the place of the injury**.
- **Swelling at the place of the injury**.
- Look for signs of a fracture: see page 137.
- Look for signs of a sprain or of a dislocation: see page 135, or of a contusion: see page 137.

2. PYOMYOSITIS

- Pain for some days in the muscles of the leg.
- **Thick swelling in a group of muscles**.
- **Pain made worse by every movement of these muscles**:
  - Pain when the patient uses these muscles.
  - Pain when you move the leg of the patient.
- Tenderness at the place of the pain.
- No sign of pus: fluctuation, or changes of the skin. The pus is deep inside the muscles. You cannot find it by palpation.

- Thick pus found by sterile puncture and aspiration of the affected muscles.
- Often fever, especially during the evening.

3. THROMBOPHLEBITIS

- **Swelling of the ankle and of the lower leg**.
- **Pain and tenderness in back of the lower leg made worse by walking**.
- Pain made worse by **bending the foot up, in "dorsi-flexion."** We call this "Homan's sign."
- Often fever.

4. CELLULITIS

- **Pain and tenderness in the skin and in the subcutaneous tissues**.
- **Heat and swelling of the skin and subcutaneous tissues in the affected region**.
- Often a small wound or ulcer at the lower end of the affected region.
- Often fever and a rapid pulse.
- Often tender lymph nodes in the inguinal or femoral regions.

5. FILARIASIS

- **Swelling lasting for weeks or months with no pitting**. Often this starts at the inguinal region and moves down the leg.
- **Skin thick with loss of elasticity and no pitting**.
- No tenderness or fever. Tenderness or fever indicates an infection, or cellulitis, in the region.
- Often big lymph nodes in the inguinal or femoral regions.
- **Microfilaria in the blood at night, from 22 hr to 2 hr**: (Wuchereria).
- Or **microfilaria in the skin fluid** found by the skin scratch test: (Onchocerciasis)

6. CHRONIC LYMPHADENITIS

- **Swelling lasting for weeks or months with no pitting**.
- No tenderness or fever unless there is also cellulitis.
- Big inguinal or femoral lymph nodes.
- **No microfilaria**.
- To find the cause of the big lymph nodes, see the strategy on BIG LYMPH NODES on page 550.

7. VARICOSE VEINS

- **Swelling for weeks or months, with no pitting**.
- **Big veins, like serpents, under the skin**.
- Sometimes pain in the leg made worse by walking.

8. BAD CIRCULATION

- No signs of general or local disease.
- Sometimes shallow ulcers of the skin of the lower leg. These ulcers have no signs of infection.

SYMPTOMATIC TREATMENT OF SWELLING OF ONE LEG

1. Do not give a diuretic medicine. This will not help the swelling at all.

2. If the patient has much pain and tenderness, put him in bed until the pain and tenderness are gone. If he has signs of infection, give him penicillin or another antibiotic.

3. Treat every ulcer or sore of the lower leg.

   ● Daily dressings.

   ● Elastic bandage.

   ● Antibiotics in case of infection.

TO MAKE THE DIAGNOSIS

In the history, ask:

- When did your leg start to swell?
- Does the leg hurt?
- Does it hurt to touch it? To walk on it? To move it?
- Have you just had an accident and hurt your leg?
- Do you have a wound, a sore, or an ulcer on the leg?
- Do you have fever?

In the physical exam, look for:

- Where the swelling is.
- Pitting edema where the leg is swollen.
- Tenderness. If so, where is it? Is it deep? Is it in the skin or just under the skin?
- Pain on movements of the leg.
- Heat in the swollen region. Feel the skin with the back of your hand. Feel the skin of the other leg with the back of your hand. Compare the temperature of the two legs.
- Thick swelling in one muscle group.
- Pain on extension (dorsi-flexion) of the foot - "Homan's sign."
- Fever, rapid pulse.
- Big inguinal or femoral lymph nodes. If so, are they tender?
- If there has been an accident, look for signs of a fracture, of a sprain, of a dislocation, or of a contusion. See pages 135 and 137.
- Big swollen veins, like serpents, under the skin.
- Wound, ulcer, sore on the lower leg.

In the laboratory, do:

- A fresh blood drop exam during the night, from 22 hr to 2 hr to look for the microfilaria of Wuchereria.
- A skin scratch test to look for the microfilaria of Onchocerciasis.
- A sterile puncture and aspiration if there is a group of thick tender muscles.

SWELLING OF ONE LEG

Possible causes

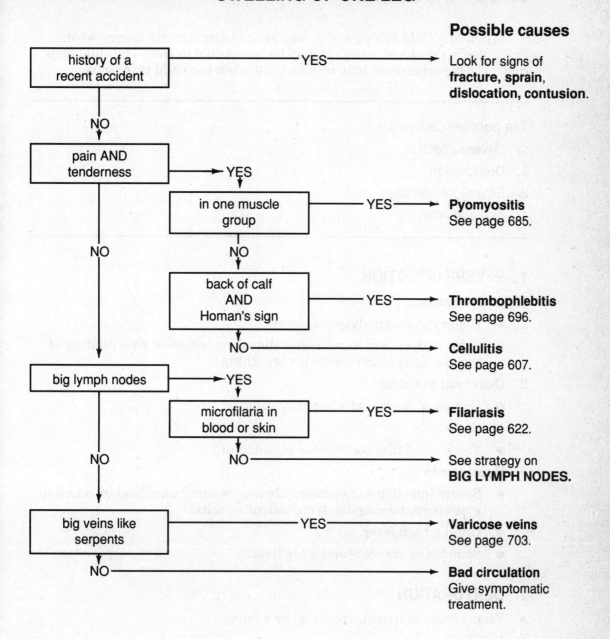

history of a recent accident	—YES→	Look for signs of **fracture, sprain, dislocation, contusion**.

↓ NO

pain AND tenderness	→YES→ in one muscle group	—YES→ **Pyomyositis** See page 685.

NO ↓ (in one muscle group) ↓ NO

	back of calf AND Homan's sign	—YES→ **Thrombophlebitis** See page 696.

↓ NO————→ **Cellulitis** See page 607.

big lymph nodes	→YES→ microfilaria in blood or skin	—YES→ **Filariasis** See page 622.

NO ↓ ↓ NO————→ See strategy on **BIG LYMPH NODES.**

big veins like serpents	—YES→	**Varicose veins** See page 703.

↓ NO————————————→ **Bad circulation** Give symptomatic treatment.

SHOCK IN A CHILD

Shock in a child is a sign of a very serious disease. He is very weak. The pulse is rapid and weak. It may be impossible to feel. The child feels cold. The consciousness may be clear, but often the child is in coma.

The possible causes are:

1. Severe infection
2. Dehydration
3. Severe hemorrhage
4. Acute anemia

1. SEVERE INFECTION

1. Pneumonia

- History of cough, dyspnea, fever.
- Signs of dyspnea: rapid respirations, retraction of ribs, dilating of the openings of the nose with breathing.

2. Cerebral malaria

- History of fever and often convulsions.
- Coma.
- Thick blood film positive for plasmodium.

3. Septicemia

- Severe infection somewhere: abscess, wound, umbilical infection in a newborn, meningitis, lymphadenitis, otitis.
- Often a high fever.
- Sometimes jaundice and a big liver.

2. DEHYDRATION

- From severe diarrhea, vomiting, or a burn.
- Extreme weakness.
- **Mouth dry**.
- **Skin dry**, with many folds, and with loss of elasticity.
- **Eyes dry**, sunken deep in the eye sockets, with no tears.
- Little or no urine for many hours.

3. SEVERE HEMORRHAGE

- An injury, a wound, or a big burn.
- An intestinal hemorrhage, with black or red stools.
- An accident with internal injuries.
- A snake bite.

4. ACUTE ANEMIA

- From malaria or sickle cell anemia.
- A rapid fall in hemoglobin can cause shock. A slow progressive fall in hemoglobin does not often cause shock.
- **Pale color of mucous membranes**.
- Often jaundice.
- Often a big spleen.
- **Hemoglobin below 5 g**.

TREATMENT OF SHOCK IN A CHILD

1. Put the child in bed with no pillow under his head.
2. Cover him well to keep him warm. The mother, or another parent, must stay with him at all times.
3. The child needs sugar, at least one teaspoonful per kilo of weight. Dissolve the sugar in a glass of water. Give this to him to drink. If he cannot drink, pass a naso-gastric tube. Be sure the end of the tube is in the stomach. Then give the sugar water by the tube.
4. He also needs much water. Give him much water to drink. If he cannot drink, give him liquids by an IV or a rectal infusion.
5. In case of infection, give him antibiotics in big doses.
6. In case of dehydration, follow the instructions on pages 322-325.
7. In case of severe hemorrhage or severe anemia, a transfusion may be necessary. If you cannot give it, send the child to hospital.
8. After you have given urgent treatment, try to send him to hospital.

TO MAKE THE DIAGNOSIS:

In the history, ask the parents:

- Has the child had a fever, a cough, or trouble breathing?
- Has he had convulsions?
- Does he have an infection somewhere? A tender swelling or lump?
- Does he have a wound or a sore, or pus coming from somewhere?
- Has he had severe diarrhea, or vomiting?
- Has he just had an accident, a burn, or a snake bite?
- Has the child just lost much blood from a wound? Or from the nose? Or in the stools?

In the physical exam, look for:

- Fever.
- Signs of dyspnea.
- Delirium or coma.
- Abscess, infected wound, pus coming from somewhere, tender lymph nodes.
- Jaundice, or a pale color of the mucus membranes.
- Signs of dehydration.
- Bleeding from somewhere.
- A big liver or a big spleen.
- In case of an accident, look for:
  - Signs of a fracture.
  - Severe tenderness or rebound tenderness in the abdomen.
  - A big wound or a burn.

In the laboratory, do:

- A hemoglobin exam.
- A thick blood film to look for plasmodium.
- A fresh blood drop exam to look for sickle cells.

SHOCK IN A CHILD

Possible causes

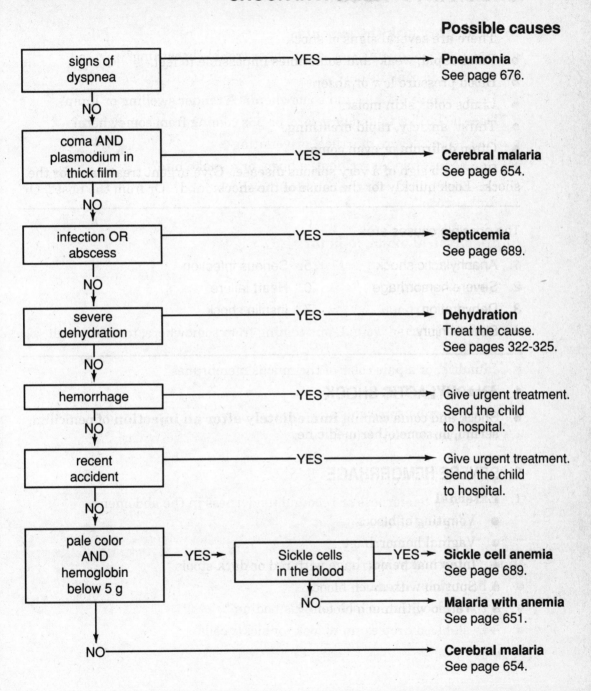

- signs of dyspnea — YES → **Pneumonia** See page 676.
- NO ↓
- coma AND plasmodium in thick film — YES → **Cerebral malaria** See page 654.
- NO ↓
- infection OR abscess — YES → **Septicemia** See page 689.
- NO ↓
- severe dehydration — YES → **Dehydration** Treat the cause. See pages 322-325.
- NO ↓
- hemorrhage — YES → Give urgent treatment. Send the child to hospital.
- NO ↓
- recent accident — YES → Give urgent treatment. Send the child to hospital.
- NO ↓
- pale color AND hemoglobin below 5 g — YES → Sickle cells in the blood — YES → **Sickle cell anemia** See page 689.
  - NO → **Malaria with anemia** See page 651.
- NO → **Cerebral malaria** See page 654.

SHOCK IN AN ADULT

There are several signs of shock:

- Pulse rapid, weak, and sometimes impossible to feel.
- Blood pressure low or absent.
- Limbs cold: skin moist.
- Thirst, anxiety, rapid breathing.
- Often delirium or even coma.

Shock is a sign of a very serious disease. Give urgent treatment for the shock. Look quickly for the cause of the shock.

The possible causes are:

1. Anaphylactic shock
2. Severe hemorrhage
3. Dehydration
4. Severe injury
5. Serious infection
6. Heart failure
7. Insulin shock

1. ANAPHYLACTIC SHOCK

- Shock and coma coming **immediately after an injection** of penicillin, serum, or some other medicine.

2. SEVERE HEMORRHAGE

1. **External**
   - Vomiting of blood.
   - Vaginal hemorrhage.
   - Intestinal hemorrhage with red or dark stools.
   - Sputum with much blood.
   - Wound with much bleeding.

2. **Internal**.
- Ruptured ectopic pregnancy.
  - Severe abdominal pain.
  - Rebound tenderness in the abdomen.
  - Often a history of absence of menstrual periods for one or more months.
- Premature separation of the placenta.
  - Pregnancy in the last trimester.
  - Sudden strong pain in the abdomen.
  - Uterus very hard and very tender.
  - No fetal movements or fetal heart sounds.

3. DEHYDRATION
- From severe diarrhea, vomiting, or a big burn.
- **Mouth dry**.
- **Skin dry**, with many folds, and with loss of elasticity.
- **Eyes dry**, sunken deep into eye sockets, with no tears.
- Little or no urine for many hours.

4. SEVERE INJURY
- Rupture of an abdominal organ: much pain and rebound tenderness in the abdomen.
- Rib fractures: bleeding into the chest, or collapse of a lung.
- Fracture of a big bone: femur, or the spine.
- A recent snake bite or a recent severe burn.
- Severe pain. A very strong pain can, by itself, cause shock.

5. SERIOUS INFECTION
- Peritonitis, meningitis, septicemia, severe pneumonia, infected abortion, cerebral malaria.
- **Fever**. The fever may go away after the shock comes.
- **Signs of the infection**.

6. HEART FAILURE - SEE CHAPTER 3 ON PAGE 93

- The shock comes in the final stage of heart failure.
- Pulse very rapid or absent, respirations very rapid, many crackles in the lungs, big tender liver, edema, swollen veins in the neck.

7. INSULIN SHOCK

- **History of diabetes**.
- **History of an injection of insulin a few hours before**. The patient has eaten little or nothing since the insulin injection.
- Loss of consciousness and often convulsions.
- Pulse slow and strong.
- Pupils dilated, skin moist.

SYMPTOMATIC TREATMENT OF SHOCK IN AN ADULT

1. Put the patient in bed with no pillow under his head.

2. Cover the patient to keep him warm. Someone must stay with him at all times.

3. Start immediately an IV infusion of normal saline. Give this rapidly, even up to 100 drops/minute. Use normal saline. 5% dextrose does not help. But do not give an IV infusion to a patient with heart failure.

4. If the cause of the shock is a severe hemorrhage, the patient will need a transfusion. If you cannot give a transfusion, send him to hospital after giving urgent treatment.

5. If the only cause of shock is severe pain, give meperidine or morphine.

6. Look at the patient very often. After you have given urgent treatment, try to send him to hospital as quickly as possible.

TO MAKE THE DIAGNOSIS

In the history, ask the patient or someone else with him:
- Has he just had an injection? If so, of what medicine?
- Has he just had much bleeding?
  - Vomiting blood? Vaginal bleeding? In the stools? In the sputum?
  - From a big wound?
- In a woman, is she pregnant? If so, how many months?
- Is there much pain in the abdomen?
- Has there been much diarrhea, or vomiting?
- Has there just been a serious accident, a burn, or a snake bite?
- If so, what happened? What part of the body was injured, or burned, or bitten?
- Has there been fever, trouble breathing, or swelling?
- Does the patient have diabetes?
- If so, has the patient just had an injection of insulin?

In the physical exam, look for:
- The state of consciousness: clear? Delirium? Coma?
- Hemorrhage: From the mouth, the vagina, the rectum, or from a wound.
- Tenderness, or rebound tenderness in the abdomen.
- A pregnancy. Of how many months? Is the uterus hard and tender?
- Signs of dehydration.
- A big burn.
- After an accident, look for:
  - Much tenderness of the chest.
  - Much tenderness of the abdomen.
  - Fracture of the femur or of the spine.
  - A snake bite, with much swelling.
  - Strong pain.

- Signs of a serious infection, such as:
  - Fever, stiff neck, dyspnea, crackles in the lungs.
  - Much pain in the abdomen; swelling of the abdomen.
  - Secretions with a very bad odor coming from the vagina.
- Signs of heart failure:
  - Rapid pulse, rapid respirations, crackles in the lungs.
  - Swelling of the feet and legs, big tender liver.
  - Swollen veins in the neck.

In the laboratory, do:

- A hemoglobin exam. Remember that after a severe hemorrhage, the hemoglobin will not go down immediately. It takes up to 6 hours for the hemoglobin to diminish. But in the meantime, the patient is in shock because of loss of blood. So do not depend on a hemoglobin exam right after the hemorrhage to tell you how serious the hemorrhage is. Depend rather on the signs of the patient: pulse and blood pressure.
- A thick blood film to look for plasmodium.

SHOCK IN AN ADULT

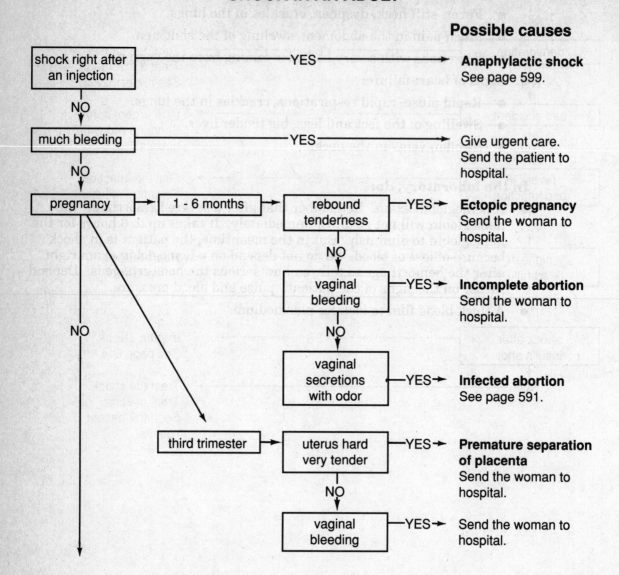

Possible causes

shock right after an injection → YES →	**Anaphylactic shock** See page 599.
much bleeding → YES →	Give urgent care. Send the patient to hospital.
pregnancy → 1 - 6 months → rebound tenderness → YES →	**Ectopic pregnancy** Send the woman to hospital.
vaginal bleeding → YES →	**Incomplete abortion** Send the woman to hospital.
vaginal secretions with odor → YES →	**Infected abortion** See page 591.
third trimester → uterus hard very tender → YES →	**Premature separation of placenta** Send the woman to hospital.
vaginal bleeding → YES →	Send the woman to hospital.

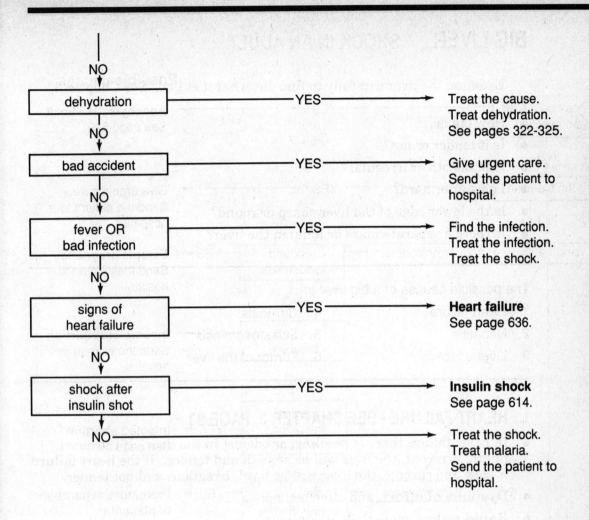

NO

| dehydration | —YES——→ | Treat the cause.
Treat dehydration.
See pages 322-325. |

NO

| bad accident | —YES——→ | Give urgent care.
Send the patient to
hospital. |

NO

| fever OR
bad infection | —YES——→ | Find the infection.
Treat the infection.
Treat the shock. |

NO

| signs of
heart failure | —YES——→ | **Heart failure**
See page 636. |

NO

| shock after
insulin shot | —YES——→ | **Insulin shock**
See page 614. |

NO————————————→ Treat the shock.
Treat malaria.
Send the patient to
hospital.

BIG LIVER

Examine the liver carefully to find out what it is like. See Chapter 3, page 105.

- How big is it?
- Is it tender or not?
- Is it smooth or irregular?
- Is it soft or hard?
- Is the lower edge of the liver sharp or round?
- Is there a separate mass or lump in the liver?

The possible causes of a big liver are:

1. Heart failure
2. Hepatitis
3. Liver abscess
4. Cirrhosis
5. Schistosomiasis
6. Tumor of the liver

---

1. HEART FAILURE - SEE CHAPTER 3, PAGE 93

- In heart failure there is swelling, or edema, in the liver. If the heart failure is recent, the liver will be smooth and tender. If the heart failure is slow and chronic, the liver will be hard, irregular, and not tender.
- **Dyspnea of effort**, and often orthopnea.
- **Rapid pulse**: more than 100/minute.
- Crackles in the lungs, especially at the bases of the lungs.
- **Swelling** of the feet, the legs, and even of the lower abdomen.
- Often cough with sputum. The sputum may be clear, or it may have small amounts of red-brown blood.
- Frequent urination during the night.
- Swollen veins in the neck.

2. HEPATITIS

- The liver is **tender and smooth, and a little big**.
- **Pain in the right upper quadrant**.
- Often **jaundice**.

- Fever at the beginning going away after a few days.
- Often vomiting and loss of appetite.
- The urine becomes dark, and often the stools become pale.

3. LIVER ABSCESS

- **The liver is tender** or has a separate tender mass in it.
- Often a history of recent diarrhea.
- **Fever**, which can go up to 40°.
- Rarely jaundice.
- High white blood cell count.
- Improvement after treatment with metronidazole and chloramphenicol.

4. CIRRHOSIS

- **The liver is big, hard, irregular and usually not tender**.
- No fever.
- Signs of weight loss.
- Often ascites.
- Sometimes swelling of the feet, the legs, and even the lower abdomen.
- Sometimes vomiting of blood.
- No jaundice except when the cirrhosis is very severe.

5. SCHISTOSOMIASIS

- The aspect of the liver is like that of cirrhosis.
- History of blood in the stools or in the urine.
- **Eggs of Schistosoma mansoni in the stools, or of Schistosoma hematobium in the urine.**

6. TUMOR OF THE LIVER

- The liver is big and tender with sometimes a big mass in it.
- No fever.
- Signs of weight loss.
- No jaundice.
- Sometimes vomiting of blood.
- It is often impossible to distinguish between cirrhosis and liver tumor.

TO MAKE THE DIAGNOSIS

In the history, ask:

- Do you feel pain in the right upper part of your abdomen? If so, when did the pain start?
- Do you have a cough?
- Do you have sputum? If so, what is it like?
- Do you have trouble breathing? If so, when?
- How many times do you urinate during the night?
- Have you had a fever, jaundice, vomiting, or dark urine?
- Have you had diarrhea, or blood in your stools or urine?
- Have you lost weight?

In the physical exam, look for:

- The aspect of the liver. Examine it carefully.
- Signs of heart failure:
  - Rapid pulse, dyspnea, crackles at the bases of the lungs.
  - Swelling of the feet, the legs, or the lower abdomen.
  - Swollen veins in the neck.
- Fever.
- Jaundice.
- Ascites.

In the laboratory, do:

- A stool exam and a urine exam to look for eggs of schistosomes.
- If the patient has a high fever, do a white blood cell count.

BIG LIVER

In every patient with a big liver, always look carefully for signs of heart failure.

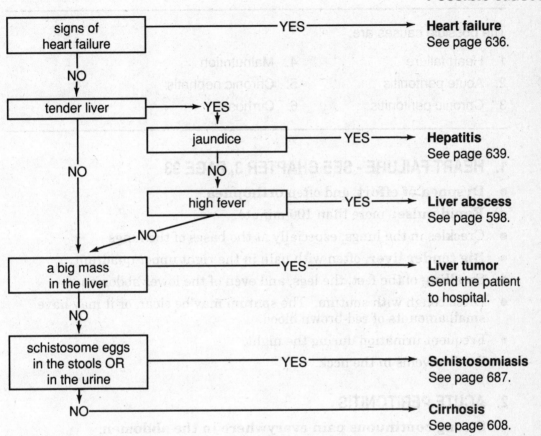

Possible causes

signs of heart failure —YES→ **Heart failure** See page 636.

NO

tender liver →YES→ jaundice —YES→ **Hepatitis** See page 639.

NO

high fever —YES→ **Liver abscess** See page 598.

NO

a big mass in the liver —YES→ **Liver tumor** Send the patient to hospital.

NO

schistosome eggs in the stools OR in the urine —YES→ **Schistosomiasis** See page 687.

NO→ **Cirrhosis** See page 608.

ASCITES

Ascites is the accumulation of liquid inside the abdominal cavity. To find out how to examine the patient for ascites, read page 110 in Chapter 3.

The possible causes are:

1. Heart failure
2. Acute peritonitis
3. Chronic peritonitis
4. Malnutrition
5. Chronic nephritis
6. Cirrhosis

1. HEART FAILURE - SEE CHAPTER 3, PAGE 93

- **Dyspnea of effort**, and often **orthopnea**.
- **Rapid pulse**: more than 100/minute.
- Crackles in the lungs, especially at the bases of the lungs.
- **Big tender liver**, often with pain in the right upper quadrant.
- **Swelling** of the feet, the legs, and even of the lower abdomen.
- Often cough with sputum. The sputum may be clear, or it may have small amounts of red-brown blood.
- Frequent urination during the night.
- Swollen veins in the neck.

2. ACUTE PERITONITIS

- **Strong continuous pain everywhere in the abdomen**.
- **Fever**, rapid pulse, breathing only with the chest muscles.
- **Much tenderness in the abdomen, with rigid muscles**.
- **Rebound tenderness in the abdomen**.
- **Swelling of the abdomen**.
- No sounds of peristalsis in the abdomen: a "silent abdomen."
- No stools or gas passed since the beginning of the abdominal pain.
- High white blood cell count.

3. CHRONIC PERITONITIS

- **Fever which is irregular and chronic**.
- Abdominal colicky pain.
- **Tenderness of the abdomen**, but with little or no muscle rigidity.
- No rebound tenderness.
- Loss of weight.
- Diarrhea for some days, then constipation for some days.

4. MALNUTRITION

- **Loss of weight**.
- **Swelling** of the feet, the legs, and often of the face.
- **Changes in the color of the skin and the hair**.
- Weakness and no energy to work or play.

5. CHRONIC NEPHRITIS

- Loss of weight, weakness.
- Signs of anemia: pale color of the mucus membranes, hemoglobin below 10 g.
- Swelling of the feet, the legs, and often of the face.
- Sometimes high blood pressure.
- **Protein and often white or red blood cells in the urine**.

6. CIRRHOSIS

- **The liver is big, hard, irregular, and usually not tender**.
- Sometimes, if there is much ascites, it is impossible to feel the liver.
- Signs of weight loss.
- Sometimes swelling of the feet, the legs, and even of the lower abdomen.
- Sometimes vomiting of blood.
- No jaundice except when the cirrhosis is very severe.
- No fever.

TO MAKE THE DIAGNOSIS

In the history, ask:
- When did your abdomen start swelling?
- Do you have a cough?
- Do you have sputum? If so, what is it like?
- Do you have trouble breathing? If so, when?
- How many times do you urinate during the night?
- Do you have pain in the abdomen? If so, where? Since when?
- Have you lost weight?
- Have you had a fever, diarrhea, constipation, or vomiting?
- Have you passed gas or stools today? Yesterday?

In the physical exam, look for:
- Signs of heart failure:
  - Rapid pulse, dyspnea, crackles at the bases of the lungs.
  - Big tender liver, swelling of the feet and legs.
  - Swollen veins in the neck.
- Fever.
- Tenderness of the abdomen, with rigid muscles.
- Rebound tenderness in the abdomen.
- Sounds of peristalsis: are they present or absent?
- Signs of malnutrition:
  - Signs of weight loss.
  - Changes in the color of the skin and the hair.
  - Swelling of the feet, the legs, the face.
- Pale color of the mucous membranes.
- High blood pressure.
- Liver that is big, hard, irregular and not tender.

In the laboratory, do:
- A hemoglobin exam.
- A urine exam to look for protein and white or red blood cells.

ASCITES

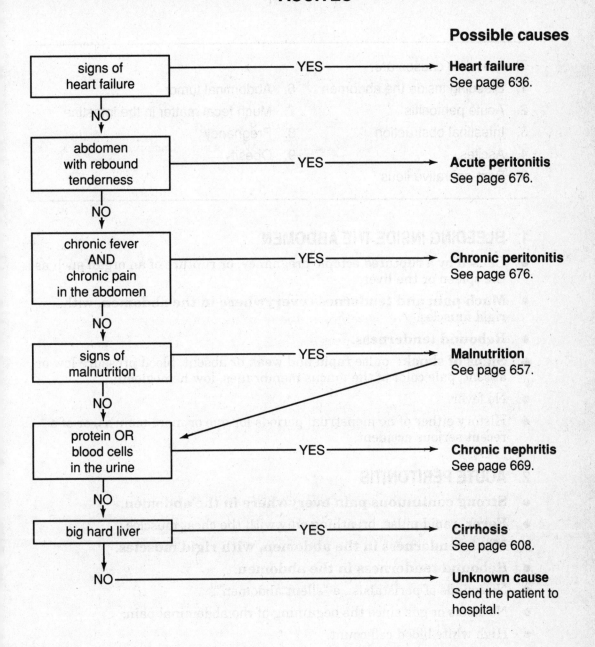

Possible causes

signs of heart failure — YES → **Heart failure** See page 636.

NO

abdomen with rebound tenderness — YES → **Acute peritonitis** See page 676.

NO

chronic fever AND chronic pain in the abdomen — YES → **Chronic peritonitis** See page 676.

NO

signs of malnutrition — YES → **Malnutrition** See page 657.

NO

protein OR blood cells in the urine — YES → **Chronic nephritis** See page 669.

NO

big hard liver — YES → **Cirrhosis** See page 608.

NO → **Unknown cause** Send the patient to hospital.

SWELLING OF THE ABDOMEN

The possible causes are:

1. Bleeding inside the abdomen
2. Acute peritonitis
3. Intestinal obstruction
4. Ascites
5. Post-operative ileus
6. Abdominal tumor
7. Much fecal matter in the intestine
8. Pregnancy
9. Obesity

1. BLEEDING INSIDE THE ABDOMEN

- Caused by a ruptured ectopic pregnancy, or rupture of an organ such as the spleen or the liver.
- **Much pain and tenderness everywhere in the abdomen**, with rigid muscles.
- **Rebound tenderness**.
- **Signs of shock**: pulse rapid and weak or absent, blood pressure low or absent, pale color of the mucus membranes, low hemoglobin.
- No fever.
- History either of no menstrual periods for one or more months, or of a recent serious accident.

2. ACUTE PERITONITIS

- **Strong continuous pain everywhere in the abdomen**.
- **Fever**, rapid pulse, breathing only with the chest muscles.
- **Much tenderness in the abdomen, with rigid muscles**.
- **Rebound tenderness in the abdomen**.
- No sounds of peristalsis: a "silent abdomen".
- No stools or gas since the beginning of the abdominal pain.
- High white blood cell count.

3. INTESTINAL OBSTRUCTION - SEE CHAPTER 3, PAGE 112

- **Intermittent pain (colic) everywhere in the abdomen for some hours or days**.
- **Vomiting** of liquid with bile, or brown liquid that smells like fecal matter.
- **No stools or gas for some hours or days**.
- Visible waves of peristalsis going across the abdomen.
- **Loud sounds of peristalsis** heard through the stethoscope. These sounds come and go. They come when there is a visible wave of peristalsis and when the patient feels strong pain.

4. ASCITES - SEE CHAPTER 3, PAGE 110

- General swelling of the abdomen without pain.
- **Dullness to percussion in the flanks and the lower abdomen**.
- **Resonance around the umbilicus**.
- **Change in the limit between dullness and resonance** when the patient turns on his side or stands up - see page 111.
- Often swelling of the feet and legs.
- Often a big liver.

5. POST-OPERATIVE ILEUS - SEE CHAPTER 3, PAGE 112

- This is normal after a major operation on the abdomen. The intestines fill with gas, and there is no peristalsis.
- **Resonance everywhere in the abdomen**.
- **No sounds of peristalsis**.
- No stools or gas.

6. ABDOMINAL TUMOR

- **One or more masses in the abdomen**.
- Loss of weight.
- Often pain in the abdomen.
- Often vomiting, constipation or diarrhea.

7. MUCH FECAL MATTER IN THE INTESTINE

- **History of constipation and very hard stools**.
- Many small lumps in the abdomen which move and are not tender. The lumps move or go away after a good enema.
- By rectal exam, much fecal matter in the rectum. We call this a "fecal impaction."

8. PREGNANCY

- **History of no periods for several months**.
- **Presence of a fetus inside the uterus**. You can feel it move, and hear the sounds of its heart.

9. OBESITY

- **The patient is overweight**.
- Much fat in the limbs, on the chest, and in the abdomen.

TO MAKE THE DIAGNOSIS

In the history, ask:
- When did your abdomen start to get big?
- Did it start slowly or quickly?
- Have you had pain in the abdomen? If so, where? What is it like?
- Have you had a fever, diarrhea, vomiting, or constipation?
- Have you had a severe accident recently with a blow to your abdomen?
- In a woman: Are you pregnant? If so, how many months? Have you missed any periods? If so, how many?
- Have you passed stools or gas today or yesterday?
- If not, how long has it been since you passed stools or gas?

In the physical exam, look for:
- Tenderness of the abdomen, or rigid muscles.
- Rebound tenderness.
- Fever.
- Signs of shock:
  - Pulse rapid and weak, blood pressure low or absent.
  - Pale color of the mucus membranes.
- Visible waves of peristalsis.
- Sounds of peristalsis: Are they normal? Absent? Very loud and strong?
- Signs of ascites.
- Resonance everywhere in the abdomen, or only around the umbilicus.
- Big liver.
- Masses or lumps in the abdomen: Where? Hard or soft? Fixed or mobile?
- Much fecal matter in the rectum.
- Signs of loss of weight.
- Swelling of feet or legs.
- Pregnancy.
- Much fat everywhere.

In the laboratory, do:
- A hemoglobin exam.
- A white blood cell count.

SWELLING OF THE ABDOMEN

Possible causes

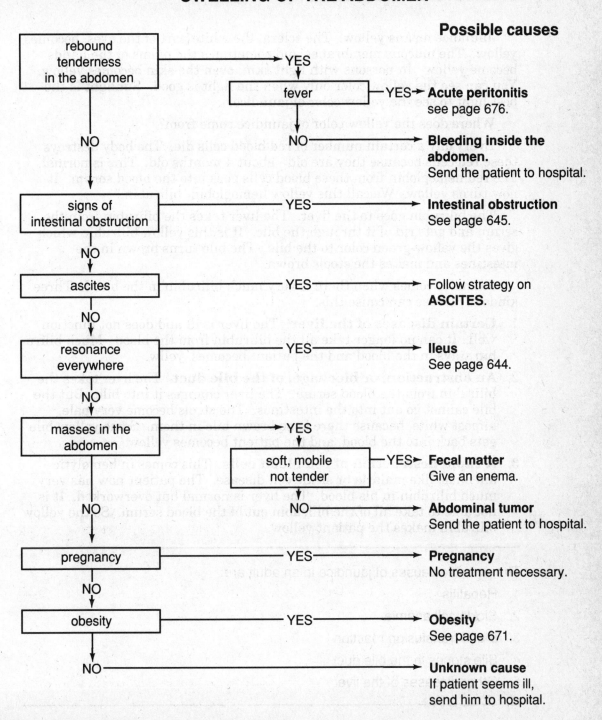

rebound tenderness in the abdomen → YES →

fever — YES → **Acute peritonitis**
see page 676.

NO → **Bleeding inside the abdomen.**
Send the patient to hospital.

rebound tenderness — NO ↓

signs of intestinal obstruction → YES → **Intestinal obstruction**
See page 645.

NO ↓

ascites → YES → Follow strategy on **ASCITES**.

NO ↓

resonance everywhere → YES → **Ileus**
See page 644.

NO ↓

masses in the abdomen → YES →

soft, mobile not tender — YES → **Fecal matter**
Give an enema.

NO → **Abdominal tumor**
Send the patient to hospital.

NO ↓

pregnancy → YES → **Pregnancy**
No treatment necessary.

NO ↓

obesity → YES → **Obesity**
See page 671.

NO → **Unknown cause**
If patient seems ill,
send him to hospital.

JAUNDICE IN AN ADULT

Jaundice means yellow. The sclera, the white part of the eyes, becomes yellow. The mucous membranes and sometimes the palms of the hands become yellow. In persons with light skin, even the skin becomes yellow. You can see the yellow color only when the light is good. Sunlight is the best light to see the yellow color of jaundice.

Where does the yellow color of jaundice come from?

Every day a certain number of red blood cells die. The body destroys these red cells because they are old - about 4 months old. This is normal. The red hemoglobin from these blood cells goes into the blood serum. It now turns yellow. We call this yellow hemoglobin "bilirubin."

The bilirubin goes to the liver. The liver takes the bilirubin from the serum and gets rid of it through the bile. It is this yellow bilirubin which gives the yellow-green color to the bile. The bile turns brown in the intestines and makes the stools brown.

Jaundice comes when there is very much bilirubin in the blood. Three kinds of disease can cause this.

1. **Certain diseases of the liver**. The liver is ill and does not function well. It can no longer take all the bilirubin from the blood. Much bilirubin stays in the blood and the patient becomes yellw.

2. **An obstruction, or blockage, of the bile duct**. The liver takes the bilirubin from the blood serum. The liver changes it into bile. But the bile cannot go out into the intestines. The stools become very pale, almost white, because there is no brown bile in them. Some yellow bile gets back into the blood, and the patient becomes yellow.

3. **A rapid destruction of red blood cells**. This comes in hemolytic anemias, like malaria or sickle cell disease. The patient now has very much bilirubin in his blood. The liver is normal but overworked. It is not able to take all of the bilirubin out of the blood serum. So the yellow bilirubin makes the patient yellow.

The possible causes of jaundice in an adult are:
1. Hepatitis
2. Sickle cell anemia
3. Blood transfusion reaction
4. Bile stones in the bile duct
5. Other diseases of the liver

1. HEPATITIS

- **Liver tender, smooth, soft, and a little big**.
- **Pain in the right upper quadrant**.
- Fever at the beginning of the illness, before the jaundice comes. The fever goes away in a few days.
- Often **vomiting and loss of appetite**.
- The jaundice comes 4 to 6 days after the beginning of the illness.
- Dark urine and pale stools.

2. SICKLE CELL ANEMIA

- This is a hemolytic anemia of children and young adults.
- **History of attacks of anemia and jaundice**.
- Often a history of frequent attacks of pain in the limbs and in the abdomen.
- **Signs of anemia**: pale color of the mucus membranes, hemoglobin below 8 g.
- Big spleen.
- **Sickle cells in the blood, seen in a fresh blood drop exam**.

3. BLOOD TRANSFUSION REACTION

- **Rapid development of jaundice in a few hours after a blood transfusion**.
- Sometimes signs of shock:
  - Pulse rapid and weak.
  - Blood pressure low or absent.
- Little or no urine since the transfusion.
- Liver not big.

4. BILE STONES IN THE BILE DUCT

- **Strong intermittent pain (colic) in the right upper quadrant**.
- Vomiting.
- Sometimes fever.
- **Tenderness in the right upper quadrant**.
- Sometimes a small, soft, very tender mass just below the middle of the liver. This is the swollen gall bladder.

5. OTHER DISEASES OF THE LIVER

- Such as cirrhosis, tumor of the liver, schistosomiasis.
- Jaundice is a late sign and a sign that the patient is very ill.
- Big liver.

TO MAKE THE DIAGNOSIS

In the history, ask:

- When did the jaundice first come?
- Did you have a fever at the beginning of the illness?
- Did you vomit?
- Are you eating well?
- Did you have pain in the abdomen? If so, where?
- Is your urine dark?
- Are your stools pale, or a very light color?
- Have you had jaundice in the past?
- Have you had attacks of anemia in the past?
- Have you had attacks of much pain in the legs, the arms, or the abdomen in the past?
- Have you just had a blood transfusion?

In the physical exam, look for:

- Big liver: what is it like?
- Fever.
- Signs of anemia: pale color of the mucous membranes.
- Signs of shock: pulse fast and weak, blood pressure low or absent.
- Big spleen.
- A soft tender mass just below the middle of the liver (the gall bladder).

In the laboratory, do:

- A hemoglobin exam.
- A fresh blood drop exam to look for sickle cells.

JAUNDICE IN AN ADULT

Possible causes

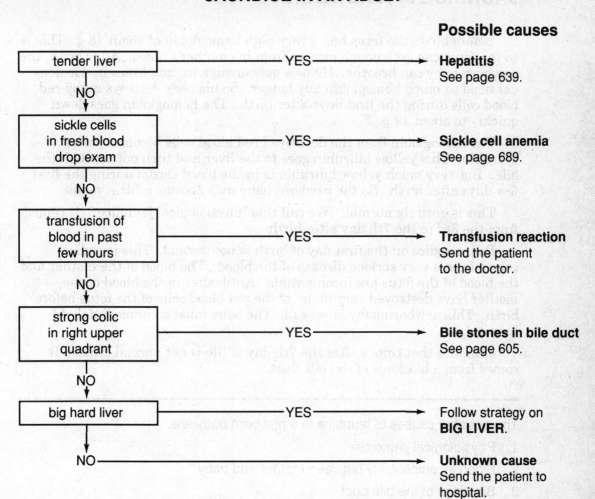

tender liver ——————YES——————→ **Hepatitis**
See page 639.

NO

sickle cells
in fresh blood ——————YES——————→ **Sickle cell anemia**
drop exam   See page 689.

NO

transfusion of
blood in past ——————YES——————→ **Transfusion reaction**
few hours   Send the patient
                                       to the doctor.

NO

strong colic
in right upper ——————YES——————→ **Bile stones in bile duct**
quadrant   See page 605.

NO

big hard liver ——————YES——————→ Follow strategy on
                                       BIG LIVER.

NO——————————————————————————→ **Unknown cause**
                                       Send the patient to
                                       hospital.

JAUNDICE IN A NEWBORN

Before birth, the fetus has a very high hemoglobin of about 18 g. This is so the fetus can get enough oxygen from his mother's blood. After birth, the newborn baby can breathe. He now gets enough oxygen himself. He does not need so much hemoglobin any longer. So his body destroys many red blood cells during the first days after birth. The hemoglobin goes down quickly to about 12 g.

The hemoglobin from the destroyed red blood cells becomes yellow bilirubin. This yellow bilirubin goes to the liver and then out through the bile. But very much yellow bilirubin is in the blood serum during the first few days after birth. So the newborn baby may become a little yellow.

This is entirely normal. We call this "physiological jaundice." It comes from the 3rd to the 7th day after birth.

But jaundice on the first day of birth is not normal. This jaundice comes from a very serious disease of the blood. The blood of the mother and the blood of the fetus are incompatible. Antibodies in the blood of the mother have destroyed very many of the red blood cells of the fetus before birth. This newborn baby is very ill. The baby must go immediately to hospital.

Jaundice that comes after the 7th day of life is not normal either. It comes from a blockage of the bile duct.

The possible causes of jaundice in a newborn baby are:

1. Physiological jaundice
2. Blood incompatibility between mother and baby
3. Blockage of the bile duct

The diagnosis is easy. You must simply find out what day the jaundice began.

JAUNDICE IN A NEWBORN

Possible causes

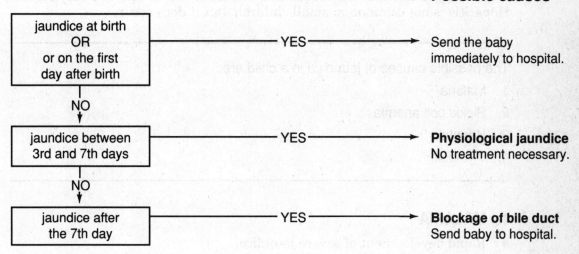

jaundice at birth OR or on the first day after birth	─── YES ───▶	Send the baby immediately to hospital.
NO ↓		
jaundice between 3rd and 7th days	─── YES ───▶	**Physiological jaundice** No treatment necessary.
NO ↓		
jaundice after the 7th day	─── YES ───▶	**Blockage of bile duct** Send baby to hospital.

JAUNDICE IN A CHILD

Hemolytic anemias are frequent in children. Often they are very serious. Hepatitis is not common in small children, but it does occur.

The possible causes of jaundice in a child are:

1. Malaria
2. Sickle cell anemia
3. Hepatitis
4. Cirrhosis

---

1. MALARIA

- Rapid development of severe jaundice.
- **High fever**, up to 40^0. But the fever can be absent if the child is very weak.
- Sometimes convulsions: sometimes diarrhea.
- Sometimes a big spleen.
- **Signs of anemia**: rapid pulse, pale color of the mucous membranes, hemoglobin below 6 g.
- **Thick blood film positive for plasmodium**.

2. SICKLE CELL ANEMIA

- **History of frequent attacks of anemia and jaundice**.
- Often a history of frequent attacks of pain in the limbs or in the abdomen.
- Swelling of the back of the hands or the top of the feet.
- **Signs of anemia**: rapid pulse, pale color of the mucous membranes, hemoglobin below 6 g.
- Often a big spleen.
- **Sickle cells in the blood seen on a fresh blood drop exam**.

3. HEPATITIS

- **Liver tender, smooth, soft, and a little big**.
- **Pain in the right upper quadrant**.
- Fever at the beginning of the illness. The fever goes away in a few days.
- Often vomiting and loss of appetite.

4. CIRRHOSIS

- **Liver big, hard, and irregular**. It may be tender.

TO MAKE THE DIAGNOSIS

In the history, ask the parents:

- When did the jaundice start?
- Has the child had a fever?
- Has he had convulsions, diarrhea, vomiting, or loss of appetite?
- Has he had attacks of anemia or jaundice in the past?
- Has he had attacks of pain in the legs, the arms, or the abdomen in the past?
- Has he had swelling of the back of the hands or the top of the feet?

In the physical exam, look for:

- Fever.
- Big liver: What is it like?
- Big spleen.
- Signs of anemia: rapid pulse, pale color of the mucous membranes.

In the laboratory, do:

- A hemoglobin exam.
- A fresh blood drop exam to look for sickle cells.
- A thick blood film to look for plasmodium.

JAUNDICE IN A CHILD

Possible causes

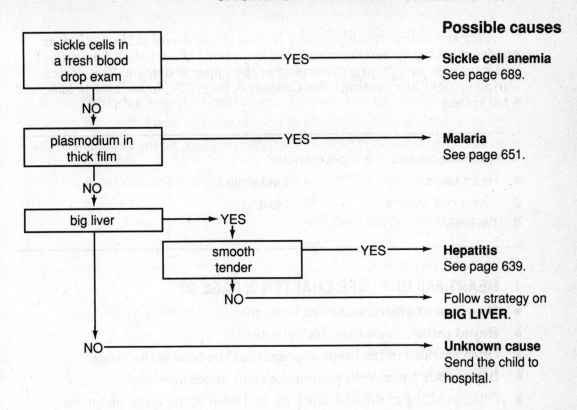

sickle cells in a fresh blood drop exam —— YES ——▶ **Sickle cell anemia** See page 689.

NO

plasmodium in thick film —— YES ——▶ **Malaria** See page 651.

NO

big liver —— YES

    smooth tender —— YES ——▶ **Hepatitis** See page 639.

    NO ———▶ Follow strategy on **BIG LIVER**.

NO ———▶ **Unknown cause** Send the child to hospital.

BIG SPLEEN

A big spleen can cause pain or a feeling of heaviness in the left upper quadrant. A big spleen can also cause symptoms of gastritis. The patient will have pain or a feeling of burning in the upper abdomen. This comes during or right after eating. See Chapter 3, page 107, to see how to look for a big spleen.

The possible causes of a big spleen are:

1. Heart failure
2. Sickle cell anemia
3. Cirrhosis
4. Leukemia
5. Malaria

---

1. HEART FAILURE - SEE CHAPTER 3, PAGE 93

- **Dyspnea of effort**, and often orthopnea.
- **Rapid pulse**: more than 100/minute.
- Often crackles in the lungs, especially at the base of the lungs.
- **Big tender liver**, with pain in the right upper quadrant.
- Often swelling of the feet, the legs, and even of the lower abdomen.
- Cough with sputum. The sputum may be clear, or it may have small amounts of red-brown blood.
- Frequent urination during the night.
- Sometimes swollen veins in the neck.

2. SICKLE CELL ANEMIA

- This is a disease of children and young adults.
- **History of frequent attacks of anemia and jaundice**.
- Often a history of frequent attacks of pain in the limbs and the abdomen.
- **Signs of anemia**: pale color of the mucous membranes, hemoglobin below 10 g.
- Sometimes jaundice.
- **Sickle cells in the blood, seen in a fresh blood drop exam**.

3. CIRRHOSIS - SEE CHAPTER 3, PAGE 106

- **The liver is big, hard, irregular, and usually not tender**.
- Signs of weight loss.
- Sometimes swelling of the feet, the legs and even of the lower abdomen.
- Often ascites.
- Sometimes vomiting of blood.
- No jaundice except when the cirrhosis is very severe.

4. LEUKEMIA

- This is a malignant tumor of the blood-forming cells.
- **Very many white blood cells: more than 50,000/mm3**.
- Weakness, weight loss.
- Sometimes an irregular fever.

5. MALARIA

- **Frequent attacks of malaria with fever**.
- **Thick blood film positive for plasmodium during the attacks**.
- Sometimes anemia: hemoglobin below 10 g.

TO MAKE THE DIAGNOSIS

In the history, ask:

- Do you have a cough? If so, do you bring up sputum? What is it like?
- Do you have trouble breathing? If so, when?
- Do you have swelling of the feet or legs?
- How many times do you urinate during the night?
- Do you often have fever?
- Have you lost weight?
- Do you often have attacks of anemia or of jaundice?
- Do you often have attacks of pain in the arms, the legs, or in the abdomen?
- In a child: does the child often have swelling of the back of the hands or of the top of the feet?

In the physical exam, look for:

- Signs of heart failure:
  - Rapid pulse, dyspnea, crackles in the lungs especially at the base.
  - Big tender liver, swelling of the feet and legs.
  - Swollen veins in the neck.
- Pale color of the mucous membranes, jaundice.
- Big hard irregular liver.
- Signs of weight loss.
- Ascites.

In the laboratory, do:

- A hemoglobin exam.
- A fresh blood drop exam to look for sickle cells.
- A white blood cell count.
- A thick blood film to look for plasmodium.

BIG SPLEEN

Possible causes

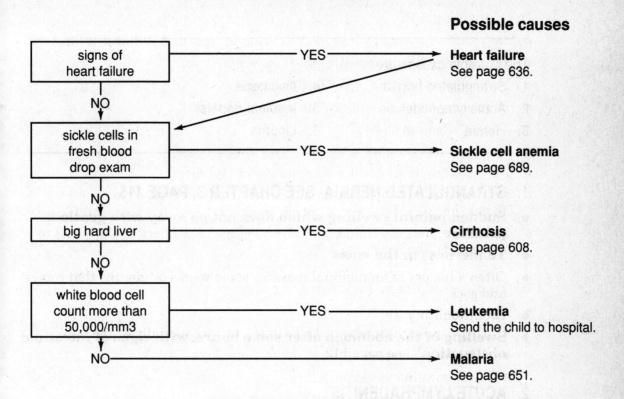

signs of heart failure	—YES→	**Heart failure** See page 636.
↓ NO		
sickle cells in fresh blood drop exam	—YES→	**Sickle cell anemia** See page 689.
↓ NO		
big hard liver	—YES→	**Cirrhosis** See page 608.
↓ NO		
white blood cell count more than 50,000/mm3	—YES→	**Leukemia** Send the child to hospital.
↓ NO		**Malaria** See page 651.

MASS IN THE INGUINAL REGION

The possible causes are:

1. Strangulated hernia
2. Acute lymphadenitis
3. Hernia
4. Iliac node
5. Inguinal node(s)
6. Lipoma

1. STRANGULATED HERNIA- SEE CHAPTER 3, PAGE 115

- **Sudden painful swelling which does not go away with gentle pressure**.
- **Tenderness in the mass**.
- Often a history of an inguinal mass for some weeks or months that comes and goes.
- Often vomiting.
- **Swelling of the abdomen after some hours, with signs of intestinal obstruction** - see page 112.

2. ACUTE LYMPHADENITIS

- **Painful swelling that develops over 1 or 2 days**.
- **Tenderness and heat in the mass**.
- Often fever.
- No vomiting.
- Often a sore on the leg, the buttocks, the scrotum or the vulva.
- If you cannot tell if the mass is a lymphadenitis or a strangulated hernia, send the patient immediately to hospital.

3. HERNIA - SEE CHAPTER 3, PAGE 113

- **Soft mass that comes when the patient stands, coughs, or pushes**.
- **The mass goes away with gentle pressure, or when the patient lies down**.
- No tenderness or heat in the mass.
- Mass often present for some weeks, months, or even years.

4. ILIAC NODE - SEE CHAPTER 3, PAGE 116

- **Firm mass fixed to the pelvis just to the outside of the iliac artery**. You can easily feel the pulse of this artery as it goes across the inguinal ligament. It is just inside the iliac node, toward the middle.
- The mass is **deep inside the muscles of the lower abdomen**.
- The mass is sometimes tender.
- Sometimes the patient has a low irregular fever.
- The cause may be tuberculosis, or it may be a tumor. Send the patient to hospital.

5. INGUINAL NODE(S) - SEE CHAPTER 3, PAGE 116

- **Small movable lumps just under the skin in front of the inguinal ligament**.
- The lumps do not go away with gentle pressure.
- Sometimes a little tenderness. Tenderness is a sign of infection.
- Often sores on the leg, the buttocks, the scrotum, or the vulva.

6. LIPOMA

- **Large soft mass just under the skin**, often present for months or years.
- **The mass does not go away with gentle pressure**.
- No tenderness, heat, or fever.

TO MAKE THE DIAGNOSIS

In the history, ask:
- When did the mass come?
- Did it start suddenly or slowly?
- Does it hurt?
- Does the mass go away when you lie down? Or when you push on it?
- Have you had fever or vomiting?

In the physical exam, look for:
- The aspect of the mass:
  - Is it hard or soft?
  - Is it tender or not? Is it hot or not?
  - Does it go away when you push gently on it? Never push hard.
  - Is it fixed? Or can you make it move?
- Where it is? Just under the skin? Or inside the muscles?
- Swelling of the abdomen.
- Fever.
- Sores on the leg, the buttocks, the scrotum, or the vulva.

MASS IN THE INGUINAL REGION

Possible causes

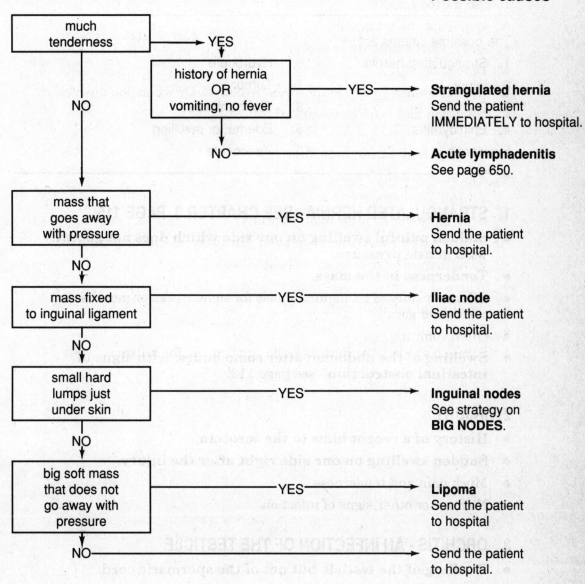

much tenderness → YES → **history of hernia OR vomiting, no fever** → YES →	**Strangulated hernia** Send the patient IMMEDIATELY to hospital.
NO →	**Acute lymphadenitis** See page 650.
mass that goes away with pressure → YES →	**Hernia** Send the patient to hospital.
mass fixed to inguinal ligament → YES →	**Iliac node** Send the patient to hospital.
small hard lumps just under skin → YES →	**Inguinal nodes** See strategy on **BIG NODES**.
big soft mass that does not go away with pressure → YES →	**Lipoma** Send the patient to hospital
NO →	Send the patient to hospital.

MASS IN THE SCROTUM

The possible causes are:

1. Strangulated hernia
2. Injury
3. Orchitis
4. Epididymitis
5. Hernia

6. Hydrocele
7. Tumor
8. Elephantiasis
9. Edema, or swelling
10. Varicocele

1. STRANGULATED HERNIA - SEE CHAPTER 3, PAGE 115

- **Sudden painful swelling on one side which does not go away with gentle pressure.**
- **Tenderness in the mass.**
- Often a history of an inguinal mass for some weeks or months that comes and goes.
- Often vomiting.
- **Swelling of the abdomen after some hours, with signs of intestinal obstruction** - see page 112.

2. INJURY

- **History of a recent blow to the scrotum.**
- **Sudden swelling on one side right after the injury.**
- Much pain and tenderness.
- No fever or other signs of infection.

3. ORCHITIS - AN INFECTION OF THE TESTICLE

- **Swelling of the testicle but not of the spermatic cord.**
- **Much pain and tenderness.**
- Often fever and sometimes vomiting.

4. EPIDIDYMITIS - AN INFECTION OF THE SPERMATIC CORD

- **Sudden swelling, pain, and tenderness of the spermatic cord and testicle**.
- Often a recent history of pain on urination or of pus coming from the urethra.
- Often fever.
- The prostate is often tender on rectal exam.

5. HERNIA - SEE CHAPTER 3, PAGE 113

- **Soft mass that comes when the patient stands, coughs, or pushes**.
- **The mass goes away with gentle pressure, or when the patient lies down**.
- No tenderness or heat in the mass.
- Mass often present for some weeks, months, or even years.
- **The testicle is outside the mass, and you can feel that it is separate from the mass**.

6. HYDROCELE

- **A firm mass inside the scrotum on one or both sides**.
- **No pain or tenderness**. The patient may have a feeling of heaviness.
- **The mass does not go away with gentle pressure or when the patient lies down**.
- The testicle is inside the mass, and you cannot feel it.
- Use a strong light and hold it against the mass. You will be able to see some light through the hydrocele. This is because there is liquid in the hydrocele.

7. TUMOR

- **Hard mass in one testicle or in the spermatic cord**.
- No pain or tenderness.

8. ELEPHANTIASIS

- **Swelling of both sides of the scrotum for weeks or months**, with no pitting.
- **Skin very thick and moist**.
- It is difficult or impossible to feel the testicles or spermatic cords inside the scrotum.
- Often big inguinal lymph nodes.

9. EDEMA

- From heart failure, cirrhosis, kidney disease or malnutrition.
- **Soft swelling of both sides of the scrotum, with pitting**.
- Pitting edema of the feet, the legs, and even the lower abdomen.
- **Other signs of heart failure, cirrhosis, kidney disease or malnutrition**.

10. VARICOCELE

- This means varicose veins in the spermatic cord.
- **Mass of twisted veins like big worms in the spermatic cord on one side of the scrotum**.
- Feeling of heaviness.
- No pain, tenderness, or fever.

See the section about the male organs in Chapter 3 on pages 119.

TO MAKE THE DIAGNOSIS

In the history, ask:

- When did the swelling come?
- Did it start slowly or suddenly?
- Does it hurt?
- Have you vomited? Or had much pain in the abdomen?
- Have you had an accident with a blow to the scrotum?
- Have you had fever?
- Have you had pain on urination? Or pus coming from the urine opening?
- Does the mass go away when you push on it? Or when you lie down?
- Have you had a cough, or trouble breathing, or other swelling?

In the physical exam, look for:

- The aspect of the mass:
  - Is it hard or soft? Tender or not?
  - Does it go away when you push gently on it?
  - Is it in the testicle, or in the spermatic cord?
  - Is it in the skin, or in the subcutaneous tissue?
- Swelling of the abdomen, or other signs of intestinal obstruction.
- Fever.
- Tenderness of the prostate by rectal exam.
- Swelling of the skin of the scrotum. Is it thick? Is there pitting?
- Pitting edema of the feet, the legs, or the lower abdomen.
- Signs of heart failure or of malnutrition.
- Big hard liver.
- Twisted veins, like worms, in the spermatic cord.

In the laboratory, do:

- A fresh blood drop exam to look for microfilaria.
- A urine exam to look for protein or white blood cells.

MASS IN THE SCROTUM

Possible causes

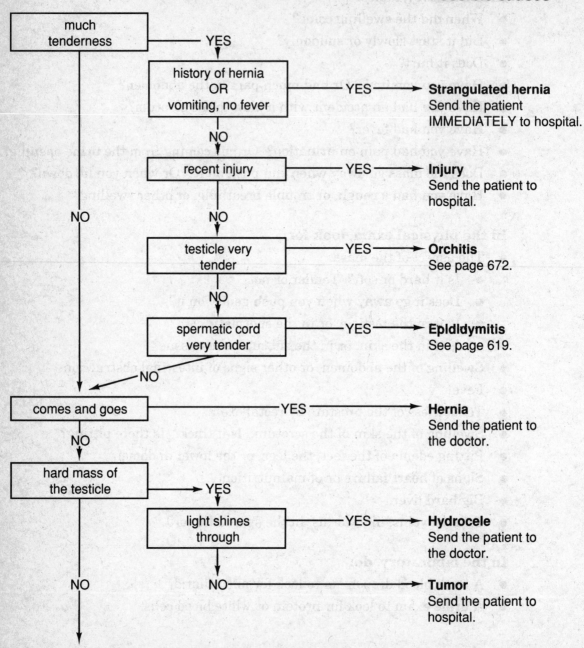

much tenderness — YES →

history of hernia OR vomiting, no fever — YES → **Strangulated hernia**
Send the patient IMMEDIATELY to hospital.

NO ↓

recent injury — YES → **Injury**
Send the patient to hospital.

NO ↓

testicle very tender — YES → **Orchitis**
See page 672.

NO ↓

spermatic cord very tender — YES → **Epldldymitis**
See page 619.

NO →

comes and goes — YES → **Hernia**
Send the patient to the doctor.

NO ↓

hard mass of the testicle — YES →

light shines through — YES → **Hydrocele**
Send the patient to the doctor.

NO → **Tumor**
Send the patient to hospital.

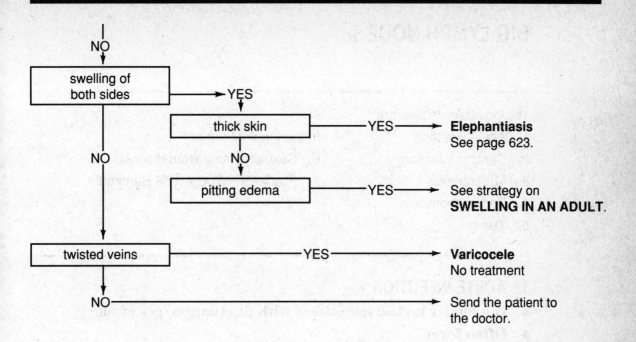

NO
↓

| swelling of both sides | → YES ↓ |

thick skin —— YES ——→ **Elephantiasis**
See page 623.

NO ↓

pitting edema —— YES ——→ See strategy on **SWELLING IN AN ADULT**.

NO ↓

| twisted veins | —————— YES ——————→ **Varicocele**
No treatment

NO ——————————————————→ Send the patient to the doctor.

BIG LYMPH NODES

The possible causes are:

1. Acute infection
2. Chronic infection
3. Tuberculosis
4. Trypanosomiasis
5. Tumor

In the inguinal region:

6. Sexually transmitted disease
7. Filariasis - Wuchereria Bancrofti

1. ACUTE INFECTION

- **Big tender nodes, sometimes with fluctuation** (pus inside).
- **Often fever**.
- Usually an acute infection in the region: abscess, cellulitis, tonsillitis, eczema.
- Some infectious diseases cause a general enlargement of lymph nodes. The big lymph nodes go away after the infection is finished.

2. CHRONIC INFECTION

- Such as scabies, chronic sores, infected fungus infection of the skin.
- The lymph nodes in the region of the infection are **big and a little tender**.

3. TUBERCULOSIS

- Big nodes in one or more regions
- **Some pain and a little tenderness in the nodes**.
- **Often several nodes stuck together**.
- The main regions for tuberculous lymph nodes are:
  1. **The neck**: just above the clavicles, or the posterior chain in back of the sternomastoid muscle.

2. **The abdomen**:
   - In the mesentery. They are small, tender, mobile lumps in the abdomen.
   - In the iliac region. The nodes are fixed to the inguinal ligament just to the outside of the iliac artery. They are inside the muscles of the lower abdomen.
3. **The armpit**.
4. **The inguinal and femoral regions**. Most often big nodes in these regions come from an ordinary infection, or from filariasis. But sometimes tuberculosis can cause big lymph nodes in these regions.

- Chronic irregular fever.
- **Often a history of a member of the family who has, or who has had tuberculosis**.
- It is necessary to do a surgical biopsy to confirm the diagnosis of tuberculous nodes. Send every patient to hospital who you think may have tuberculosis of the lymph nodes.

4. TRYPANOSOMIASIS - AFRICAN SLEEPING SICKNESS

- This disease exists only in Central and West Africa.
- **One or more small separate nodes in the posterior part of the neck**.
- **No pain or tenderness in the nodes**.
- Low chronic fever.
- Rapid pulse.
- **Moving trypanosomes in the liquid taken from a node by node puncture and aspiration**.

5. TUMOR

- One or more groups of big nodes.
- **Nodes big, hard, not tender, and often stuck together**.
- Sometimes a mass or tumor in the region.

6. SEXUALLY TRANSMITTED DISEASE

- Syphilis and lymphogranuloma venereum cause **big nodes in one or both inguinal regions**.
- **Big nodes with some pain and tenderness**.
- Sometimes fluctuation, and sometimes rupture with formation of a fistula.
- Chronic swelling around the nodes.
- Usually the first lesion on the penis or the vulva has disappeared.

7. FILARIASIS - WUCHERERIA BANCROFTI

- Big inguinal or femoral lymph nodes.
- **Nodes hard with no pain or tenderness**.
- Often **chronic swelling** of the leg, the vulva or the scrotum with the skin becoming very thick. We call this "elephantiasis."
- **Microfilaria in the blood between 20 hr and 24 hr.**

See the section on lymph nodes in Chapter 3 on pages 116-117.

TO MAKE THE DIAGNOSIS

In the history, ask:

- When did the nodes first start to become big?
- Do they hurt?
- Have you had fever? Or a sore or an infection in that area?
- Is there someone in your family who has, or who has had tuberculosis?
- Is there swelling or a lump around or near the big nodes?
- Do you have a sore on the penis? Or on the vulva?
- Was there a sore before the nodes came?

In the physical exam, look for:

- The region or the regions where the big nodes are.
- What the nodes are like: Size, hard or soft, fixed or mobile, tender or not tender, separate or stuck together, just under the skin, or inside the muscles.
- Another infection in the region: Scabies, sore, fungus infection, eczema, abscess.
- Fever. Sometimes it is necessary to take the temperature of the patient three times a day for several days to see if there is fever and to see what it is like. Write down the temperature each time.
- Rapid pulse.
- A mass or tumor in the region.
- Chronic swelling of the leg, the vulva, or the scrotum.

In the laboratory, do:

- A fresh blood drop exam between 20 hr and 24 hr to look for microfilaria.
- In Central or West Africa, a node puncture of any posterior neck nodes to look for trypanosomes.
- A thick blood film to look for microfilaria and trypanosomes.

BIG LYMPH NODES

Possible causes

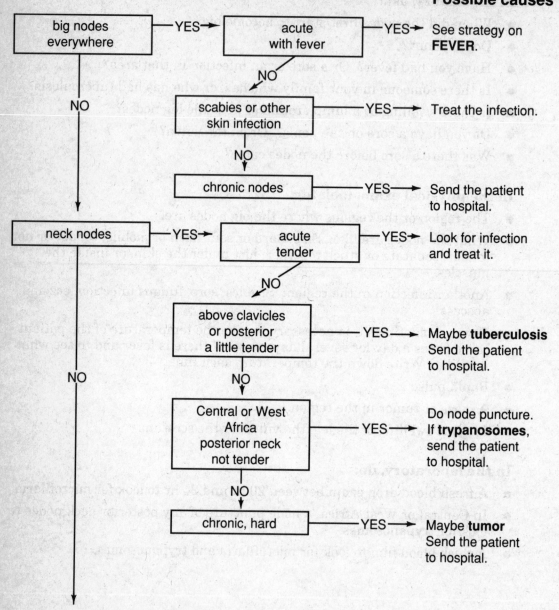

big nodes everywhere	—YES→ acute with fever	—YES→ See strategy on **FEVER**.
	NO	
	scabies or other skin infection	—YES→ Treat the infection.
	NO	
	chronic nodes	—YES→ Send the patient to hospital.
neck nodes	—YES→ acute tender	—YES→ Look for infection and treat it.
	NO	
	above clavicles or posterior a little tender	—YES→ Maybe **tuberculosis** Send the patient to hospital.
	NO	
	Central or West Africa posterior neck not tender	—YES→ Do node puncture. If **trypanosomes**, send the patient to hospital.
	NO	
	chronic, hard	—YES→ Maybe **tumor** Send the patient to hospital.

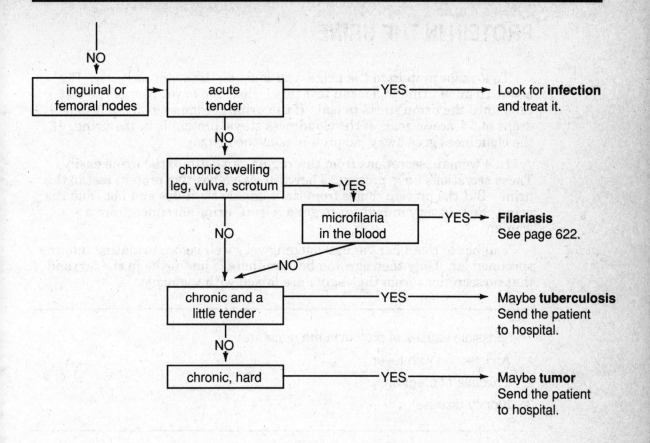

PROTEIN IN THE URINE

To look for protein in the urine, you must do the exam correctly. Put about 10 ml of urine in a clean test tube. Heat the lower part of the test tube until the urine starts to boil. If the urine becomes cloudy, put in 3 drops of 3% acetic acid. If the cloudiness stays, protein is in the urine. If the cloudiness goes away, no protein is in the urine.

In a woman, secretions from the vagina can get into the urine easily. These secretions have protein. They will give a positive protein test to the urine. But the protein comes from the vaginal secretions and not from the urine. So it is very important to get a "clean" urine specimen from a woman.

Tell her to clean her vaginal opening very well before urinating into the specimen jar. Only then can you be sure there is just urine in the jar, and that no secretions from the vagina are mixed with the urine.

The possible causes of protein in the urine are:

1. An infection with fever
2. Toxemia of pregnancy
3. Kidney disease

---

1. INFECTION WITH FEVER

● Such as malaria, pneumonia, typhoid fever.

● If the patient has protein in the urine AND a fever, look for other symptoms and signs of infection. Follow the strategy of each one.

2. TOXEMIA OF PREGNANCY

● **Pregnancy in the last 3 months - the last trimester.**

● **Swelling** of the feet, the legs, the face and even of the hands.

● Often **high blood pressure: above 130/90**.

● Protein in the urine during the first six months of pregnancy comes from a kidney disease and not from toxemia.

● Protein in the urine during the last trimester with no swelling and no high blood pressure also comes from a kidney disease and not from toxemia.

3. KIDNEY DISEASE

- Such as nephritis, pyelonephritis, or nephrosis.
- Often **swelling** of the feet, the legs, and even the lower abdomen.
- Often high blood pressure.
- Sometimes a fever.
- Often **white or red blood cells in the urine**.

TO MAKE THE DIAGNOSIS

In the history, ask:
- Do you have difficulty urinating?
  - Pain on urinating, frequent urination, or much urine?
  - Do you have trouble passing the urine? Or blood or pus in the urine?
- Have you had fever?
- Have you had swelling of the feet or the legs?
- In a woman: are you pregnant? If so, how many months?

In the physical exam, look for:
- Fever. If present, look for other signs of infection.
- A pregnancy in the last trimester.
- Swelling of the feet, the legs, the abdomen.
- High blood pressure.

In the laboratory, do:
- A complete urine exam to look for red and white blood cells.
- Other lab exams necessary to see if another infection is present.

PROTEIN IN THE URINE

Possible causes

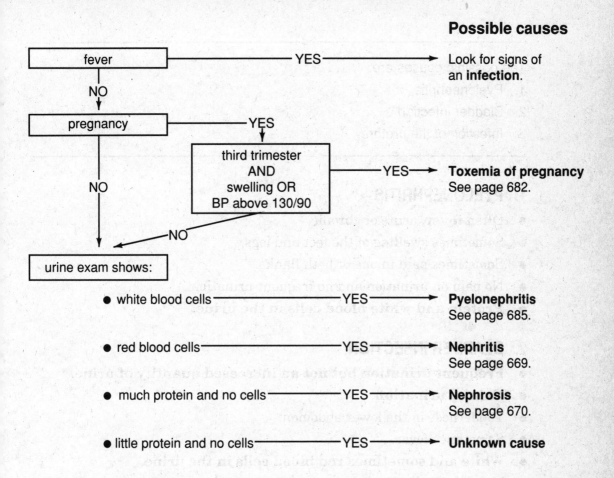

fever ——————YES——————→ Look for signs of
an **infection**.

NO

pregnancy ————YES

NO

third trimester
AND
swelling OR
BP above 130/90 ———YES→ **Toxemia of pregnancy**
See page 682.

NO

urine exam shows:

● white blood cells ——————YES——————→ **Pyelonephritis**
See page 685.

● red blood cells ——————YES——————→ **Nephritis**
See page 669.

● much protein and no cells ——————YES——————→ **Nephrosis**
See page 670.

● little protein and no cells ——————YES——————→ **Unknown cause**

If the cause is unknown and the patient has no symptoms, give no
treatment. Tell the patient to drink much water. Repeat the urine exam
after one or more weeks. If protein is still in the urine, send the patient to
hospital.

WHITE BLOOD CELLS IN THE URINE

The possible causes are:
1. Pyelonephritis
2. Bladder infection
3. Infection of the urethra

1. PYELONEPHRITIS

- Often **fever**, acute or chronic.
- Sometimes swelling of the feet and legs.
- Sometimes pain in one or both flanks.
- No pain on urination and no frequent urination.
- **Protein and white blood cells in the urine.**

2. BLADDER INFECTION

- **Frequent urination but not an increased quantity of urine**.
- **Painful urination**.
- Tenderness in the lower abdomen.
- Sometimes fever.
- **White and sometimes red blood cells in the urine.**
- **No protein in the urine.**

3. INFECTION OF THE URETHRA

- This is rare in a woman.
- **Often a history of gonorrhea in the past**.
- Pain on urination.
- Sometimes **pus coming out of the urethra between urinations**. In this case, make a smear of the pus on a microscope slide. If possible, do a gram stain and look for gram-negative diplococci inside the white blood cells. If they are present, the cause is gonorrhea.

TO MAKE THE DIAGNOSIS

Give 3 urine specimen jars to the patient. Tell him to urinate in each one in the following way.

- A small quantity at the beginning of urination is to go into the first jar.
- Then, most of the urine is to go into the second jar.
- The last small quantity is to go into the third jar.

Examine the urine in all three jars. This exam will tell you the cause of the white blood cells in the urine.

- White blood cells only in the first jar ——→ **Infection of the urethra**
  Give treatment for
  bladder infection,
  page 605.

- Many white blood cells in the third jar
  and few cells in the first and second jars——→ **Bladder infection**
  See page 605.

- The same number of white blood cells
  in all three jars ————————————————→ **Pyelonephritis**
  See page 685.

BLOOD IN THE URINE (HEMATURIA)

Blood in the urine is a sign of a very serious disease. The possible causes are:

1. Injury of the urethra
2. Hypertrophy of the prostate
3. Bladder infection
4. Kidney stone
5. Schistosomiasis of the bladder
6. Kidney disease
7. Tumor in the urinary system
8. Tuberculosis in the urinary system

Do not confuse hematuria with "black water fever." This is a complication of malaria. It causes the urine to become very red like blood. But in black water fever, there are no red blood cells in the urine. There is only hemoglobin.

In a case of red urine, look at the urine under the microscope. If there are many red blood cells, it is hematuria. If there are no red blood cells, the red color comes from hemoglobin. The patient has black water fever. For the treatment, see page 654.

The only possible cause of hematuria that you can find and treat in a health center is schistosomiasis. If the patient with hematuria does not have schistosomiasis, send the patient **immediately** to hospital.

A serious accident can cause an injury to the urethra or the bladder. This can cause hematuria. Send the patient immediately to hospital. **Do not try to pass a catheter into the bladder**. This could make the injury much worse.

The patient may have a bladder full of urine. You will then be able to feel the full bladder in the lower abdomen. In this case, before you send the patient to hospital, make a sterile puncture of the bladder through the wall of the lower abdomen. Take out the urine by aspiration.

The injured patient may have much tenderness in the lower abdomen, in the back, or at the pelvis. In this case there may be a fracture of the pelvis. Find a solid stretcher, or even a long board. Put a mattress, or blankets, on it. Send the patient to hospital on this solid stretcher. Give the patient a big dose of an antibiotic before the journey.

STIFF NECK

The possible causes are:

1. Tetanus
2. Acute meningitis
3. Chronic meningitis
4. Arthritis of the neck

1. TETANUS

- **Frequent muscle spasms caused by noise or by movements.**
- **Inability to open the mouth.** The teeth are tightly shut together. We call this "trismus."
- **Stiffness of the neck and of the whole back.**
- Fever. The fever is sometimes absent.
- No delirium or coma. The consciousness is clear.
- There is often a wound, a sore, a burn, chiggers, or an open fracture.

2. ACUTE MENINGITIS

- **High fever.**
- Convulsions.
- In a small baby, a swollen fontanel.
- **CSF cloudy**, with many white blood cells.

3. CHRONIC MENINGITIS

- **Chronic headache and chronic pain in the neck.**
- **Irregular fever**, high at night and absent during the day.
- **CSF clear, but with some white blood cells: from 10 to 1000/mm3.**

- Loss of weight.
- Sometimes difficulty speaking, walking, or seeing.
- Sometimes delirium or coma.

4. ARTHRITIS OF THE NECK

- **Pain in the neck made worse by movement**.
- No fever.
- No signs of tetanus or of meningitis.

TO MAKE THE DIAGNOSIS

In the history, ask the patient or a member of the family:
- When did the stiff neck begin?
- Did it begin quickly or slowly?
- Have you had a fever, convulsions, muscle spasms, loss of consciousness, or headache?
- Can you open your mouth?

In the physical exam, look for:
- Muscle spasms caused by noise or by movements.
- Trismus.
- Fever.
- Consciousness: Clear? Delirium? Coma?
- Wound, burn, chiggers, open fracture.
- In a baby, a swollen fontanel.
- Signs of weight loss.
- Pain on movements of the neck: extension, flexion, turning.
- Limitation of movements of the neck.

In the laboratory, do:
- A lumbar puncture on any patient with:
  - High fever and a stiff neck or a swollen fontanel.
  - Fever and convulsions.
  - Chronic headache and chronic fever.

STIFF NECK

Possible causes

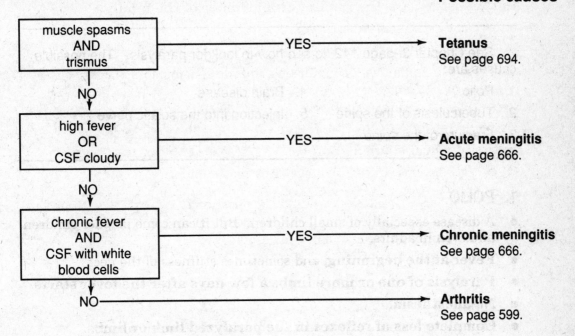

muscle spasms AND trismus —YES→ **Tetanus** See page 694.

NO

high fever OR CSF cloudy —YES→ **Acute meningitis** See page 666.

NO

chronic fever AND CSF with white blood cells —YES→ **Chronic meningitis** See page 666.

NO→ **Arthritis** See page 599.

PARALYSIS OF ONE OR BOTH LEGS

See Chapter 3, page 142, to see how to look for paralysis. The possible causes are:

1. Polio
2. Tuberculosis of the spine
3. Fracture of the spine
4. Brain disease
5. Injection into the sciatic nerve

1. POLIO

- A disease especially of small children. But it can come in older children and even in adults.
- **Fever at the beginning,** and sometimes stiffness of the neck.
- **Paralysis of one or more limbs a few days after the fever starts.**
- **No anesthesia.**
- **Complete loss of reflexes in the paralyzed limb or limbs.**

2. TUBERCULOSIS OF THE SPINE - POTT'S DISEASE

- **Chronic pain in one spot on the spine.**
- Often **a tender bony swelling at the painful spot.**
- After some weeks, progressive weakness of the legs.
- Also **progressive anesthesia** of the legs and even the abdomen.
- **Loss of reflexes in the legs.**

3. FRACTURE OF THE SPINE

- **History of a fall or a severe injury to the back** followed by paralysis of both legs and often anesthesia.
- Often a **deformity of the spine at the place of the fracture.**
- Loss of reflexes in the legs for some months. Then the reflexes come back and are very strong.

4. BRAIN DISEASE

- Brain hemorrhage, brain tumor, brain abscess.
- **Paralysis of the arm and the leg on one side of the body**.
- **No anesthesia**.
- Often difficulty with speech and delirium or coma.

5. INJECTION OF THE SCIATIC NERVE

- **History of an injection in one buttocks followed by paralysis of all or part of that leg**.
- Sometimes anesthesia.
- Sometimes loss of one or both reflexes: knee jerk and ankle reflex.

SYMPTOMATIC TREATMENT OF LEG PARALYSIS

Passive exercises of each paralyzed limb are very important. They keep the joints mobile, and protect them from becoming stiff. They also help the circulation of the limb. Show someone in the family of the patient how to do these exercises. Explain the importance of doing them every day.

1. Do all the movements of each joint of the paralyzed limb: extension, flexion, rotation. Show the family member how to do this.

2. Try to move each joint in the complete range of motion: full extension, full flexion, etc. The patient may already have stiffness of one or more joints. If so, it is necessary to try to overcome this stiffness. Pull or push quite hard. Try to pull or push the joint a little more each day. After some days or weeks, the stiffness will go away.

3. Do these exercises at least 3 times a day.

4. Make each movement of each joint at least 20 times during each session of exercises.

5. Encourage the family to take the patient to the doctor regularly for more instructions and help.

TO MAKE THE DIAGNOSIS

In the history, ask:
- When did the paralysis start?
- Did it start slowly or suddenly?
- Did you have a fever at the beginning? A stiff neck?
- Did you fall or have an accident that caused the paralysis?
- Did you get an injection in the buttocks just before the paralysis?

In the physical examination, look for:
- Fever.
- Anesthesia of the paralyzed limb or limbs.
- Presence or absence of reflexes of the paralyzed limb or limbs. Compare the strength of the reflexes of the two legs or arms.
- A deformity of the spine.
- A tender bony swelling of the spine.
- High blood pressure.
- Difficulty with speech, or delirium, or coma.

PARALYSIS OF ONE OR BOTH LEGS

Possible causes

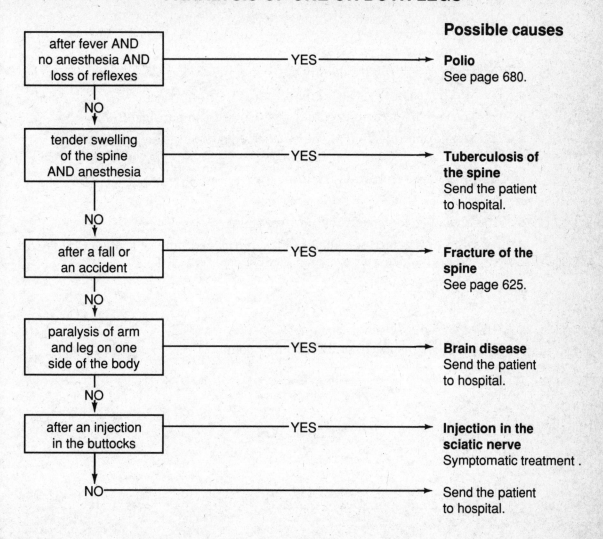

after fever AND no anesthesia AND loss of reflexes — YES → **Polio**
See page 680.

NO

tender swelling of the spine AND anesthesia — YES → **Tuberculosis of the spine**
Send the patient to hospital.

NO

after a fall or an accident — YES → **Fracture of the spine**
See page 625.

NO

paralysis of arm and leg on one side of the body — YES → **Brain disease**
Send the patient to hospital.

NO

after an injection in the buttocks — YES → **Injection in the sciatic nerve**
Symptomatic treatment .

NO → Send the patient to hospital.

Chapter 10
THE PRINCIPLES OF TREATMENT

10.1 Know your patient

10.2 Give urgent treatment quickly

10.3 Specific treatment

10.4 Symptomatic treatment

10.5 Make sure the patient gets well and stays well

10.6 Keep good records of all the diseases you treat

10.1 Know your patient

THE PATIENT AS A PERSON

At the beginning of the consultation find out who your patient is. The patient is a person like yourself. He has a name. Find out what it is. Try to remember it. Call him by name each time you see him.

Find out where he lives. Ask him what kind of work he does. Ask questions about his family. Ask about his living conditions.

This is very important. This will show the patient that you are interested in him as a person. You are interested not just in the illness but in him as a person. This will help you gain his confidence. It will help him work with you in the treatment. The treatment will work better and he will be more sure to get well.

THE PATIENT HAS NEEDS

Find out the needs of your patient. Give attention to these needs. He certainly needs treatment. But he also needs good care, good instructions, and an understanding of the illness.

Be sure you know what disease the patient has. You can give good treatment only if you know the disease you are treating. That is why a good history and a complete physical examination are very important.

The patient may also have needs for food, clothing, or other personal matters. You cannot give him food or clothes. But you can talk to him about this. You can also talk to his family.

Sometimes a patient has no one to help him. In this case, you can talk to other persons in his community. You can ask them to help him.

In many health services, patients pay money for their treatment and care. In this case, you will probably receive money from the patient or from his family. But remember that you are trying to help him get well. This is your first interest. Do not work just to get more money from him. Our work is to serve our patients. But we must not use them just to get more money for ourselves.

WE ARE NOT HEALERS

Sometimes we think we are healers. This is a false idea. We are simply helpers. Our medicine and our care are only helps for our patients.

As persons, we have many abilities in our bodies and minds to get well and to stay well. These abilities work together to heal us when we are ill. Our task is to help these natural abilities make our patients well. It is these abilities that do the real healing. Our job is to give our patients the medicines, the care, and the instructions that can help them get well.

10.2 Give urgent treatment quickly

Some diseases are very serious. Other diseases are not serious. Read again in Chapter 1 how to tell if a disease is serious or not. Serious diseases will take much time and work. It may be necessary to leave some of your other work for a short time to care for a seriously ill patient. But then go back to your other work later to finish that as well.

Some conditions require treatment quickly. You must treat them immediately, often before you take a full history or do a complete physical examination. You will complete the history and the physical examination later. These are the conditions that need immediate treatment.

1. Obstruction of the breathing.
2. Shock.
3. Severe hemorrhage.
4. Convulsions.
5. A big open wound, especially of the chest, of the abdomen, or of a bone.
6. A fracture.

1. OBSTRUCTION OF THE RESPIRATION

1. Remove all secretions from the mouth. Use a bulb syringe, a piece of gauze, or even your fingers.
2. Remove any object from the mouth - food, loose teeth, foreign body.
3. Pull the lower jaw forward. This will open the back of the throat so that air can go through.
4. If possible, turn the patient on his side, or at least the head to one side.

2. SHOCK

For the treatment of shock, see the strategies on SHOCK IN A CHILD and SHOCK IN AN ADULT on pages 500 and 504.

3. HEMORRHAGE

If the hemorrhage is from a wound, put a sterile or clean gauze or cloth on the wound. Then press strongly on the wound to stop the hemorrhage. If you can find a pulse above the wound, press strongly on this pulse to close the artery. This will also help stop the bleeding. Do not use a tourniquet. This is dangerous and may cause gangrene. If the hemorrhage does not stop, or if it starts again, send the patient to hospital as quickly as possible.

If the hemorrhage is inside the body, in the stomach, the intestines, the vagina, the lungs, the nose, or the abdomen, keep the patient quiet. Start an infusion. The patient will probably need a transfusion. If you cannot give a transfusion, send the patient quickly to hospital.

4. CONVULSIONS

For the treatment of convulsions, see the strategies on CONVULSIONS IN A CHILD and CONVULSIONS IN AN ADULT on pages 422 and 428.

5. OPEN WOUND

Of the chest

For an open wound of the chest through which air passes, cover the wound immediately with a clean or sterile dressing. If the hospital is far away, close the wound by sutures. Give antibiotics. Then send the patient to hospital.

Of the abdomen

For an open wound of the abdomen, wash the skin very carefully around the wound. Cover the wound with a clean or sterile dressing. Give the patient antibiotics. Send him to hospital. He needs an operation to see if he has serious wounds inside the abdomen.

Of a fracture

For an open wound of a fracture, wash the skin very carefully around the wound. Cover the wound with a clean or sterile dressing. Do not close the wound with sutures. Give the patient antibiotics. Immobilize the fracture with a splint and send the patient to hospital.

After urgent treatment

After you have completed the urgent treatment, take a good history from the patient or from his family. Finish the physical examination. Look for other injuries or diseases. Do any necessary laboratory exams. Write on the patient's record the history of the disease or the accident. Write down all the signs you have found. Then decide on the treatment he needs.

10.3 Specific treatment

Specific treatment is treatment for the cause of the disease. It is the treatment you give the patient to get rid of the disease. For example:

- Chloroquine is a specific treatment for malaria.
- Penicillin is a specific treatment for pneumonia.
- Piperazine is a specific treatment for ascaris.
- Dapsone is a specific treatment for leprosy.

In this section of the book you will find the specific treatment for the diseases we have listed in the book. Learn the treatment for each disease. Follow the instructions carefully. This will help the patient get well quickly.

Specific treatment for a certain disease can change. Sometimes doctors find new medicines that work better. So you no longer use the old medicine. It is possible that your health service does not use a medicine listed in this book. So learn well the medicine your health service does use. If a new medicine comes, find out all about it. Learn to use it well.

10.4 Symptomatic treatment

In addition to the specific treatment to cure the disease, the patient needs treatment for his symptoms. This is to help him feel better. You will find the treatment for each symptom in the strategy for that symptom. Give the patient this treatment until the symptom goes away.

Remember, however, that symptomatic treatment will not cure the disease. So give specific treatment to cure the disease and symptomatic treatment to help the patient feel better.

10.5 Make sure the patient gets well and stays well

See the patient again when the treatment is finished. Find out if he has any more signs or symptoms of disease. If so, decide if he needs more of the same treatment. Or perhaps you will need to change the treatment.

When your patients are well, it will no longer be necessary to see them again often. But many of your patients live in one of the communities you serve. Try to see them again from time to time. See if they are following the health education you gave. See if they have other problems that need education or care. Encourage them to do all that is necessary to stay well and to keep from becoming ill again.

10.6 Keep good records of all the diseases you treat

Keep a register of the patients you treat. In this register, write the name, sex, age, and address of each patient and the date he came to your health center. Write also the diagnosis, the treatment you gave him, and the result. When this register is full, be sure to keep it in a safe place. This register is very important, and you should keep it for many years.

At the end of each month, make a list of all of the different diseases you have seen during that month and the number of cases of each disease. Send this list to the doctor in charge of your health center. The doctor will then be able to let the government authorities know all of the different diseases in your area and the number of cases of each one. In this way the authorities of the Ministry of Health will know what the important diseases are that affect the health of the people.

Chapter 11
THE ADMINISTRATION OF MEDICINES

11.1 Different names for the same medicine

11.2 Different forms of the same medicine

11.3 Always be sure you give the correct medicine

11.4 Always give the correct dose

11.5 How to find out the correct dose of each medicine

11.6 Always give a complete cure

11.7 Signs of toxicity and what to do

11.1 Different names for the same medicine

Each medicine has a generic name. This is the real name of the medicine. But the drug companies who make medicines often give their own name to each medicine. This is the commercial name of the medicine. If more than one drug company make a certain medicine, that medicine will have more than one commercial name.

For example, several drug companies make chloroquine to treat malaria. Chloroquine is the real, or generic, name of this medicine. But chloroquine has several commercial names: Nivaquine, Resochine, Aralen, Avloquine. Be sure you know the generic name for each medicine you use. Learn also the common commercial name, or names, of this medicine.

In this book we use the generic name of most medicines. If we give the commercial name, we put an * in front of that name. Remember, however, that chloroquine and *Nivaquine are exactly the same medicine.

11.2 Different forms of the same medicine

Many medicines come in different forms: liquid, solid, or for injection. Know the different forms for each medicine. Know when and how to use each different form.

Often we use the liquid form for babies and young children. This is because babies and young children have difficulty in swallowing tablets or capsules.

We use the injection form if the patient is very ill, or if the patient cannot swallow. Some medicines, however, come only in injectable form, like streptomycin, or insulin.

11.3 Always be sure you give the correct medicine

Before you give a medicine, look carefully at the name of the medicine on the bottle, the ampoule, or the vial. If there is no name, or if you cannot read the name, do not use that medicine. Throw it away. You cannot be sure what medicine is inside. If you use this medicine anyway, you can do much harm to the patient. The medicine may be the wrong medicine for the patient.

For this reason, make sure each bottle of medicine has a label on it. Write the name of the medicine clearly. Keep the labels clean. If the label becomes dirty, make a new label to put on the bottle.

Also, before giving a medicine to a patient, be sure you know what medicine you must give. Look at the patient's record to see again the medicine to give. Then look at the label on the medicine bottle, or ampoule, or vial. Be sure it is the same medicine as the medicine written on the record.

11.4 Always give the correct dose

The correct dose helps the patient get well. If the dose is too small, it will not give much help. The patient may not get well. If the dose is too big, it may make him very sick. It can even kill him.

So always give the correct dose. You must know how to calculate, or find, the correct dose. Often the dose depends on the weight of the patient. This is true especially with children. So weigh the patient before you calculate the dose to give.

11.5 How to find the correct dose of each medicine

First of all, learn how much medicine to give for each kilogram of weight. In most cases, you will find this on the label of the bottle. If not, look in this book to find the number of milligrams or milliliters to give for each kilogram of weight.

Then weigh the patient. Write down the number of milligrams or milliliters to give for each kilo. Multiply the number of milligrams per kilo (mg/kg) or milliliters per kilo (ml/kg) by the weight of the patient in kilograms. This will give you the total number of milligrams or milliliters to give the patient.

mg/kg X weight of patient in kg = dose to give in milligrams

ml/kg X weight of patient in kg = dose to give in milliliters

Now look at the medicine bottle or vial again. See how many milligrams there are in each tablet or in each milliliter of solution.

Write down the total number of milligrams in the dose you want to give the patient. Divide this by the number of milligrams in one tablet, or in one milliliter of solution. This will show you how many tablets or how many milliliters of solution to give your patient.

$$\frac{\textbf{dose to give}}{\textbf{mg/tablet}} = \textbf{number of tablets to give}$$

$$\frac{\textbf{dose to give}}{\textbf{mg/ml}} = \textbf{number of milliliters to give}$$

For example, the dose of streptomycin for tuberculosis is 20mg/kilo. Your patient weighs 30 kg. Multiply 20 by 30. This gives you 600 mg. That is the dose of streptomycin to give your patient.

A vial of streptomycin has 5 g of streptomycin in 10 ml of solution. So one milliliter of solution has 0.5 g, or 500 mg, of streptomycin. Write down 600 mg. Divide this by 500 mg. This will give you 1.2. That is the number of milliliters of streptomycin to give your patient.

Here is another example. A small child has malaria. You have a solution of chloroquine with 100 mg in 1 ml of solution. The normal dose is 5mg of chloroquine per kilo for one dose. The child weighs 6 kg.

5 mg/kg X 6 kg = 30 mg to give in each dose

$$\frac{30 \text{ mg}}{100 \text{ mg/ml}} = 0.3 \text{ ml of solution to give for each dose}$$

Look at Table 6 on page 587. This gives the dose in milligrams for the weight of your patient in kilos. The column on the left gives the weight in kilos. Across the top is the dose to give in mg/kg. Find the dose to give in mg/kg. Go down that column until you come to the line which gives the weight in kg of your patient. You will then see the total number of milligrams to give your patient.

11.6 Always give a complete cure

The patient must take the medicine for a certain number of days, weeks, or months. He must do this in order to get well. You must know how long he must take the medicine. Be sure he knows and understands this.

If the cure is too short, the patient will not get well. The disease may come back. It will then be difficult to treat. This is true with the treatment of infections by antibiotics like penicillin or chloramphenicol. It is especially true for tuberculosis.

A cure that is too short will permit the bacteria to become resistant to the antibiotics. The antibiotics will no longer work against these bacteria. The patient may then become very seriously ill and die.

So be sure the patient knows this. Tell him he must complete the cure even if the symptoms go away before the end of the cure.

11.7 Signs of toxicity and what to do

Most medicines are dangerous. They can cause much harm to the patient if the dose is too high. Some can cause problems even when the dose is normal. We call these problems toxicity from the medicine. Digitalis preparations, streptomycin, penicillin, and many other medicines can cause toxic signs or symptoms.

You must know the toxic signs and symptoms of each medicine you give. If a patient develops a sign or symptom of toxicity while taking a medicine, you must either

- Stop the medicine immediately, or

- If the sign or symptom is not serious, diminish the dose of the medicine.

Explain to the patient the symptoms and signs of toxicity of each medicine you give. Tell the patient to stop taking the medicine if one of these symptoms or signs comes and to come back to see you immediately. Then you can decide whether or not to stop the medicine completely, or just to diminish the dose.

Table 6 - Doses of medicines per kilogram of weight

Weight in kilos	mg per kilogram							
	2 mg	3 mg	4 mg	5mg	10 mg	20 mg	25 mg	50 mg
4 kg	8 mg	12 mg	16 mg	20 mg	40 mg	80 mg	100 mg	200 mg
5 kg	10 mg	15 mg	20 mg	25 mg	50 mg	100 mg	125 mg	250 mg
6 kg	12 mg	18 mg	24 mg	30 mg	60 mg	120 mg	150 mg	300 mg
8 kg	16 mg	24 mg	32 mg	40 mg	80 mg	160 mg	200 mg	400 mg
10 kg	20 mg	30 mg	40 mg	50 mg	100 mg	200 mg	250 mg	500 mg
12 kg	24 mg	36 mg	48 mg	60 mg	120 mg	240 mg	300 mg	600 mg
14 kg	28 mg	42 mg	56 mg	70 mg	140 mg	280 mg	350 mg	700 mg
16 kg	32 mg	48 mg	64 mg	80 mg	160 mg	320 mg	400 mg	800 mg
18 kg	36 mg	54 mg	72 mg	90 mg	180 mg	360 mg	450 mg	900 mg
20 kg	40 mg	60 mg	80 mg	100 mg	200 mg	400 mg	500 mg	1.00 g
25 kg	50 mg	75 mg	100 mg	125 mg	250 mg	500 mg	625 mg	1.25 g
30 kg	60 mg	90 mg	120 mg	150 mg	300 mg	600 mg	750 mg	1.50 g
35 kg	70 mg	105 mg	140 mg	175 mg	350 mg	700 mg	875 mg	1.75 g
40 kg	80 mg	120 mg	160 mg	200 mg	400 mg	800 mg	1.00 g	2.00 g
45 kg	90 mg	135 mg	180 mg	225 mg	450 mg	900 mg	1.125 g	2.25 g
50 kg	100 mg	150 mg	200 mg	250 mg	500 mg	1.00 g	1.25 g	2.50 g
60 kg	120 mg	180 mg	240 mg	300 mg	600 mg	1.20 g	1.50 g	3.00 g
70 kg	140 mg	210 mg	280 mg	350 mg	700 mg	1.40 g	1.75 g	3.50 g
80 kg	160 mg	240 mg	320 mg	400 mg	800 mg	1.60 g	2.00 g	4.00 g

Chapter 12
THE TREATMENT FOR SPECIFIC DISEASES

ABORTION

An abortion is when the uterus pushes the fetus and placenta out of the uterus sometime during the first six months of the pregnancy. If this happens after the sixth month, we call it a premature delivery. There are different kinds of abortion.

Threatened abortion

The woman has strong colicky pain in the lower abdomen with little or no bleeding from the vagina. The treatment is:

- Bed rest.
- Analgesics: aspirin or paracetamol.
- Hormone treatment such as progesterone does not help.

Incomplete abortion

The woman has much pain and considerable bleeding. The opening of the uterus (cervix) is open. Some of the pregnancy may have come out already.

Check the general condition and vital signs of the woman. If she has had much bleeding, she may be in shock. Start an infusion. She will need a transfusion.

Often a curettage is necessary to complete the abortion. In this case, send the woman to hospital. However, if the bleeding and pain have stopped, the abortion may now be complete.

Septic abortion

The woman has signs of an incomplete abortion and signs of a serious infection in the uterus: much tenderness, high fever, rapid pulse, and often a bad odor coming from the vagina.

1. Start an infusion of normal saline solution.
2. Give a big dose of penicillin, ampicillin IV, or chloramphenicol IV.
3. Send the woman immediately to hospital.

If the hospital is far away, keep the woman in bed. Give her high doses of one of the above antibiotics for several days until all fever, pain, tenderness, and vaginal secretions are finished. If the fever and pain continue, find a way to send her to hospital.

ABSCESS

Incision and drainage

An incision and drainage under local anesthesia are necessary to let out the pus. In most cases, an incision is sufficient to cure the abscess. If the abscess is deep or in a dangerous place like the neck or face, send the patient to hospital.

Local care

1. Complete rest for the part of the body where the abscess is.
2. Warm compresses to help the inflammation go away.
3. Daily dressings as long as pus continues to come out.

Antibiotics

Antibiotics alone are not sufficient. Often the bacteria in an abscess are resistant to antibiotics. Give antibiotics only in these cases.

1. The patient has a fever of more than $38°C$.
2. He has tender lymph nodes near the abscess.

In these cases, give him antibiotics for 7 days: penicillin, trimethoprim-sulfamethoxazole, ampicillin, or tetracycline.

AIDS

Treatment

The cause of AIDS is a virus. We have no specific treatment for it because we have no medicine that can kill the AIDS virus. We can give symptomatic treatment for these conditions.

Severe weight loss

Patients must try to eat foods with much protein. They should eat 3 or more meals a day and eat only a small or moderate amount of food at each meal.

Diarrhea

We have no specific treatment for the diarrhea of AIDS. Do not give antibiotics or antidiarrhea medicines. They may make the patient worse. If he has dehydration, give him oral rehydration solution. He should eat soft foods that have protein and carbohydrates but only a little fat or oil.

Severe cough or signs of pneumonia

Give the patient trimethoprim-sulfamethoxazole for 7 days. Look for TB bacilli in his sputum. Send him to the doctor."

● If the cough or signs of pneumonia continue after the treatment is finished.

● If you find TB bacilli in the sputum.

Big lymph nodes

We have no specific treatment for them. If the patient has fever or much weight loss, send him to the doctor. He may have tuberculosis.

Mouth sores

Tell a patient who has mouth sores to do these things:

1. Wash the inside of your mouth several times a day with salt water, or water with sodium bicarbonate.

2. Gargle at the same time.

3. After each mouth wash, take a small spoonful of honey. Let the honey stay in the sore parts of your mouth for a minute before swallowing it.

Precautions in treatment

Do not isolate patients with AIDS. However, you must use certain precautions to prevent the spread of the AIDS virus to others including yourself. This is very important.

Injections

If there are persons suffering from AIDS in your area, be very careful with syringes and needles. If possible, use only plastic disposable syringes and needles. Throw them away immediately into a deep hole after one use.

If you use glass syringes and metal needles, you must clean them well and sterilize them by boiling before using them again.

1. After the injection, rinse the syringe and needle in water. Throw this water away.
2. Separate the parts of the syringe and needle.
3. Put them into a solution of bleach (sodium hypochlorite) for at least 10 minutes. Make a fresh solution of bleach each morning. To do so, use a strong solution of bleach as follows:

Strong bleach	Clean water	To make
10 ml	90 ml	100 ml of solution
20 ml	180 ml	200 ml of solution
50 ml	450 ml	500 ml of solution
100 ml	900 ml	1 liter of solution

4. After at least 10 minutes in the bleach solution, rinse the syringe and needle in clean water to remove all bleach.
5. Boil the syringe and needle for 15 minutes before using them again.

Secretions

The AIDS virus is in blood, sexual secretions, and stomach juices. If any of these secretions touch your skin, you can get the AIDS virus. You must wear rubber or plastic gloves every time you do these things.

1. Treat an open wound.
2. Do any surgical or dental procedure.
3. Draw blood from a patient.
4. Examine a patient's mouth with your fingers.
5. Do a vaginal or rectal examination.
6. Help a mother deliver a baby.
7. Clean up after a delivery.
8. Clean anything that has blood, vaginal secretions, or vomit on it: instruments, basins, linens, bed, other furniture, the floor.

If you have an open wound or sore on your hand, cover it completely with a bandage before touching any patients.

Education

Give much education to your people about the spread of AIDS. The virus of AIDS is spread by these ways.

- Sexual relations.
- Dirty or non-sterile syringes and needles.
- A transfusion of blood from a person with the AIDS virus.
- A mother who has AIDS can give it to her newborn baby.

Tell your people to follow these rules. If they do so, they will not get AIDS.

Injections

Permit no one to give you an injection unless you are absolutely sure the syringe and needle are new disposable ones, or the glass syringe and metal needle have been carefully boiled just before the injection.

One sexual partner

If married, be faithful to your spouse. If not married, do not have sexual relations until you are ready for marriage.

Avoid having sexual relations with different persons. A man who has sexual relations with different women can get AIDS easily. He can then give the AIDS virus to other women including his own wife.

A woman who has sexual relations with different men can get AIDS easily. She can then give the AIDS virus to other men including her own husband.

Condoms

Using a condom does not give complete protection against AIDS. Do not count on them to protect you from AIDS.

Blood transfusions

Accept a blood transfusion only when absolutely necessary. The blood should come from a spouse or parent, or from someone else who has no possibility of having the AIDS virus. Doctors in hospitals do everything possible to make sure that blood for transfusions does not have the AIDS virus.

ALLERGY

An allergy, or "allergic reaction," can cause one of three things:

- Shock: See Anaphylactic shock on page 598.
- An acute attack of asthma: See Asthma on page 601.
- Big bumps on the skin with much itching, called "urticaria."

Treatment

For urticaria, give an antihistamine such as promethazine or chlorpheniramine until the symptoms go away. These medicines can make a person sleepy. A person taking one of them must not drive a vehicle or operate dangerous machines.

Find the cause

Try to find out the cause of the allergy. Ask the patient about any medicines taken, any foods eaten, or any soap or perfume used just before the reaction started. The cause may be a medicine, like penicillin or a sulfa drug. It may be a new food like a fruit. If the patient has taken, eaten, or used something new, tell him not to do this again. If so, he may have another allergic reaction, perhaps a severe one.

Prevention

Patients who have an allergic reaction from a medicine like penicillin or a sulfa drug must never take that medicine again. Give each patient a small card. Write on the card ALLERGIC TO _____. The patient must keep this card and show it to the doctor or other health worker every time he needs treatment.

AMEBIASIS

You must find moving ameba in the fresh stools of the patient to be sure the diagnosis is correct. Give specific treatment only if you are sure of the diagnosis. Most cases of diarrhea do not come from amebiasis. Do not give treatment for amebiasis to a person who has diarrhea only. Give treatment for amebiasis only if you find ameba in the stools.

General treatment

1. Rehydration if the patient is dehydrated. See page 322.
2. Good nutrition. See page 658.

Specific treatment

1. Metronidazole (*Flagyl), tablets of 250 mg.
   - For an adult, 750 mg 3 times a day for 7 days.
   - For a child, 15 mg/kg 3 times a day for 7 days.
   - This acts against ameba in the wall of the intestine.
2. Also give one of the following medicines:
   - Diloxanide, 500 mg 3 times a day for 10 days.
   - Diiodohydroxyquinoline 600 mg 3 times a day for 21 days.
   - Tetracycline, 500 mg 4 times a day for 10 days for an adult. Do not use tetracycline for children less than 8 years old.

These medicines act against ameba in the canal of the intestine. They act together with metronidazole to get rid of all ameba and to cure the patient.

Other treatment

1. Bed rest during the treatment.
2. A soft or liquid diet until there is no more diarrhea.

Prevention

The transmission of ameba is by contaminated water and food. Flies can also transmit ameba on their feet. Give these instructions to the patient and to the family.

1. Drink only clean, or potable, water.
2. Protect the water source or the well from contamination.
3. Always wash your hands before eating, before preparing food, and after passing stools.
4. Protect all food from flies.

5. Make a good latrine, and keep flies from living in it.

6. Keep the kitchen clean.

7. Wash dishes, pots, and pans after each use.

Amebiasis is a transmissible disease. Send a report of each case to your doctor and the local government authorities.

AMEBIASIS OF THE LIVER - liver abscess

If possible, send the patient to hospital. If this is not possible, give this specific treatment.

1. Metronidazole, as above, for 10 days.

2. Diloxanide, as above, for 10 days.

3. Chloroquine, 300 mg daily for 14 days.

4. If the patient is not better 3 days after the start of this treatment, give 2-dihydroemetine, 80 mg IM once a day for 10 days for an adult or, for a child, 1 mg/kg once a day for 10 days.

5. Strict bed rest during the treatment.

If signs of infection continue, send the patient to hospital. It may be necessary for the doctor to drain the abscess.

ANAL FISSURE

Treatment

1. Analgesic ointment, or vaseline to put on the skin around the anus.

2. Antibiotics only if there is swelling and much tenderness, or fever.

Instructions to the patient

1. Take a bath every day.

2. Sit in a basin of warm water with soap, morning and evening. This will help very much.

3. Keep the skin clean and dry around the anus. Clean it carefully every time after passing stools.

4. Eat foods with much fiber or residue every day to prevent constipation. These foods are fruits such as papaya, pineapples, mangoes, and green leafy vegetables. Corn, millet, and groundnuts are also good.

5. Drink much water and do much exercise. All of this will help keep the stools soft and easy to pass.

ANAPHYLACTIC SHOCK

This comes very suddenly right after the patient has taken a medicine or been stung by a bee. The cause is usually a medicine such as penicillin or a sulfa drug, or the substance in the bee sting. Treat the patient immediately because he can die in 5 minutes or less without treatment.

1. Epinephrine (adrenaline), 0.5 ml IV immediately.

2. Artificial respiration if the patient has stopped breathing.

3. Infusion of normal saline solution, given rapidly.

In most cases, if you give treatment immediately, the patient will recover in a few minutes. But observe him for 24 hours to make sure the recovery is complete.

Find the cause of the shock. If it is a medicine, the patient must never take that medicine again. See Allergy, page 596. If it is a bee sting, the patient must stay away from bees.

ANKYLOSTOMIASIS - see page 753

APPENDICITIS

The patient needs a surgical operation immediately. Otherwise, the appendix will rupture in 24 to 48 hours and cause peritonitis.

If your health center is far from the nearest hospital:

1. Start an infusion of normal saline.

2. Give the patient a dose of an antibiotic like penicillin, ampicillin IV, or chloramphenicol IV.

3. If he has much pain, give an analgesic by injection.

4. He must eat nothing. Do not give him an enema.

5. Then send him to hospital as quickly as possible with a letter telling what treatment you have given him.

ARTHRITIS

There are three aspects in the treatment of arthritis.

● Analgesics to relieve the pain.

● Rest, or less activity, for the joint or joints affected.

● Heat to the affected joint or joints.

Analgesics

1. Aspirin, 4 times a day with food until the pain is gone.
2. Indomethacin, 3 times a day with food. It can cause headache, heart burn, stomach ulcers, or skin eruptions. Do not give aspirin and indomethacin together to the same patient.

Rest, or less activity

If the patient has much pain, put the joint, or joints, at rest. If the arthritis is in the arm or hand, put the arm in a cloth sling. Tell the patient not to use the arm. If the arthritis is in the neck, the back, or the leg, put the patient in bed. He must not walk or work until the pain and swelling are gone.

Too much weight makes the arthritis worse. Tell the patient to eat less and do more exercise in order to lose weight. The arthritis will improve or go away when his weight becomes normal.

Heat

Heat to the joint increases the blood flow. This will relieve the pain and help the inflammation of the joint to heal. Use hot baths or hot compresses. Do this 3 times a day.

If the pain of the arthritis does not go away in 2 weeks, send the patient to hospital.

ARTHRITIS WITH INFECTION - Septic arthritis

Send the patient immediately to hospital. If this is not possible, give the following treatment.

Treatment

1. Put the patient in bed and keep the joint from moving. If necessary, use a splint or even a plaster cast.
2. Give antibiotics: penicillin or ampicillin for at least two weeks.
3. If there is pus inside the joint, like the knee, take it out.
   - Use a sterile syringe and a big sterile needle.
   - Clean the skin very carefully with an antiseptic solution.
   - Draw out all of the pus with the syringe.
4. If the pus comes back, find a way to send the patient to hospital.

ARTHRITIS AFTER INJURY - Traumatic arthritis

1. Keep the joint from moving. Use a splint or a plaster cast.
2. Give the patient analgesics to relieve the pain.
3. Do not do an aspiration of the joint. This can cause an infection.
4. When the pain and swelling are gone, have the patient start doing exercises. He must start slowly, but use the joint more and more each day.

ASCARIASIS - see page 708

ASTHMA

The disease

In asthma the bronchial tubes become small. Air comes in, but it is difficult for it to go out. Patients must work hard to push air out of the lungs. Many thick secretions accumulate in the bronchial tubes, and it is difficult to cough them out. The treatment for asthma must help to relax and open up the bronchial tubes. The air can then come in and go out easily. For this we use medicines called "broncho-dilators."

Treatment

Broncho-dilators

1. Epinephrine (adrenaline) sub-cutaneously, in a 1:1000 solution.
   - In a very severe attack, give 0.2 to 0.3 ml.
   - Give it again after one hour if the asthma is still bad.
   - For a child, give 0.1 to 0.2 ml.
   - Do not give more than 3 injections in one day.
2. Aminophylline, in ampoules for injection IV and in tablets of 100 or 200 mg.
   - In a severe attack, give aminophylline 250 mg IV in 10 ml of solution very slowly.
   - Or else put 500 mg in 250 ml of normal saline and give it IV over 2 hours.
   - For a child, give 5 mg/kg IV in normal saline.

- Never give aminophylline IM.
- When the patient is better, start giving aminophylline 200 mg by mouth 4 times a day, or 5 mg/kg 4 times a day to a child. Continue giving this until the attack has stopped completely.

3. Salbutamol (*Ventolin), in tablets of 2 mg.

- Give 1 or 2 tablets every 6 hours.
- Do not give both salbutamol and aminophylline to the patient at the same time. Use one or the other.

4. Broncho-dilators by inhalation.

- These act when the patient inhales them in a fine spray.
- Isoproterenol, metaproterenol, and salbutamol are good, but they cost a lot.
- These medicines come with a small plastic "inhaler."
- If you have them with inhalers, read carefully the instructions that come with them. Ask your doctor about them.
- Show the patient how to use them.
- The patient should use the inhaler with one of these medicines at the beginning of an attack. Often this will stop the attack before it becomes severe.

SUMMARY

1. In a severe attack, give epinephrine immediately subcutaneously. If this helps, then give aminophylline or salbutamol by mouth.

2. If the epinephrine does not help after three injections, give aminophylline IV.

3. When the patient is better, give the aminophylline or salbutamol by mouth until the attack has stopped.

4. If the patient is not better in 12 hours, send him to hospital.

5. If the attack is not severe, start giving aminophylline or salbutamol by mouth.

Hydration

Give much liquid to drink to every asthma patient. This will make the secretions more liquid and easy to cough out. If a patient cannot drink, give normal saline, or 5% dextrose IV. It is important to keep him well hydrated.

Antibiotics

Give an antibiotic, like penicillin, only if there is fever or other signs of lung infection. Most cases of asthma do not need antibiotics.

Cortisone

Do not give cortisone, or other cortisone preparations, for they are dangerous. Only the doctor can know when to prescribe these medicines.

IMPORTANT NOTE

NEVER give morphine or phenobarbital. These can stop the respirations and the patient will die.

Other diseases

Always look carefully for other diseases in patients with asthma.

1. High blood pressure. In this case, give only small doses of epinephrine and use aminophylline.

2. Heart failure: crackles at the bottom of the lungs, big liver, swelling. If the patient has heart failure, give him treatment for it. Do not give him epinephrine or salbutamol. Give only aminophylline. Send him to hospital as soon as possible.

3. Tuberculosis: low fever for weeks or months, chronic cough, loss of weight, blood in the sputum, crackles at the top of the lungs. Look for TB bacilli in the sputum. If you think the patient may have tuberculosis but you cannot find TB bacilli in the sputum, send him to the doctor.

Prevention of attacks

Give aminophylline 200 mg 3 times a day every day during the season when the patient has frequent attacks. Aminophylline can sometimes cause heart burn. So tell the patient to take the aminophylline during meals.

Instructions to the patient

1. Try to find out what brings on an attack. It could be things like much dust, much smoke, cold weather, certain flowers or foods. Try to stay away from anything that brings on an attack.

2. Strong emotions, like anger or jealousy, can sometimes cause an attack of asthma. If this is true in your case, try to keep these strong emotions from coming.

3. No smoking. Tobacco smoke will make the asthma worse.

4. You can continue to work. But certain working conditions, such as dust or smoke, can make the attacks come. In this case, try to change these conditions or stay away from them.

5. Drink much water. This will keep the bronchi in good condition. If an attack comes, the secretions will be more liquid and easy to cough out.

6. Come to the consultation if you get:

- A fever.
- Much difficulty in breathing.
- Sputum with pus or blood.
- Much pain in your chest.

ASTHMATIC BRONCHITIS

The disease

Sometimes bronchitis can cause spasms in the bronchial tubes. The patient will have wheezes just like those of asthma. It is easy to tell if a patient really has asthma or only asthmatic bronchitis.

- A patient with asthma has had attacks of dyspnea and wheezing in the past.
- A patient with asthmatic bronchitis has not had dyspnea and wheezing in the past. Do not tell this patient the disease is asthma because this can cause fear and worry. Probably the disease is not asthma and therefore will not come again.

Treatment

1. Give the patient treatment for bronchitis.

2. Give him aminophylline by mouth, or salbutamol.

3. If the patient has fever, give him penicillin for 5 to 7 days. Do not give him penicillin if he has no fever.

4. The attack will finish in one to three days and will not come back. If another attack does come, then the patient is probably developing asthma. In this case, give him aminophylline to prevent attacks - see page 603.

BILE STONES

1. If the patient has much pain in the right upper quadrant, give him:
   - An analgesic: aspirin or paracetamol.
   - An antispasmodic such as propantheline.
2. If the patient has fever, start giving him ampicillin or chloramphenicol.
3. Send the patient to hospital as quickly as possible.

BLADDER INFECTION - Cystitis

In a man

1. The patient must drink much water.
2. Give him one of these antibiotics: trimethoprim-sulfamethoxazole, ampicillin, or nitrofurantoin. See the table on page 710 for the dose.
3. If the symptoms continue after this treatment, or the patient still has white blood cells in the urine, send him to hospital.

In a woman

1. One single big dose of an antibiotic will cure most bladder infections in women. Give her either:
   - Trimethoprim-sulfamethoxazole, 8 tablets immediately, or
   - Ampicillin, 3 g immediately.
2. Tell the woman to drink much water.
3. If after one week she still has symptoms or white blood cells in the urine, repeat the treatment.
4. If the second treatment does not cure her, send her to hospital.

BLACK WATER FEVER - see page 654

BRAIN HEMORRHAGE

This is very serious. It can cause death quickly. Send the patient to hospital as quickly as possible. In the meantime, keep him very quiet and flat in bed. Do not move him more than necessary. If he is in coma, give him the treatment for coma shown on page 440.

BRONCHITIS

Treatment

Medicines

1. Give the patient an expectorant for 7 days - see page 257.
2. If he has dyspnea with wheezing, give him aminophylline or salbutamol.

Examine the sputum

If the patient has sputum, look carefully at his sputum.

1. Clear sputum is probably simply saliva.
2. Thick white or green sputum comes probably from bronchitis. It can also come from pneumonia or tuberculosis.
3. Red-brown liquid sputum comes probably from heart failure.
4. Sputum with blood can come from bronchitis, pneumonia, or tuberculosis.
5. Do a sputum exam 3 times to look for TB bacilli. If you find them, send the patient to hospital with a letter of reference and with the slide of the sputum. If you cannot do a sputum exam, give him treatment for bronchitis.

Treatment for pneumonia

Give the patient treatment for pneumonia if he has:

- Much pus in the sputum.
- A fever.
- Crackles in the lungs with no signs of heart failure.
- A cough continuing after 7 days of treatment with an expectorant.

This is the treatment to give.

1. Give him penicillin for 7 days.
2. Continue giving him the expectorant.
3. Do sputum exams if possible.

Refer the patient

If the cough continues after 7 days of treatment with penicillin, send the patient to hospital. He could have tuberculosis or another serious disease.

Instructions to the patient

1. Drink much water. This will make the bronchial secretions liquid and help them come out easily. The cough will then soon go away.

2. Do not smoke. The smoke of cigarettes causes an irritation of the bronchial tubes and makes a chronic cough.

3. When coughing, cover your mouth with your hand or with a cloth handkerchief.

4. If you have sputum, cough the sputum into a small bottle or can and keep it closed.

5. Do not spit on the ground. This can spread disease to other persons.

CELLULITIS

1. Give the patient an antibiotic - penicillin or ampicillin - for 7 days.

2. Put the infected part of the body to rest:
   - Arm or hand: put the arm in a cloth sling. The patient must not use the arm or hand.
   - Leg or foot: put the patient in bed. Raise his leg on a pillow. He must not stand or walk.
   - Chest, back, or abdomen: put the patient in bed.
   - The rest must continue until the pain and swelling are gone.

3. If the patient has much pain, give him aspirin.

4. Put hot compresses on the infected area. This will help the infection to go away quickly.

5. Look for signs of pus in the tissues: fluctuation. If fluctuation is present, an incision under local anesthesia is necessary to let out the pus.

6. If the infection does not go away in 7 days, send the patient to hospital. He may have a serious infection or other disease in the deep tissues.

CIRRHOSIS

Causes of cirrhosis

Look for the cause.

1. Heart failure can cause cirrhosis. Always examine the heart in every patient with cirrhosis. Look for signs of heart disease with heart failure. If he has signs of heart disease or failure, give him treatment for this - see page 636.

2. Alcohol can cause cirrhosis. Does the patient drink much alcoholic drinks? If this is the case, tell him to stop drinking all alcoholic drinks: beer, wine, and whisky.

3. Schistosomiasis can cause cirrhosis. If you are in a region with much schistosomiasis, do a stool and a urine exam. Look for Schistosome eggs. If you find them, treat the schistosomiasis - see page 687.

4. Malnutrition can cause cirrhosis after some years. Look for signs of malnutrition. Ask about malnutrition in the past.

5. Some forms of hepatitis. Ask the patient if he has had jaundice in the past.

6. In many cases, you will not find a specific cause for the cirrhosis. But in every case, look for heart failure, alcoholism, schistosomiasis, malnutrition, and a history of hepatitis.

Treatment for cirrhosis

We have no specific treatment for cirrhosis.

Food rich in protein

The most important treatment is good food with much protein and little fat or oils. Protein helps the liver make new liver cells. In this way the liver can get better. Tell the patient to eat foods that have much protein - see page 658. Tell him not to eat the fat of meat or food with much oil, like palm oil, groundnut oil, or corn oil.

Edema and ascites

If he has much edema or ascites, tell him not to eat any salt or any foods that have much salt, like salted fish. If he has much ascites and trouble breathing, it will be necessary to take out the ascites liquid by needle aspiration. Send him to hospital for this.

Anemia

If he has anemia, look for the cause. See page 474. Treat each cause.

Bleeding

If he has bleeding from the stomach, with vomiting of blood, or bloody or black stools, send him immediately to hospital. But check his condition first. If he has signs of shock, start an infusion. Give him vitamin K, 10 mg IM. He will need a transfusion.

COMMON COLD

1. Give the patient aspirin 3 times a day.
2. If he has thick secretions coming from the nose and trouble breathing through the nose, give him nose drops such as:

   ● Phenylephrine (*Neosynephrine) 1/4%, 2 drops in each side of the nose 3 times a day, or

   ● Ephedrine 1/2%, 2 drops in each side of the nose 3 times a day.
3. If the symptoms become serious, with fever, much cough, and trouble breathing, look for signs of pneumonia.

CONJUNCTIVITIS

1. Always examine the vision first - see page 71. If the vision is not normal, send the patient immediately to the doctor.
2. If the vision is normal, put an antibiotic eye ointment into the eye 3 times a day for 5 days. Do not use an ointment with cortisone.
3. If the pain and redness do not go away in 5 days, send the patient to the doctor. He may have a more serious eye disease.
4. Tell the patient not to rub his eyes and not to put anything into them other than the eye medicine.

CONTUSION

1. Give the patient aspirin if he has much pain.
2. Put the injured part of the body to rest until the pain and swelling go away.

3. Hot compresses can help the pain and swelling go away.

4. If the pain and swelling do not go away in one or two days, send the patient to the doctor. He may have a more serious injury.

CROUP

The disease

Croup is a very severe infection of the larynx. The vocal cords become swollen and thick. It usually comes in small children. The child can breathe only with much difficulty. If the swelling continues, the larynx may become completely closed. The child will die quickly.

Treatment

1. Send the child immediately to hospital. The doctor may have to do an operation on the trachea - tracheotomy - to let him breathe.

2. Before you send the child, give him a big dose of one of these antibiotics:

   ● Ampicillin, 50 mg/kg of weight IM or IV.

   ● Chloramphenicol, 50 mg/kg IV in an infusion.

   ● Crystalline penicillin, 5,000,000 u.

3. If the hospital is more than 6 hours away, the child may die on the way. In this case, treat him yourself. Keep on giving the antibiotic, a dose every 6 hours. Help the child drink much water.

CYSTITIS - see BLADDER INFECTION on page 605

DIABETES

Diabetes is a serious chronic disease. It requires the care of a doctor. The doctor must examine all diabetic patients carefully. Only he can decide the correct treatment for each patient. He needs to see each patient regularly. So send every new case of diabetes to the doctor for examination and treatment.

When the doctor has prescribed the correct treatment, the patient may come to your health center to continue care and treatment. So you must know how to care for diabetic patients.

We have no cure for diabetes. A patient must follow instructions and often take treatment for the rest of his life. He must come regularly to the clinic for examination and control of the disease. Consult with the doctor if possible whenever you have a problem with one of your diabetic patients. Follow these important rules in the treatment of diabetes.

Treatment

Food and diet

Instructions about eating are very important for a patient with diabetes. Give him these instructions about food.

1. Try to eat three meals a day. Eat a normal quantity of food each time. Do not eat very big meals. This is because a big meal will require much insulin.

2. Do not eat sugar. Soft drinks and alcoholic drinks like beer have much sugar, so do not drink them. There are certain pills which are like sugar. You can use them in tea or coffee. Do not eat candy, sweet pastry, or sweet conserves like jam.

3. You can eat foods with starch, such as maize, rice, cassava, bananas, potatoes, sweet potatoes, millet, sorghum, soya, and beans.

4. Plant foods with protein are good, such as groundnuts, soya, beans, and maize.

5. Animal foods with protein are also good, such as meat, fish, eggs, and milk. But do not eat large quantities of meat.

6. Eat many fruits and green vegetables.

7. You can eat oil from maize, groundnuts, palm nuts, and soya. But do not eat large quantities of these oils.

8. Try not to eat animal fat, butter, and cream.

9. Eat many different kinds of food. This will give you plenty of protein, vitamins, and different kinds of starch.

Ideal weight

Diabetes often comes in patients who are obese. The extra weight and fat require more insulin. The body cannot make enough insulin, so the patient develops diabetes. An obese patient with diabetes must lose weight until his weight becomes normal. In this way he will need less insulin.

The body can often make enough insulin if the weight is normal, and the diabetes will go away. So tell each patient to keep a normal weight. A patient can do 2 things to lose weight:

- Eat less food.
- Do more physical work or activities.

Infections in diabetes

In diabetes the body cannot fight well against infections. Infections come frequently. They make the diabetes more serious. Look for signs of an infection somewhere in the body in every case of diabetes. Look in these places.

- On the skin for furuncles or for cellulitis.
- On the feet and legs.
- On the hands and arms.
- In the ears and in the mouth.
- In the lungs and in the abdomen.
- In the urine. Do a urine exam in every diabetic patient.
- In the prostate. Do a rectal exam in every man with diabetes.
- Look also for signs of tuberculosis.

Infections stay longer and are difficult to treat in patients with diabetes. Treat every infection you find in a diabetic patient. Treat it until all signs of infection are gone. Give also insulin. If the infection does not become better soon, or if the diabetes becomes more severe, do not wait. Send the patient to hospital quickly.

Insulin

Insulin is the specific treatment for diabetes. The patient has diabetes because the body does not make enough insulin. But too much insulin can be dangerous. It can cause shock and even death. Only the doctor can prescribe insulin. The doctor will follow each patient for some days to see if the dose is correct. The patient may then come back to you to continue the treatment.

Long acting insulin (NPH, Lente, or PZI) is best. Give it in the morning and tell the patient to eat well during the day. If he cannot eat that day, do not give the insulin. If he follows carefully the instructions about eating and takes insulin regularly, the blood sugar will probably remain normal. He must come back to see you quickly if:

- The polyuria comes again.
- An infection or other illness comes.
- He loses much weight.

Pills for high blood sugar

We have medicines in pill form that make the sugar in the blood and urine become normal. We use these pills only in patients who:

- Are older adults.
- Do not have severe diabetes.
- Have no serious infection.

We cannot use them in children or young adults, or in patients who have severe diabetes. Use one of these pills:

1. Tolbutamide (*Orinase), tablets of 0.5 g. Give 1 tablet 3 times a day before each meal.

2. Chlorpropamide (*Diabenase), in tablets of 100 or 250 mg. Give 100 mg or 250 mg 1 time a day, in the morning.

3. Tolazamide (*Tolinase), in tablets of 100, 250, or 500 mg. The patient takes 1 tablet of 100, 250, or 500 mg each morning.

4. Acetohexamide (*Dymelor), in 250 or 500 mg tablets. Give 250 mg to 1.5 g each day in one or two doses.

5. Cyclohexylurea (*Daonil), 5 mg. Give 5 to 10 mg each morning.

6. Glyburide (*Glibenclamide), in 1.25, 2.5 or 5 mg tablets. Give 5 to 10 mg each morning.

7. Glipizide (*Glucotrol), in 5 or 10 mg tablets. Give 5 to 10 mg each morning one half hour before eating.

General treatment

1. 1 multivitamin a day for some weeks.

2. If the patient has anemia, look for the cause and treat each cause.

3. Look for intestinal worms. If the patient has worms, give worm medicine.

4. Look for malaria. If the patient has plasmodium in the thick blood film, treat the malaria.

Insulin shock

This is very serious. It comes from an over-dose of insulin. The sugar in the body becomes very low. The patient has convulsions, coma, and often shock because he does not have enough sugar in the brain. Without treatment he will die in a few hours.

Give him sugar immediately. If he can eat, give him a banana, some bread, or some sugar. If he can drink, put 4 big spoonfuls of sugar in a glass of water and tell him to drink it all quickly.

If he is unconscious, pass a stomach tube into his stomach. Put 4 big spoonfuls of sugar in water and pass this through the tube into the stomach. The convulsions will soon stop and he will recover. If he does not wake up in a few minutes, give the same amount of sugar in water again.

If you have 50% dextrose or glucose for IV injection, give 100 ml of this immediately but slowly into the vein. This will stop the convulsions. When the patient has recovered, send him to the doctor. The doctor will examine him to find out exactly how much insulin he needs.

Talk to every diabetic patient about the possibility of insulin shock. It begins suddenly with dizziness and weakness. If this happens, he must immediately eat some food with starch or sugar. In this way, the sugar in the blood will go up quickly and insulin shock will not develop. So a diabetic patient must have some food or sugar with him at all times.

Pills for diabetes can also cause insulin shock. Warn a patient taking one of these medicines about the dangers of insulin shock. This is very important if the patient is old or has heart or liver disease. Insulin shock in such a patient can quickly cause death.

Diabetic coma

This comes when the patient has very much sugar in his blood. It is very serious, and he can die quickly. Treatment for diabetic coma can be given only in hospital. The patient must receive much insulin and liquids by IV infusion. So send him immediately to hospital. The doctor will examine his blood every few hours to find out the amount of sugar in the blood. He must do this to know how much insulin to give.

Records

Keep a good record of every one of your diabetic patients. Each time you see a patient, write down the general condition and the instructions and treatment you give him. When the doctor comes, show him the record of each patient and talk about the case with him. Have the doctor see every diabetic patient who is not doing well.

DRUG ABUSE

Causes

Several drugs can cause addiction or drug abuse.

1. Alcohol: The patient drinks much wine, whisky, or other alcoholic beverages.
2. Drugs: Morphine, cocaine.
3. Marijuana, heroin.

Symptoms

Patients with drug abuse prefer to drink, smoke, or take drugs. They do not like to work. When they work, they do not work hard or well. Often they drink or take drugs to forget their work, their problems, or their responsibilities.

Treatment

The treatment is difficult. Talk to the patient about the dangers of drug abuse to his health. Tell him the effect of the drug abuse on his family, his work, and his life. He should use for his family the money he spends on alcoholic drinks or on drugs. He can live much better if he stops drinking and taking drugs.

Talk to the families of drug abuse patients about this. Ask other leaders in the community, like clan leaders, religious leaders, educated persons, to help you with these patients.

DYSENTERY, ACUTE

Dysentery is an infection of the intestines causing severe diarrhea. Acute dysentery comes from ameba, certain bacteria like Shigella or Salmonella, or cholera. Chronic dysentery comes from tuberculosis, certain parasites, or sometimes from AIDS.

Look for the cause of the dysentery. Look at a liquid stool carefully and quickly for ameba and parasites. If you find ameba in the stools, give treatment for amebiasis - see page 596.

Rehydration

The most important treatment is rehydration. Follow the instructions for rehydration on page 322. Examine the patient several times a day. See if the signs of dehydration are going away.

Antibiotics

For a patient with acute dysentery who has no ameba in the stools, give him one of the following antibiotics for 7 days:

- Trimethoprim-sulfamethoxazole.
- Tetracycline.
- Chloramphenicol.
- Ampicillin.
- Sulfadiazine.

Trimethoprim-sulfamethoxazole is the best treatment. Tetracycline and chloramphenicol are very good. If possible, use one of them. If you do not have them, use ampicillin or sulfadiazine. Do not use iodochlorhy-droxyquin (*Entero-vioform). It does not work well.

Care

Put the patient in bed. If he is weak, put a bedpan near the bed. Someone must empty it into the latrine after each use and then wash it very carefully with water and disinfectant. This person must then wash his hands very carefully with soap and water. Tell the family to boil all drinking water for the patient and for the whole family.

Food

A patient with dysentery can start eating when the diarrhea becomes less frequent and when the fever comes down. At first he must eat only soft foods, like rice, bread, bananas, eggs. He must not yet eat maize, millet, beans, cassava, groundnuts, green leafy vegetables, fruits, or meat. After 3 days with no diarrhea, he can eat any foods.

DYSENTERY, CHRONIC

Look for the cause

1. Look for signs of tuberculosis: Loss of weight, low fever every after-noon or evening.

2. Do a stool exam several times to look for worm eggs, ameba, and other parasites.

3. Look also for signs of malnutrition. Tell the patient to eat food with much protein.

4. Send the patient to the doctor:
   - If you cannot find the cause.
   - If he has lost much weight.
   - If he has a fever.

Treatment

1. Give the patient specific treatment for every cause you find.

2. Give him instructions about eating.
   - Eat much food with protein.
   - Drink much water.
   - Until the diarrhea stops, avoid foods with much fiber, such as pineapples, mangoes, maize, beans, and green leafy vegetables.

Health education

Talk to each patient and the family about the disease, where it comes from, and how to keep from getting it again. Give them these instructions.

1. Every house in the community must have a good latrine. Every person must use the latrine every time.

2. Protect the water source or the well. Protect it by a fence, a wall, or a cover. No one must get into the water source, take a bath in it, or put anything into it. No animals must get into the source.

3. Be sure all latrines are at least 50 meters from the source or well.

4. Make all drinking water pure by boiling it, by putting a chemical into it, or by filtering it. This is very important, especially for the drinking water of babies and young children.

5. Always wash your hands before eating, before preparing food, after work, and after using the latrine.

Report every case of dysentery immediately to the health authorities.

DYSMENORRHEA

Dysmenorrhea is pain in the lower back or abdomen right before, during, or just after the monthly menstrual period. It comes often from a disease in the female organs. Look for signs of infection in the female organs: much tenderness in the lower abdomen, fever, sometimes pus coming from the vagina, or a high white blood cell count. If the woman has signs of infection, treat her for a pelvic infection. See page 674.

If she has no signs of infection, give her aspirin during the days she has pain. Send her to the doctor:

- If the pain is serious.
- If the pain continues for more than two monthly periods.

The doctor can do other exams to find the cause.

EAR INFECTION - Otitis

Acute ear infection

1. Give the patient an antibiotic for 7 days: penicillin, penicillin V, ampicillin, or amoxicillin.
2. Give him aspirin 3 or 4 times a day as long as the pain and fever last.
3. A hot water bottle under the ear will make the pain diminish.
4. Do not put medicines or drops in the ear canal.
5. If the patient has pus coming from the ear, keep the outside of the ear clean. Put vaseline or an antiseptic ointment on the skin outside the ear canal. This will protect the skin.
6. If the fever or pain continue for more than 2 days, send the patient to hospital. He may have a serious infection, such as meningitis or an infection of the bone around the ear (mastoiditis).

Chronic ear infection

In a chronic ear infection, secretions come from the ear during some weeks or months. The patient may have pain and some fever.

1. Give him treatment for an acute ear infection.
2. Often a patient with a chronic ear infection has already had many antibiotics and still has the infection. In this case, give him an antibiotic he has not yet had. Give it to him for 3 weeks.
3. Send the patient to hospital:
   - If the pain, fever, or secretions continue after your treatment.
   - If the pain or fever become more severe.
   - If you do not have an antibiotic different from those he has already taken.

ECLAMPSIA - see TOXEMIA OF PREGNANCY on page 682

ECZEMA

1. Give the patient an antibiotic for 7 days: penicillin, penicillin V, ampicillin, or amoxicillin.

2. Keep the infected skin very clean. Clean it every day with an antiseptic solution. If possible, leave the infected skin open. Put on a dressing only if the lesion is very big, or if you cannot keep it clean.

3. Every day look at the eczema and the lymph nodes in the region. Look for fluctuation. If you find fluctuation, an incision under local anesthesia is necessary to drain the pus.

ENTERITIS

1. The cause is usually a virus. We have no specific treatment for it. Do not give antibiotics. Do not give medicines to try to stop the diarrhea.

2. The important treatment is rehydration. Follow the instructions on page 322.

3. If the patient has a fever, do a thick blood film to look for malaria parasites. If the thick film is positive, or if you cannot do it, give him treatment for malaria.

4. Keep the patient in the health center until the diarrhea stops. Look for signs of dehydration. Be sure you give enough liquid to rehydrate him.

5. Talk to the patient and to his family about the cause of enteritis and how to keep from getting it again. Give the health education listed in the treatment for dysentery - see page 617.

EPIDIDYMITIS

1. Bed rest. The patient must remain in bed until the pain and fever are gone. Keep the scrotum elevated.

2. The cause is usually gonorrhea. Give the patient an antibiotic for 7 days, or until all pain and fever are gone. Use either penicillin, penicillin V, or ampicillin.

3. To treat the pain, give him aspirin. A hot water bottle on the scrotum will diminish the pain.

4. If the pain or fever do not go away after this treatment, send the patient to hospital.

EPILEPSY

The disease

Be very careful about making this diagnosis. The word "epilepsy" brings much fear to people, especially to parents of little children. Many small children have convulsions when they have a high fever. This is NOT epilepsy. They may have convulsions with malaria, or with another disease. This is NOT epilepsy.

Epilepsy means repeated attacks of convulsions with no fever and no other cause.

Ask many questions about when the convulsions come. Do certain things seem to bring on the convulsions, like certain foods, certain emotions, or certain events?

Sometimes convulsions come when the patient has gone many hours without eating. Those convulsions are not epilepsy. They come from low blood sugar. In this case, the patient must eat regularly and not go many hours without eating. This will keep the blood sugar normal, and convulsions will not come.

If you think a child or an adult has epilepsy, send him to the doctor. He will do many exams to look for the cause. Only the doctor can make the diagnosis of epilepsy and give the correct treatment. He may then send the patient back to you to continue the treatment.

Treatment

A patient with epilepsy must take medicine every day. He must continue to do so for many years. This will keep the convulsions from coming. If he stops the medicine, the convulsions will come back. Use one of these medicines for a patient with epilepsy to keep the convulsions from coming.

1. Diphenylhydantoin (*Dilantin, *Phenytoin), 100 mg pills.

   ● For an adult, 1 pill 1 to 3 times a day.

   ● For a child, 2.5 mg/kg 1 to 3 times a day.

   ● This can cause bleeding and overgrowth of the gums. It is not serious.

2. Phenobarbital: The same dose as for diphenylhydantoin. For each patient, the doctor will determine how much to give. Follow the doctor's instructions carefully.

3. For the treatment of a severe attack with many convulsions, slowly give diazepam IV , 1 mg/kg for a child, or 10 to 20 mg for an adult.

For the treatment of the convulsions, see the strategies on CONVULSIONS on pages 422 and 428.

Instructions

A patient with epilepsy must not do dangerous things. He must not make a fire, sit or sleep near a fire, use a gun, or drive a vehicle or motorcycle. He must not climb trees or high mountains, or go to dangerous places. A patient who has a convulsion in a dangerous place or while doing something dangerous can injure himself or other people seriously.

Talk to the patient and the family about the disease. A patient can grow and live quite normally with this disease. But he must take the prescribed medicine regularly, every day. He should eat and sleep well and stay away from all dangerous activities and places.

EPISTAXIS - Nose bleed

The disease

Most cases of epistaxis are not serious. But always take the vital signs of a patient with nose bleed. Look for signs of shock. Bleeding from the nose can make the patient afraid. Tell the patient that the bleeding will soon stop.

Treatment

1. Put the patient in bed with his head raised a bit.
2. Press on the sides of his nose and on the upper lip until the bleeding stops.
3. If he is very nervous, give him diazepam or phenobarbital.
4. After the bleeding stops, examine the nose to find the cause of the bleeding. Look for a tumor or an ulcer of the lining of the nose.
5. Send the patient to hospital:
   - If he has much bleeding.
   - If most of the bleeding is in the back of the nose and goes down the throat.
   - If the bleeding continues in spite of your treatment.
   - If the patient has repeated attacks of nose bleed.

FILARIASIS

Loa Loa, Wuchereria bancrofti

Diethylcarbamazine citrate (*Hetrazan, *Carbilazine, *Banocide)

This is the specific medicine for these filaria. It works against the adult worms and the microfilaria. It comes in pills of 50 mg. The medicine is not dangerous and toxic reactions to it are rare. The individual dose is 2 mg/kg. Give this dose 3 times a day.

However, in the beginning of the treatment, many microfilaria die quickly. This causes much itching and sometimes a fever. So start with a very small dose. Follow the dose schedule in table 7.

Table 7. Start of diethylcarbamazine treatment for adults			
Day	Dose	Number of pills	Number of doses per day
1	25 mg	1/2	1
2	25 mg	1/2	2
3	25 mg	1/2	3
4	25 mg	1/2	3
5	50 mg	1	3
6	50 mg	1	3
7	100 mg	2	3

For a child from 6 to 12 years, give him one half the adult dose. In children under 6 years old, filariasis is uncommon.

If the patient has much itching, give him an antihistamine.
See ALLERGY on page 596 for the medicine and the dose.

Onchocercus Volvulus - Onchocerciasis

The treatment of onchocerciasis is difficult. Diethylcarbamazine kills the microfilaria, but it does not kill the adult worms. During the treatment with diethylcarbamazine, the patient has much itching. If many microfilaria are in the eyes, the eyes become inflamed. The patient can lose the vision in one or both eyes. For this reason, a patient with onchocerciasis must go to hospital.

We have a new medicine, *Ivermectin, which is very good for onchocerciasis. Only the doctor can prescribe it.

Dipetalonema Perstans

1. This filaria usually gives no symptoms. Do not give treatment for it.
2. If the patient has much itching, look for another cause of the itching, like another filariasis, scabies, an allergic reaction, or another disease. See the strategy on ITCHING, page 448.

FOOD POISONING

The patient has much vomiting, often with diarrhea, and sometimes with pain in the abdomen. Often other persons who ate the same food the patient ate also have vomiting. This is the treatment:

1. Bed rest.
2. Rehydration, either by rehydration solution as for dehydration from diarrhea (see page 322), or by infusion.
3. Medicine to stop the vomiting, such as:
   - Chlorpromazine, 25 mg IM.
   - Thiethylperazine (*Torecan), 10 mg IM.
   - Cyclizine (*Marezine), 50 mg IM.
4. Do not give antibiotics. If the patient has much fever, he has another serious disease. Send him to hospital.
5. If the vomiting does not stop after 1 day of treatment, send the patient to hospital.

FOREIGN BODY IN THE EYE

1. If it is a small object on the conjunctiva, take it out with a small piece of cotton. Then put in one dose of antibiotic ointment. No further treatment is necessary.

2. If the object is inside the upper lid, turn the upper lid out by using a small stick. See page 70. You can then take out the foreign body with a small piece of cotton.

3. If the foreign body is on the cornea, this is serious. It can cause a bad infection in the eye. Or it can make a permanent scar on the cornea. Send the patient immediately to the doctor. He will take out the foreign body under local anesthesia.

FRACTURE

Signs of a fracture

Several signs indicate a new fracture.

1. Much pain and tenderness where the bone is broken.
2. Often swelling and sometimes a dark blue color of the skin where the bone is broken. We call this ecchymosis.
3. Impossibility to use the part of the body where the bone is broken.
4. Change in the length or shape of the arm or leg where the bone is broken.
5. A feeling of "cracking," or "crepitations" when you move the injured part gently. This comes because the broken ends of the bone rub together. But move this part very gently. It is very painful.

Immobilisation

A patient who may have a fracture must go to hospital to have an X-ray and treatment for the fracture. But first immobilize the injured part to make certain that it cannot move during the trip.

A fracture of the hand, the arm, or the shoulder

1. Put the arm in a sling bandage.
2. Put another bandage around the arm and chest to hold the arm against the chest. This will keep it from moving.

Fracture of the foot or the lower leg

1. Put a long board in back of the leg.
2. Put soft cloths, a pillow, or blankets between the leg and the board.
3. Tie the leg firmly to the board, but not too tightly.
4. This will keep the leg and the fracture from moving during the trip to hospital.

Fracture of the back, the neck, or the upper leg

1. Prepare a hard bed or a wide board.
2. Cover it with soft cloths, pillows, or blankets.
3. Tie the patient firmly to the board. This will keep the broken bones from moving.
4. DO NOT put the patient in a chair.
5. Do not let him sit up.
6. Sitting will injure and perhaps cut the nerves in the back or the muscles and nerves in the lower leg.

   Before sending a patient with a fracture to hospital, give him medicine to calm the pain.

Rib fracture

1. Do not put a bandage around the chest.
2. See if the patient can breathe well.
3. If he can breathe well, do not send him to hospital.
4. Give him aspirin for pain.
5. The fracture will heal without treatment.
6. Send the patient immediately to hospital:
   - If he cannot breathe well.
   - If he has crackles in the lungs.
   - If he has no breath sounds in the lungs on the side of the injury.
   - If he has signs of shock. In this case, start an infusion before sending him.

Open fracture

An open fracture is when the patient has a wound where the bone is broken.

1. Wash the wound carefully with soap and water and then with a disinfectant solution.
2. If the ends of the bone come out through the wound, do not push them back in. If you do, this will cause an infection in the bone.
3. Put a sterile bandage over the wound.
4. Give the patient penicillin or another antibiotic.
5. Immobilize the injured part.
6. Send the patient immediately to hospital.

Fracture of the head

A fracture of the head (skull) gives one or more of these signs:

- Blood or clear water coming out of an ear.
- Clear water coming from the nose.
- Unconsciousness.
- Paralysis of an eye, a part of the face, or part of the body.
- Change in the size of the pupil of one eye.

In such a case, if the hospital is nearby, send the patient there. But if your health center is far from the hospital, do not move him. Care for him yourself. This requires these things.

1. Bed rest, with a good mattress.
2. Turn the patient from one side to the other every 3 hours. This will keep bed sores from coming on his skin.
3. Hydration. If he cannot drink, put down a naso-gastric tube and give him liquids through the tube. Give 2 to 3 liters of liquid every day.
4. If he cannot pass urine, or passes urine with no control, put a sterile catheter into the bladder.
5. After some days, he may become conscious. He can then eat and start moving in bed. After some more days he can start walking slowly. Gradually he can do more activities until he is completely well.

FUNGUS INFECTION OF THE SKIN

Treatment

We have many medicines for the treatment of fungus infections of the skin. They come as powders, as solutions, as ointments, or as pills.

Medicines to put on the skin

1. Benzoic acid with salicylic acid (*Whitfield's ointment).
2. Clotrimazole 1% (*Canesten or *Lotrimin).
3. Undecylenic acid, good for fungus infection of the feet - "athlete's foot."
4. Miconazole 2% (*Monistat).
5. Nystatin, for Candida infections of the vagina or the mouth.

Griseofulvin for oral use

1. It comes in pills of 125 or 500 mg.
2. Use this only for chronic fungus infections of the skin of the head, of the body, or of the finger nails.
3. Use it only when the solutions or ointments listed above do not help.
4. The dose for adults is 250 mg 2 to 4 times a day.
5. For fungus infections of the skin, give it for 6 weeks.
6. For fungus infection of the finger nails, the patient must take it for 6 months.

Instructions

Give these instructions to a patient who has a fungus infection of the skin.

1. Take a bath every day and then dry the skin well.
2. Keep the skin dry.
3. Put on one of the above medicines 2 times a day, morning and evening.
4. Continue this until the itching and the skin eruption go away.

Fungus infections get well very slowly. A patient may have to continue the treatment for a long time.

GASTRITIS

Gastritis is an inflammation of the inside of the stomach.

Acute gastritis

This can come from eating too much food, from eating too much hot spices, or from drinking too much alcoholic drinks. Give the patient antacids or an antispasmodic medicine. Tell him to:

1. Eat only soft foods with no spices until the pain goes away.
2. Stop drinking alcoholic drinks.

Chronic gastritis

Take a good history from the patient. Find out when the pain or heart-burn comes. Find out what makes the pain more severe and what, if anything, makes the pain go away. The treatment you prescribe and the instructions you give to each patient depend on the answers to these questions.

Gastritis in pregnancy

It usually comes in the first three months. The woman has heartburn, nausea, and often vomiting. Tell her these things.

1. Eat small meals 3 times a day.
2. Eat something early in the morning when getting out of bed.
3. Do not eat strong spices or drink alcoholic drinks.

Give her vitamin B-6 (pyridoxine) 50 mg 2 times a day.

In most cases, the gastritis will stop after the first trimester. But if the woman has much vomiting, or the gastritis continues into the 4th or 5th month, send her to the doctor.

Gastritis during other diseases

Gastritis can come in other diseases like diabetes, cirrhosis, or heart disease. In these cases, treat the other disease. Find out from the patient what makes the burning or the pain come. Give him instructions about eating. He must not eat things that make the pain worse. He must avoid any foods or any medicines that make the other disease worse.

Instructions to the patient about food

If certain foods make the burning or the pain come

1. Stop eating these foods or eat only very small amounts of them.
2. Avoid hot spices and alcoholic drinks like beer, wine, or whisky.

If the pain or burning comes right after eating

1. Eat less food at one time.
2. Eat three meals a day, but meals that are not big.
3. Do not eat a very big meal at one time. This can cause burning or pain.

If the pain comes before eating

1. Eat more often.
2. Do not wait many hours before eating.
3. Do not work until the afternoon without eating. This can cause burning or pain.
4. Eat three times a day, morning, noon, and night.
5. Avoid long hours between meals.

Eat slowly

Eating fast makes the stomach become full very quickly. This can cause gastritis. Eating slowly is good for the stomach and also for the digestion.

When the pain comes in the middle of the night

1. Eat a good meal in the evening, but not a very big meal.
2. Eat no hot spices.
3. If pain comes during the night, eat some food like bread or a banana, or drink some milk. This will help the pain go away.

Protein

In every case, tell the patient to eat foods with much protein. This will help him be strong and not lose weight.

Personal instructions

Many troubles in the life, work, or family of a patient can cause gastritis. Strong emotions can cause heartburn or pain in the stomach, emotions like anger, fear, jealousy, or even bad dreams. Ask the patient about this. Ask him about his family life. Is there much jealousy or anger between the husband and the wife, or between the patient and the children?

Ask about problems at work or in the community. Many worries can cause gastritis.

Ask the patient if he has bad dreams. These are a sign of conflicts, troubles, or worries. They can cause gastritis.

Talk to the patient about these difficulties. Try to help him find solutions to any problems he may have. Help him get rid of strong emotions. A patient who can find solutions to these problems will usually get well. A calm spirit is the best treatment and prevention of gastritis.

Danger signs

Tell each patient about the danger signs of gastritis:

- Much vomiting.
- Vomiting blood.
- Passing blood in the stools, or stools that are very black.
- Very strong pain in the abdomen.
- Loss of weight.

A patient who has one or more of these signs must come quickly for treatment. Usually he will need to go to hospital.

Medicines for gastritis

The most important part of the treatment of gastritis is the instructions you give to the patient. Medicines give very little help, and they cannot cure the disease. They can only help the symptoms go away for a short time. These medicines can give some help to the patient.

Antispasmodic medicines

They diminish or take away the abdominal pain for a few hours. A patient should take one kind of antispasmodic tablet before each meal.

1. Belladonna tablets: 1 or 2 tablets 3 times a day, before meals.
2. Propantheline bromide (*Probanthine): 1 tablet (15 mg) 3 times a day.
3. Phenobarbital and belladonna tablets: 1 tablet 3 times a day.
4. Clidinium bromide and chlordiazepoxide (*Librax): 1 tablet 3 times a day. This is quite expensive.

Antacids

They diminish or get rid of the heart burn. But often the heart burn comes back quickly. So antacids do not help much.

1. Aluminium hydroxide: 1 or 2 tablets 4 times a day.
2. Magnesium trisilicate with aluminium hydroxide: 2 tablets 4 times a day.
3. *Gelusil: 1 tablet 4 times a day.

Sedatives

They can sometimes be helpful. They often help in a patient who has gastritis because of strong emotions, many worries, or many troubles. But do not use them with every patient. They can cause drug abuse, especially phenobarbital. Use them only for a few days.

1. Phenobarbital: 30 mg 3 times a day for not more than 5 days.
2. Diazepam (*Valium): 2.5 to 5 mg 3 times a day.

Vitamins

Vitamins can help in a patient who has lost weight. Give him vitamin B complex.

GASTRO-ENTERITIS

This causes vomiting and diarrhea together. Look at the strategies on vomiting and on diarrhea to find the specific cause. Give the patient treatment for the cause. Give him also rehydration treatment. For this, see the instructions on page 322.

GOITER

1. Give the patient levothyroxine, 0.1 mg 1 to 3 times a day. This will make the goiter stop growing and even become small. Or give him desiccated thyroid (*Thyroid extract), 1 tablet (65 mg) 1 to 3 times a day.

2. If you do not have levothyroxine or *Thyroid extract, give the patient 5 drops a day of saturated Lugol's solution in a half a glass of water. Give him this for 3 to 6 months. The goiter will stop growing and may become small. To make Lugol's solution, put 5 g of iodine and 10 g of potassium iodide in 100 ml of water.

3. An operation is necessary only if the patient has trouble breathing, trouble swallowing, or much pain. In this case, send him to the doctor.

GONORRHEA

Treatment

Give one of the following antibiotics:

1. Penicillin, 4 million units divided in 2 or more places of injection, given at the same time, with 1 g probenecid given by mouth.

2. Tetracycline, 500 mg 4 times a day for 7 days.

3. Amoxicillin, 3 g orally in one dose, with 1 g probenecid, followed then by 7 days of tetracycline.

Treatment for resistant cases

Many cases of gonorrhea resist treatment by penicillin, tetracycline, or amoxacillin. If the symptoms continue after this treatment, give the patient one of these antibiotics:

1. Spectinomycin, 2 g IM.

2. Cefoxitin, 2 g IM with 1 g probenecid orally.

3. Cefotaxime, 1 g IM.

Sexual contacts

Ask the patient about all persons with whom he or she has had sexual contact in the last month. Try to find these persons and give them the same treatment. If the patient is married, give the same treatment to the patient's spouse.

Instructions to the patient

The patient must have no further sexual contacts until all the symptoms have gone. Tell him or her how to keep from getting the disease again.

Report

Send a report of each case to the government health authorities.

HEAD INJURY

Refer to hospital

Send the patient immediately to hospital:

1. If he has signs of shock or a skull fracture - see page 626.
2. If he is unconscious or has had convulsions.
3. If he has a big wound, or a wound of the eye, the face, or the mouth.

To send the patient to hospital

1. Prepare a hard bed or a wide board.
2. Cover it with soft cloths, pillows, or blankets.
3. Tie the patient to the bed. This will keep him from moving during the trip to the hospital.
4. If the patient is in shock, start an infusion. Let it continue slowly during the trip to hospital.

Treatment in your health center

No loss of consciousness

A head injury that does not cause coma probably is not serious. Give the patient aspirin if he has pain. Keep him quiet for a day. Observe him during this time. If after 1 day the patient feels well, he may go home.

With a short loss of consciousness

If a head injury caused coma for some minutes or more, this is more serious. Keep the patient in bed for 3 days. Give him aspirin if he has pain. Send him to hospital if he has one or more of these danger signs.

1. Bleeding from the ear.
2. Clear liquid coming from the ear or from the nose.
3. Swelling, or a very dark color, around the eyes.
4. Strong vomiting.
5. Very severe headache.
6. Very slow pulse: less than 50 per minute.
7. Paralysis of the face, of an eye, of an arm, or of a leg.
8. Loss of consciousness again.

Past head injury

If the head injury occurred some time ago, send the patient to hospital if he has one of the following conditions.

1. If he is unconscious or has been unconscious.
2. If he has had convulsions.
3. If he has trouble seeing, speaking, or hearing.
4. If he has much dizziness or severe vomiting.
5. If he has a paralysis of an eye, a part of the face, an arm, or a leg.

HEART DISEASE

The disease

Heart disease comes when there is damage to the heart valves, to the heart muscle, or to the sack around the heart, the "pericardial sack." Often the patient has a heart murmur. If the damage is not serious, the patient may have no symptoms.

A patient may have a heart murmur but no symptoms of health failure. He does not need treatment. Do not tell him he has heart disease or a heart murmur. Telling him he has heart disease will make him afraid.

A child with a heart murmur and fever

A child may have a heart murmur and fever. Look for an infection. If the child has an infection, treat it. Look for malaria parasites in a blood thick film. If he has malaria, treat it. But if the fever continues even after the treatment, he may have rheumatic heart disease. In this case, give him this treatment.

1. Penicillin or penicillin V for 10 days, and aspirin.
2. Keep the child in bed for 10 days or until all fever is gone.
3. If the fever continues, or if he has many symptoms, send him to hospital.

Heart disease during pregnancy

A pregnant woman may have a heart murmur. This can come from anemia. If she has anemia, look for the cause. Treat each cause of her anemia that you find. If she does not have anemia, she may have heart disease. Follow her very carefully during the pregnancy. Examine her every 2 weeks. When the time for delivery is near, send her to hospital to deliver. She must deliver the baby where the doctor can help her.

HEART FAILURE

Look for the cause

Several conditions can cause heart failure.

1. An infusion or transfusion which is very rapid or too much.
2. High blood pressure of more than 160/100 mm.
3. A scar on one of the heart valves. The patient will have a loud heart murmur.
4. Severe anemia, with a hemoglobin below 7 g.
5. Malnutrition.
6. A serious infection like septicemia, pneumonia, peritonitis. Such infections are even more dangerous for young children.
7. A disease of the heart muscle or of the blood vessels to the heart.

Treat the cause

Look for a cause of the heart failure. If you find a cause, like anemia, high blood pressure, malnutrition, or a serious infection, give treatment for it. Treat also the heart failure. If the cause of the heart failure is an infusion or a transfusion, stop it immediately. Then treat the heart failure.

Instructions to the patient

About diet

1. A patient with heart failure must eat food with much protein every day. A patient with anemia or malnutrition needs much protein. Do not give him vitamins. A patient receives sufficient vitamins in his food. He does not need to spend money to buy vitamin pills.
2. A patient with heart failure and who is obese must lose weight. The heart will then be able to work better. He must eat less food. But he still needs plenty of food with protein.
3. Salt causes edema and gives more work to the heart. A patient with heart failure must not eat salt. Tell him:
   - Do not add salt to your food.
   - Do not eat foods with much salt, like salted fish or salted meat.
   - Do not take medicines with sodium, like sodium bicarbonate or sodium salicylate.

About activity

In heart failure, the heart is unable to work normally. Physical work and activity make more work for the heart. So when the patient does work or physical activity, the heart is unable to meet the needs of his body for blood and oxygen. He will then have difficulty breathing, or dyspnea.

A patient with heart failure must do less work and activity. This depends on how severe the symptoms are. If he has much dyspnea and edema, bed rest is necessary. If he has only a little dyspnea or edema, he can move around. He may even be able to work a little. He can do work or other physical activity as long as he has no dyspnea. When it comes, he must rest.

Other instructions

1. Do not smoke, or drink much alcoholic drinks.

2. Come to the clinic if the dyspnea, edema, or other symptoms become more severe.

3. A woman who has had heart failure must not become pregnant again. She may die during the pregnancy or during the delivery. Talk to her and her husband about this. Tell her how to keep from becoming pregnant.

Treatment

Diuretics

A patient with edema, dyspnea, or crackles in the lungs needs a diuretic. Use hydrochlorthiazide, furosemide, or spironolactone.

The purpose of diuretics is to make the patient produce much urine. This diminishes the liquid in the body tissues. Then the patient will have less edema and less work for the heart. You can follow the progress of patients taking a diuretic by observing:

- The edema - is it diminishing?
- The dyspnea - is it less? Count the respirations each day.
- The size of the liver - is it diminishing? Is it less tender?
- Crackles in the lungs - are they going away?
- The weight of the patient - is he losing weight?

These signs will tell you if he is getting better or not.

Digoxin

Many cases of heart failure need only a good diet, more rest, and a diuretic. But if the heart failure is severe, the patient will need digoxin. Digoxin makes the heart more strong. The pulse becomes more slow. The signs and symptoms of heart failure diminish or go away.

Digoxin is a dangerous medicine. It is very toxic. Only the doctor should prescribe digoxin. If you feel a patient needs digoxin, send the patient to the doctor.

In some cases, this will not be possible. In other cases, the doctor will want you to continue giving the digoxin in your health center. So you must know how to use it. It comes in pills of 0.25 mg.

If a patient has not yet started taking digoxin, give him a big dose the first day:

- For an adult: 2 tablets every 6 hours for 3 doses.
- For a child: 0.025 mg/kg for the first dose, then 0.0125 mg/kg every 6 hours for 2 more doses.

After this, or in a patient who is already taking digoxin, give:

- To an adult, 0.25 mg (1 tablet) every morning.
- To a child, 0.01 mg/kg every morning.

Continue this treatment until the patient sees the doctor.

Remember that digoxin is very toxic. These are the signs of toxicity:

1. Loss of appetite.
2. Vomiting.
3. A slow pulse: below 60 beats per minute.
4. An irregular pulse.

Examine every day a patient who is taking digoxin. Take the pulse before giving digoxin. If his pulse is below 60, or if it is irregular, do not give the digoxin. Ask him how he is eating. If he has no appetite or has nausea or vomiting, do not give the digoxin. Send to the doctor any patient who has one or more signs of toxicity.

HEMORRHOIDS

Look for a cause

Hemorrhoids often are not serious. But they can be a sign of a tumor in the large intestine, or of cirrhosis. Look for signs of these diseases in every patient with hemorrhoids. Do a rectal exam to feel for a tumor. Examine the liver to see if it is big.

Prevent constipation

The cause of hemorrhoids is often constipation, or very hard stools. A patient with constipation needs instructions about food.

1. Eat much fruit, green leafy vegetables, maize, groundnuts and beans.
2. Drink much water. This will help make the stools soft.
3. Do much exercise. This will help the intestines work better.
4. Do not take laxatives. They keep the intestines from doing their normal work.

Small hemorrhoids

1. Give the patient some hemorrhoid suppositories. He should put a suppository in the rectum after every bowel movement.
2. Tell him to keep the skin around the anus very clean.
3. He should put ointment on the anus after every bowel movement and at night before going to bed.

Big hemorrhoids with much pain and bleeding

1. Put the patient in bed.
2. He must lie down on his side or on his abdomen. This will help the swelling of the hemorrhoids to go down.
3. Have him sit in a big basin of warm water 2 times a day. This will help the swelling to go down and the pain to go away.
4. After the swelling goes down, send him to hospital. He may need an operation to remove the hemorrhoids.

HEPATITIS

The disease

Hepatitis is a virus infection of the liver. We have no specific treatment for it. Antibiotics do not work against the virus of hepatitis.

Treatment

1. Rest is very important. A patient with hepatitis must stay in bed. He must stay in bed until all fever, nausea, and vomiting are gone, and until he is eating well.

2. If he has much vomiting, give him 5% glucose and physiologic saline by IV infusion. Or else give him liquids by rectum.

3. Do not give chlorpromazine, phenobarbital, or morphine to stop the vomiting. These can cause damage to the liver.

Instructions about eating

A patient with hepatitis loses his appetite. He does not want to eat. Do not make him eat. But when the desire to eat comes back, give him these instructions.

1. Eat foods with carbohydrates and much protein - see page 658. This will help the liver to get well.

2. Do not eat much fat or foods with oil.

3. Do not drink any alcoholic drinks.

4. Go back to work only when the jaundice is gone and when you feel well and strong again. Often this takes some months.

Isolation

Hepatitis is a contagious disease. You must follow these rules in caring for a patient with hepatitis.

1. Keep him away from other persons. Permit only 1 or 2 members of the family to stay with him.

2. Put all vomited liquid and all stools in the latrine. The hepatitis virus is in them. Wash the bedpan and all other pans and basins well with water and soap, and put this water into the latrine.

3. All persons who care for the patient must wash their hands very carefully with soap and water after caring for the patient and before caring for another patient.

4. The family must boil all drinking water for the patient and for themselves.

Injections

The virus of hepatitis can go to other persons by syringes and needles. Do not give injections to a patient with hepatitis unless it is very necessary.

If you must give a hepatitis patient an injection, use a disposable syringe and needle. Throw it away after using it. If you do not have disposable syringes and needles, boil the syringe and needle for 30 minutes before using them for another patient.

Bacterial hepatitis

A few cases of hepatitis come from bacteria. In this case, the patient has a high fever, a rapid pulse, and a high white blood cell count. The liver is very tender. If the white blood cell count is above 10,000/mm3, give the patient tetracycline 0.5 g 4 times a day for 10 days. Or give chloramphenicol, 0.5 g 4 times a day for 10 days.

Report

Report each case of hepatitis to the government health authorities.

HERNIA

Treatment

The only treatment for a hernia is a surgical operation. Send a patient with a hernia to hospital. Tell him a hernia can be dangerous. It can become strangulated, and he can die. He needs an operation as soon as possible.

Umbilical hernia

An umbilical hernia in a small baby or child does not need an operation. This hernia will cause no trouble. It will probably go away with no treatment.

Strangulated hernia

If the hernia is strangulated - see page 115 - send the patient immediately to hospital. An operation is very urgent.

HIGH BLOOD PRESSURE - Hypertension

Examination

In every patient with high blood pressure, look for:

1. Signs of heart failure.

2. Signs of kidney disease. Do a urine exam.

3. Protein in the urine and edema in a woman with a pregnancy of 7 to 9 months. These are signs of toxemia of pregnancy. See page 128.

4. Difficulties in the family, at work, or in the community and strong emotions can cause high blood pressure. Ask the patient about them.

Hospitalization

Send immediately to hospital a patient with high blood pressure who has one of these problems.

1. A diastolic blood pressure above 120 mm.

2. Severe headache, much dizziness, strong chest pain.

3. Signs of heart failure.

4. Severe kidney disease, with much protein or many cells in the urine.

5. Toxemia of pregnancy.

Treat in your health center a patient whose blood pressure is not very high and who has no severe symptoms. This is the treatment to give.

Instructions to the patient

1. Salt and sodium make the blood pressure go up. Tell a patient with high blood pressure:

   - Do not put salt in your food.

   - Do not eat salty foods like salted fish.

   - Do not take medicines with sodium, like sodium bicarbonate or sodium salicylate. They will make the blood pressure go up.

2. Being obese makes high blood pressure more serious. A patient who is obese must eat less and do more physical activity to lose weight.

3. A patient with high blood pressure should stop smoking and not drink much alcoholic drinks.

Medicines

Diuretics

A patient with a blood pressure above 140/90 needs hydrochlorthiazide 25 to 50 mg each morning, or bendriflumethiazide 5 to 10 mg each morning. This will help the blood pressure go down. He must take this every day, sometimes for several years. This will help keep the blood pressure normal so that it will not go up again. In many patients, this diuretic medicine alone is all they need.

The patient also needs some potassium. He can get this potassium by eating fresh fruits and green vegetables.

Reserpine

If a diuretic alone does not control the blood pressure, give the patient reserpine (*Serpasil) 0.1 to 0.25 mg 1 to 3 times a day. Together with a diuretic, this can make the blood pressure normal. Reserpine can also cause mental depression. In this case, stop giving it.

Other medicines

We have other medicines for high blood pressure. But they need the careful control of a doctor. Send to the doctor any patient whose blood pressure does not come down, or stay down, with the diuretic and reserpine.

The doctor may give a patient another stronger medicine and send him back to you. Follow the doctor's instructions very carefully.

Further instructions to the patient

1. You can probably continue to live and work normally.
2. Follow the instructions about diet.
3. Take your medicines regularly.
4. Continue to take these medicines for months, even years.
5. Come to the center every month for a control of your blood pressure. Come back sooner if you have symptoms of high blood pressure or heart failure.

Remember this. High blood pressure is a chronic disease. We can treat it and control it well. But we cannot often cure it.

HOOKWORM - see WORMS on page 707.

HYDROCELE

The only treatment is an operation. Send the patient to hospital. Do not try to take out the liquid from the hydrocele. This can cause a serious infection. The liquid will probably come back in a few days.

HYPERTROPHY OF THE PROSTATE

The only treatment is an operation. Follow the instructions on page 689 under the strategy DIFFICULTY IN URINATION. Then send the man to hospital. Send some members of his family with him. He may need a blood transfusion during or after the operation.

ILEUS

The intestines are full of gas. There are no sounds of peristalsis. This is normal for 2 or 3 days after a big operation on the abdomen. No specific treatment is necessary. If the patient has much pain because of the swelling in the abdomen, give an injection of a medicine to calm the pain, such as pethidine, 50 to 75 mg.

INJECTION IN THE SCIATIC NERVE

We have no specific treatment for this condition. Give the patient symptomatic treatment. See page 569 under the strategy PARALYSIS OF ONE OR BOTH LEGS.

It is very important to prevent this condition. Always be careful when you give an injection in the buttocks. Give it only in the upper outside part of the buttocks. Never give it in the lower inside part.

INJURY - OF THE ANUS

Examination

Examine the patient very carefully. Send the patient immediately to hospital:

1. If he has severe bleeding from the anus, or has signs of shock.

2. If he has severe pain in the abdomen, the lower back, or the hips.

3. If he cannot pass urine.

Look carefully at the anus and at the skin around it. Gently try to do a rectal examination. Send the patient to hospital:

1. If he has a deep wound.

2. If you can see the muscles around the anus.

3. If you find much blood inside the anus.

4. If the patient passes stools without control.

Treatment

1. If the injury is not serious, put the patient in bed.

2. Gently clean the anus and the skin around it with soap and water.

3. If the patient has pain, give him aspirin.

4. Let him sit in a basin of warm water 2 or 3 times a day.

5. Give him antibiotics only if he has definite signs of infection, like fever, much tenderness, big lymph nodes in the inguinal region, or pus coming from the wound.

INJURY - OF THE CHEST

Examine the patient carefully. Send him immediately to hospital:

1. If he has signs of shock.

2. If he has much trouble breathing.

3. If he has a big wound.

4. If air comes and goes through the wound. Put a sterile dressing on this wound before sending the patient to hospital.

Look for signs of a rib fracture - see page 82. If you find signs of a rib fracture, see page 625 for the treatment to give.

If the injury happened some time ago, no specific treatment is necessary. Give the patient aspirin if he has pain. Tell him to put a hot water bottle on the painful spot 1 or 2 times a day.

INSULIN SHOCK - see DIABETES on page 614

INTESTINAL OBSTRUCTION

This is very serious. The patient needs an operation quickly. Send him immediately to hospital. Before he goes, do these things.

1. Start an infusion. Give physiologic saline.
2. Give the patient penicillin, 800,000 u IM. If possible, give him also chloramphenicol 1 g IV, or ampicillin 1 g IV in the infusion, or tetracycline 0.5 g IM.
3. The patient must not eat or drink.
4. If possible, pass a naso-gastric tube into the stomach. Take out the liquid and gas with a big syringe.
5. Send the patient to hospital with the infusion and the naso-gastric tube.
6. Send a letter with the patient. Write the history, the physical signs you have found, and the treatment you have given.

LEPROSY

The disease

Leprosy is a serious chronic infection. Only the doctor ca make the diagnosis. If you think a patient may have leprosy, send him to the doctor. See page 139 for the signs of leprosy.

Most patients with leprosy can live at home. They do not need to be in hospital. They can get their medicines from you. Only the doctor can prescribe the treatment for leprosy patients. But the doctor may ask you to treat the leprosy patients in your area. So you must know how to use the medicines for leprosy.

Treatment

Medicines for leprosy

1. Di-amino-diphenylsulfone (*DDS, *Dapsone, *Disulfone), in tablets of 50 or 100 mg.
    - The dose for adults is 100 mg 1 time each day.
    - For children, it is 2 mg/kg 1 time each day.
    - Patients must take this medicine every day for 1 to 5 years.
    - The doctor will tell you when to stop it with each patient.

2. Clofazimine (*Lamprene), tablets of 100 mg.
   - The dose is 100 mg daily for an adult.
   - It is 2 mg/kg for a child.
3. Rifampicin, in capsules of 150 or 300 mg.
   - The dose is 600 mg for adults, or 450 mg for children.
   - Give this dose only 1 time per month.
   - Give the rifampicin yourself to each patient. Make sure he takes it in your presence.
   - Give it before he eats.
4. Ethionamide (*Prothionamide), in tablets of 125 mg or 250 mg.
   - You may use this instead of clofazimine.
   - The dose is 500 mg 1 time per month, or 250 mg 1 time per day.
   - It can cause liver disease, nerve disease, or mental difficulties.
   - If any of these come, stop the ethionamide. Send the patient to the doctor.

Most patients must take 2 or even 3 different medicines for their treatment. One medicine alone is not good because it can cause resistance to develop in the leprosy bacilli. Your doctor will tell you which medicines to give to each leprosy patient.

Reactions to the treatment

A patient on leprosy treatment can have a severe reaction. This causes a high fever, much swelling, and severe pain in the arms and legs. If this comes, stop the treatment and send the patient immediately to hospital.

Nerve damage

Leprosy destroys the nerves to the hands and feet. The patient has anesthesia and can feel no pain. He can injure himself without knowing it.

So a patient with leprosy often has sores on the skin, especially of the feet and hands. These sores come because of many small injuries. Have the doctor see every patient who has sores on the feet or hands, or who has paralysis of part of the feet or hands.

Sores

Wash each sore well with soap and water every day. Put on a clean bandage. Make the bandage thick to protect the sore from more injuries. The patient must keep the sores very clean to prevent more infection.

If a patient has shoes, look at the shoes carefully. Do they fit the feet well? Are they causing more injuries to his feet? If so, the doctor must see the patient and help him find shoes that will not cause more injuries to his feet.

Instructions to a patient with leprosy

About his hands and feet

1. Wash your feet and hands in water with soap frequently during work.
2. Soak your hands and feet for 20 minutes in water every evening.
3. Take off any dead skin with a stone or with your fingers, but never with scissors, a knife, or a razor blade.
4. Put cooking oil or vaseline on the skin after soaking your hands and feet.
5. Look carefully for sores on your hands and feet every evening. Feel for places that are painful or tender.
6. Rest the hand or foot if you have any places that are red, tender, swollen, or have any sores.
7. Do not use the hand or foot until all signs of infection or of a sore have gone.
8. Protect your hands and feet from anything that can cause a wound or sore, such as:
   - Fire, or cooking pots that are very hot.
   - Things that are sharp, like knives, broken glass, tin cans, nails.
   - Shoes that do not fit well.
   - Rocks, stones, roots, or other things where you walk.

About his eyes

Leprosy can cause damage to the eyes. You can lose the sight in one or both eyes.

1. Protect your eyes from the hot sun with a big hat, or sun glasses.
2. Do not work where there is much dust, or where there is a danger of dirt or sand going into an eye.
3. Wash your face around your eyes carefully with water every evening.
4. Keep your fingers away from your eyes.
5. Cover your eyes during sleep with a bandage to prevent injury.

About hygiene

1. Keep yourself very clean. Take a complete bath with soap and water every day.
2. Wash your clothes regularly. Always wear clean clothes.
3. Keep your house very clean inside.
4. Keep the land around your house very clean. Do not leave anything sharp on the ground. Throw all rubbish into a hole in the ground.
5. The latrine must be very clean, with a cover on the hole to keep flies away.

Family contacts

Leprosy is a contagious disease. It can go from one person to another, but only very slowly. It is not necessary to send the patient away from the other members of the family. But be certain to look at all of the other members of his family. Look for signs of leprosy. If you find any signs that look like leprosy on any of the family members, send them to the doctor. They may also have leprosy and need treatment.

LICE

The treatment for lice is hexachlorocyclohexane 1% (*Lindane, *Kwell). Explain carefully to the patient how to use it.

Head lice

1. Wash your hair carefully. Use a shampoo with hexachlorocyclohexane.
2. Leave the shampoo for 5 to 10 minutes, then wash it off. This will kill the lice.
3. If you still have living lice after 1 week, repeat the treatment.

If you have no hexachlorocyclohexane shampoo, tell the patient to shave off all his hair and wash his head with soap and water. This will get rid of the lice.

Body lice

1. Take a bath. Wash carefully and vigorously with soap and water.
2. After the bath, rub hexachlorocyclohexane solution into your skin in the parts where you have lice. Leave the lotion on for 12 hours, then wash it off.

3. At the same time, wash all your clothes and bed linens. Dry these well in the sun.

Treat the family

Lice go quickly from one person to another, especially to all those living in the same house. Treat everyone living in the house at the same time. They must wash all their clothes and bed linens. This is because lice can stay in these clothes or linens for a long time. If they do not wash them well, the lice will return to them after the treatment.

LIPOMA

This needs a small surgical operation. Send the patient to hospital.

LOA LOA - see FILARIASIS on page 622

LYMPHADENITIS

1. Give the patient an antibiotic for 7 days: penicillin, erythromycin, or ampicillin.
2. If pus comes, an incision is necessary. If you cannot do this, send the patient to hospital.
3. If the lymphadenitis does not go away after 7 days of treatment, send the patient to hospital. He may have a more serious disease causing the lymphadenitis.

MALARIA

The disease

Malaria is a serious disease for patients. It also causes many problems for the whole community.

1. It kills many young children.
2. It affects many older children and adults. They lose much time from work or school and much money for treatment.
3. It affects many pregnant mothers. It causes abortions and also makes the newborn baby weigh less.

4. It causes many serious complications, like cerebral malaria and severe anemia.

5. In many countries chloroquine does not work well any more against malaria. The malaria parasites have become resistant to chloroquine.

The fight against malaria requires four things:

1. A complete cure for every case of malaria. This requires a correct diagnosis, early treatment, and correct treatment.

2. Prevention of severe malaria in young children and in pregnant mothers.

3. Health education about how to treat malaria and how to prevent it.

4. Health education about how to get rid of mosquitoes.

To cure an attack of malaria

Make a correct diagnosis

Examine carefully each patient, and especially each child. Look for other diseases like meningitis, pneumonia, ear infection, or another infection. If possible, do a thick blood film and look for plasmodium. Give malaria treatment only to those who have plasmodium in the thick film. If you cannot do a thick blood film, then give malaria treatment to all patients who have a high fever and no signs of another infection.

Give medicines correctly

Know the amount of medicine to give to each patient. Be sure he takes it until the number of days for the cure is complete.

Medicines to treat malaria

Chloroquine (CHQ)

This is still the best medicine. BE SURE you know how many milligrams are in the tablets, solution, ampoules or vials you have. There are 2 different ways to write the dose of CHQ in mg. Some drugs companies tell you the number of mg of pure CHQ, or **chloroquine base**. Others give you the number of mg of **chloroquine salt**. This means the number of mg of chloroquine phosphate (CHQ + phosphate), or chloroquine sulfate (CHQ + sulfate).

Look carefully at the writing on the bottle of your CHQ. See if the dose is in mg of chloroquine base or of chloroquine salt.

- 60 mg of CHQ base equals 100 mg of CHQ salt.
- 100 mg of CHQ base equals 167 mg of CHQ salt.
- 150 mg of CHQ base equals 250 mg of CHQ salt.
- 600 mg of CHQ base equals 1000 mg, or 1 g of CHQ salt.

In this book we give you the dose as mg of chloroquine base, or pure chloroquine. The dose to treat malaria is 25 mg/kg of CHQ base given over 3 days.

- Day 1: 10 mg/kg in one dose, or in 2 doses of 5 mg/kg in each dose.
- Day 2: 10 mg/kg in one dose, or in 2 doses of 5 mg/kg in each dose.
- Day 3: 5 mg/kg in one dose.

For an adult, this is 600 mg the first day, 600 mg the second day, and 300 mg the third day. Be sure ALL patients complete this cure.

For a child, the dose depends on the weight of the child.

Follow these rules in using chloroquine to treat a patient with malaria.

1. Give CHQ by mouth, either in tablets or in solution.
2. Give it by injection ONLY when the patient is unconscious or has severe vomiting.
3. Stop giving it by injection as soon as the patient can take it by mouth.
4. Do not give CHQ by IM injection to babies or small children.
5. CHQ can give stomach problems - vomiting or the desire to vomit. It can also cause itching and sometimes noise in the ears.
6. Be very careful to give the correct dose to small children. An overdose can kill the child.

Amodiaquine

1. The dose is 10 mg/kg in one dose for one day only. For an adult, give 600 mg.
2. Amodiaquine often causes a severe headache and much weakness. Do not use it for small children.

Quinine

Give quinine for malaria which does not get well after 3 days of CHQ treatment. BE SURE you know how many milligrams are in the tablets, solution, or ampoules you have.

1. To an adult, give 500 mg 3 times a day for 7 days.
2. To a child, give 10 mg/kg 3 times a day for 7 days.

Tetracycline

Some doctors also give tetracycline with quinine to these patients.

- 250 mg 4 times a day for 7 days to an adult.
- 5 mg/kg 4 times a day to children over 8 years old.

Sulfadoxine-pyrimethamine (*Fansidar)

Use this for patients who cannot take CHQ or quinine. It comes in tablets of 500 mg of sulfadoxine + 25 mg of pyrimethamine.

1. The dose for an adult is 3 tablets in just one dose.
2. Give 2 tablets to children from 8 to 14 years old.
3. Give 1 tablet to children 4 to 7 years old.
4. Give half of one tablet to children under 4 years old.

Treatment of complications

Frequent complications

1. High fever: aspirin, 10 mg/kg, and a cool bath. This is very important for stopping convulsions in young children.
2. Diarrhea with dehydration: rehydration. See page 322.
3. Severe anemia. Do not give iron. Malaria destroys red blood cells but the iron is still in the body. The patient must have good food with much protein. If the anemia is very severe, a blood transfusion is necessary.
4. Convulsions. Give immediate treatment for malaria. Give aspirin for fever. Protect the patient from injury - see the strategies on CONVULSIONS, pages 422 and 428. Do not give diazepam or phenobarbital unless the convulsions continue. These medicines act slowly.

Cerebral malaria

This causes convulsions and coma. Give the patient:

1. Quinine.
   - 10 mg/kg IV in an infusion of 5% glucose over a period of 2 hours.
   - Repeat this dose after 8 hours if the patient still cannot take quinine by mouth.
   - As soon as the patient can take it by mouth, give quinine, 10 mg/kg 3 times a day for 7 days.
2. Much sugar. Patients with cerebral malaria have a very low blood sugar.
   - Give dextrose 50% IV, up to 100 ml.
   - Or give 1 to 3 large spoonfuls of sugar in water through a naso-gastric tube.
   - Do this quickly. It may save the life of the patient.

Black water fever

This is a very serious complication of malaria. It often causes death. The malaria parasites destroy many millions of red blood cells very quickly. The hemoglobin comes out in the urine. The urine is therefore red. The urine has no red blood cells in it, only hemoglobin.

1. Send a patient with black water fever immediately to hospital.
2. Before sending the patient, give chloroquine, 10 mg/kg.
3. DO NOT use quinine.
4. The patient needs blood transfusions and infusions to help keep the kidneys working well.

To keep a person from getting malaria

Prevention is very important for children from 0 to 4 years of age. They can die from malaria. It is also very important for pregnant mothers. Teach the parents of small children and also pregnant mothers the importance of taking medicine regularly to keep from getting malaria. Help them get this medicine in your clinics for small children and your prenatal clinics.

Chloroquine

Chloroquine is very good. Give 5 mg/kg 1 time a week.

Table 8. Dose of chloroquine to prevent malaria	
Age of patient	**Weekly dose**
0 to 1 year	50 mg
1 to 3 years	100 mg
4 to 6 years	150 mg
7 to 9 years	200 mg
10 to 12 years	250 mg
more than 12 years	300 mg

You can give CHQ to pregnant mothers. It will not cause an abortion or damage the unborn baby. The mother will not get severe malaria during the pregnancy. This will help the unborn baby grow bigger.

Quinine

Do not use quinine to prevent malaria. It can cause serious problems.

Attacks of malaria in spite of prevention

Persons who take medicine to keep from getting malaria can still get malaria. But they will not get it very often. It will be less serious. They must come for treatment whenever they get symptoms of malaria.

Health education about treatment

Explain to your people very carefully the importance of good treatment for malaria. They must follow the rules for taking the treatment. This will help stop malaria from becoming resistant to chloroquine and other medicines. Explain these rules to them.

1. Come for diagnosis and treatment when the illness first starts. Do not wait. If you do, the disease will be much more serious.

2. Take the full dose of CHQ: 10 mg/kg on day 1, 10 mg/kg on day 2, and 5 mg/kg on day 3. If you do not, some plasmodium will remain. They can then become resistant to treatment.

3. Finish the full cure of 3 days. If not, some plasmodium will remain and become resistant.

This is why it is important for all patients to come to the health center for diagnosis and treatment. Patients who give themselves treatment for malaria at home may not have malaria. They may have another disease. They may also not take enough CHQ. Then the plasmodium will become resistant.

Explain all of this carefully to your people. Encourage them to come quickly to the health center for a correct diagnosis and good treatment.

Fight against mosquitoes

Mosquitoes carry malaria from one person to another. If we protect ourselves from mosquitoes, we protect ourselves from malaria. Talk to your people about how to fight against mosquitoes.

Get rid of mosquitoes

Get rid of all places where mosquitoes lay their eggs.

1. They lay eggs in quiet water.

2. Get rid of all empty tin cans, pots, or any other thing that can hold water.

3. Fill all holes in the ground where rain water can stay.

4. Put a cover on all things used to collect rainwater: barrels, drums, pots, jugs.

It is not good to live near swamps or ponds where mosquitoes can lay their eggs. The community should be a kilometer or more from such water.

During the day mosquitoes hide in tall grass or other plants. Cut all tall grass around each house.

Protect the house from mosquitoes.

1. Make sure there are no holes in the walls.

2. Make sure there is no space between the walls and the roof where mosquitoes can go into the house.

3. If possible, put protective wire screens on all windows and doors. If this is not possible, be sure all windows and doors are closed after 4 o'clock in the afternoon.

4. Protect the bedrooms from mosquitoes. Make a ceiling with no holes or spaces between the ceiling and the walls. Grass mats make a good ceiling.

5. Put white paint or whitewash on the walls inside the house. Mosquitoes do not like white. You can easily see them on the white walls and kill them.

6. Clean the whole house every week.

   ● Take down all pictures and other things hanging on the walls and clean behind them.

   ● Clean behind all the furniture.

   ● Clean under the beds and tables.

   ● Use a soft broom to clean the walls and the ceiling.

   ● These things will help keep mosquitoes from staying in the house.

7. Use a mosquito net at night to cover the bed. The net must come completely down to the floor. Put it down every afternoon at 4 o'clock. Only then will it keep mosquitoes from biting you at night.

MALNUTRITION

Where malnutrition comes from

Malnutrition comes when people do not eat enough food or do not eat the right kinds of food. Our bodies need food every day. We need foods that give us energy to do work. We need foods to build the tissues of our bodies. These foods help us build bones, muscles, blood, skin, and our organs. These foods also help us keep these tissues and organs strong.

The foods we must have to build our bodies and to keep them strong are foods that have much protein. Protein is the substance the body uses to build our tissues and organs. Protein foods help keep our bodies strong and healthy.

If children do not eat enough food or enough foods with protein, their bodies will not grow well. Their tissues will become weak. Other diseases, especially infections, will come easily.

If adult persons do not eat enough food or enough protein foods, their bodies will become weak. They will get other diseases and infections. Adults and children all need good food with much protein.

Foods with protein

Protein foods come from animals and from plants.

Many protein foods come from animals.

- Milk: mother's milk, milk from animals, powdered milk.
- Fish: fresh fish, dried fish, salted fish.
- Meat: from all sorts of animals.
- Meat: from birds like chickens, ducks, birds of the forest.
- Eggs: from chickens, ducks, and other birds.
- Insects: caterpillars, termites, ants, and others.

Other protein foods come from plants.

- Beans: soya beans, dry beans.
- Groundnuts and peas.
- Maize (corn), millet, wheat, sorghum, rice, seeds of gourds.
- Dark green vegetables, like the leaves of the cassava (manioc) plant.

Other foods, like cassava root (manioc), plantain, bananas, sweet potatoes, bread, fruits, and oils are good foods. They have much starch, and they give us much energy to work and play. But they do not give us protein. So they do not help us build our bodies or keep our bodies strong.

Amino acids

Proteins are made of "building blocks" called amino acids. The body uses amino acids from our food to make proteins for our organs. Our bodies can make many amino acids.

But there are 8 amino acids our bodies cannot make. We call these "essential" amino acids. It is essential that we get these amino acids in the foods we eat. We must get all 8 of them in each meal. If we do not get them, our bodies cannot make proteins. We then become malnourished.

Animal proteins

Animal proteins have all 8 essential amino acids. Therefore we call animal proteins "complete proteins." It is good to eat one or more animal foods each day, like meat, fish, milk, or eggs. But often animal foods are hard to find. They cost much money. So we cannot always eat them.

Plant proteins

Plant proteins do not have all 8 essential amino acids. One or more of them are missing from each plant protein. If we eat only one plant protein, like maize or groundnuts, we do not get all 8 amino acids. In this case, our bodies cannot make proteins. We become malnourished.

There are two kinds of plant protein foods. One kind we call cereals. One of the 8 essential amino acids is missing from each cereal. The other kind of plant food we call grains. A different essential amino acid is missing from each grain food.

But if we eat one cereal and one grain together, we get a complete protein. The amino acid missing from the cereal is present in the grain. The amino acid missing from the grain is present in the cereal. So one cereal plus one grain give us a complete protein with all 8 essential amino acids. Table 9 shows you the different cereals and grains.

Table 9. Cereals and Grains

cereals	grains
maize (corn)	groundnuts
millet and sorghum	soya beans (soja)
wheat	dry beans
rice	seeds of gourds, or squash fruits
some green leafy vegetables	peas

Mixing cereals and grains

People with money can buy many good foods with protein. It is difficult, however, for people who are poor. But poor people can keep from getting malnutrition by eating cereals and grains together. Together they give a complete protein. A person who eats cereals and grains together in each meal will not get malnutrition. Teach this fact to your people and especially to your patients with malnutrition and to their families.

Feeding babies and small children

Babies and small children get malnutrition very easily. This is because they are growing fast. Their bodies need much protein. Here are suggestions as to how to feed babies and young children well. Children who eat these foods will not get malnutrition.

Babies from birth to 4 months of age

They need only their mother's milk. Tell their mothers not to give them powdered milk in a baby bottle. This often causes severe diarrhea which can sometimes cause death.

Babies from 4 months to 12 months

Tell the mother to give the baby every day:

1. Mother's breast milk.
2. Thin soup, or porridge, made from pounded rice, maize, sorghum, or wheat flour with 1 grain food such as:
   - Soya flour.
   - Groundnut powder or paste made from pounded groundnuts.
   - Beans, pounded and with the skins taken out.
   - Give this porridge to the baby 2 times each day.
3. Eggs. One egg 3 times a week is very good.
4. Rice. Soft rice cooked well in water is good. Give this with pounded groundnuts or beans.
5. Fish. Fish pounded well is good with the porridge or rice.
6. Porridge made from cassava flour, bananas, or maize alone is not enough. These foods do not have complete proteins. The baby cannot use them to grow and build a healthy body.

Children over one year of age

Tell the mother to give the child every day:

1. Breast milk until the age of 2 years or more.
2. Regular daily food of adults, like cassava, bananas, plantain, or sweet potatoes.
3. A cereal food and a grain food together 2 times a day.
4. A dark green leafy vegetable 1 or 2 times a day.

5. If possible, 1 egg a day.

6. If possible, she should give the child:

   ● Groundnuts: 1 cup 3 times a week.

   ● Flour from soya beans: 1 cup 3 times a week.

   ● Other beans: 1 cup 3 times a week.

   ● Fish: 2 or more times a week.

   ● Meat: 2 or more times a week.

   ● Caterpillars, termites, or other insects: 2 or more times a week.

   ● Powdered milk is good, 1 or 2 glasses a day. Make this fresh just before drinking it. It becomes sour, or bad, very quickly.

Pregnant mothers

These foods are very important for growing children. They are also very important for a pregnant mother. These foods will keep her body strong. They will help her build the body of her baby.

Sick persons

These foods are also important for sick persons. They help sick persons fight against their disease. They help the tissues of their body become strong again. They are important for persons with liver disease, tuberculosis, chronic infections, peptic ulcer, and after a big operation or serious infection.

Helping children eat

Often small children with malnutrition do not want to eat. You and the parents must help these children eat. Talk to the mothers about this. They must not "force" their children to eat. But they must encourage them to eat. Show each mother how to make porridge with a cereal and a grain. Watch her as she makes it. See that she makes it correctly. Show her how to give it to her child. Often a crushed sweet banana put in the porridge will make the child want to eat the porridge. Show her how to do this.

No medicines for malnutrition

Patients do not need medicines for malnutrition. Vitamin pills do not help. They only waste the patient's money. The only treatment is food with protein. Teach your patients to eat these foods every day and to feed them to their children.

Treating the diarrhea of malnutrition

Diarrhea is a very serious problem in malnutrition. The stools are like water. The patient has many stools a day. The diarrhea comes because the intestines are weak and cannot digest food well. The undigested food makes the diarrhea.

The only treatment is protein.

1. Feed the child foods with protein.
2. Start with soft foods, like a porridge of maize and soya, of maize and groundnuts, or of maize and pounded fish.
3. Give the child rice if possible.
4. If he is dehydrated, give him liquids for rehydration.

At first, these foods will make more diarrhea. This is normal. Do not stop giving these foods. Each day give a little more. When enough protein gets into the intestines, the diarrhea will stop. Then the child can eat more and will get well.

Do not give antidiarrhea medicines or antibiotics for this diarrhea of malnutrition.

Other diseases

Look for other diseases in every patient with malnutrition.

1. If he has intestinal worms, give him worm medicine.
2. If he has malaria, give him chloroquine.
3. If he has anemia, give him iron. But give only a little at first.
4. If he has an infection, treat it well.

Tuberculosis

Look for tuberculosis in every patient with malnutrition. Tuberculosis is hard to find in patients with malnutrition.

1. Ask if someone else in the family has, or has had, tuberculosis.
2. Ask if the patient has a low fever each evening.
3. See if he has big lymph nodes.
4. If you think the patient may have tuberculosis, send him to the doctor.

Education

The only cure for malnutrition is food with much protein. The best prevention for malnutrition is education. Talk to mothers and fathers about how to feed their children. Talk to sick persons about the foods they need to help them get well. Talk to community leaders about how to grow more foods with protein. Set a good example yourself by having a good garden, and by giving good food to your family.

MEASLES

The disease

Measles is a serious acute disease of babies and small children. It can cause death, especially in children who also have malnutrition. The cause of measles is a virus. We have no specific treatment for the virus of measles. There are 4 important parts of the general treatment for measles.

1. Treatment for the fever.
2. Liquids for hydration.
3. Good food.
4. Treatment of other infections that may come.

Treatment

Treatment for fever

For a fever over 38°C, give the child aspirin every 4 to 6 hours. For a small baby, crush the tablet and put the pieces in a teaspoonful of water. If the tablet of aspirin has 0.5 g, then 1 ml of this water will have 100 mg of aspirin. Give the baby 2 drops for every kg of weight and make the baby drink this. Save the rest for the following doses.

For a fever over 39°C, give the baby a bath in cool water. It is very important to keep the fever below 38°C. A high fever can cause dehydration and convulsions.

Liquids for hydration

Children with measles lose much water. They quickly become dehydrated. This makes their condition worse. So give much liquid to children with measles. They may not want to drink, but do your best to help them drink.

Children who cannot drink because of vomiting or sores in the mouth will need an infusion. Give this either by IV infusion, by rectum, or by naso-gastric tube.

Mother's milk is best for the small child. Water, thin soup, weak tea with sugar, and the juice of fruits are all good. Each child needs 150 ml/kg of liquid every day plus the mother's milk.

Food

Food with much protein is very important for children with measles. Measles can bring on malnutrition very quickly if the child does not eat well. When he has much fever, a child who has measles often will not eat. Wait until the fever comes down or goes away. Then tell the mother to start giving him food with much protein 2 or 3 times a day. In this way, he will not get malnutrition. See page 658 for the foods to give him.

Treatment of other infections

Look for infections that may come during the attack of measles and treat them immediately.

Pneumonia

It causes much difficulty in breathing and crackles in the lungs. Give the child penicillin or penicillin V for 7 days.

Ear infection (otitis)

The child will have pain in the ear, or pus coming from the ear. He will pull frequently on the infected ear. See page 618 for the treatment of ear infection.

Throat infection (tonsillitis)

The child will have much pain on swallowing and will not want to eat. His throat will be red and often he will have white spots on the tonsils. See page 693 for the treatment of tonsillitis.

Severe laryngitis, or croup

It can be very dangerous. If the child cannot speak or cry, or if he has severe dyspnea, give him chloramphenicol 25 mg/kg every 6 hours. If the hospital is near, send him to hospital.

Conjunctivitis

This comes from the virus of measles.

1. Keep the child in a dark room until the conjunctivitis goes away.
2. Put an antibiotic ointment in his eye or eyes 6 times a day.
3. Also put in atropine ointment 1 time a day.
4. Keep the eye or eyes closed with a dressing.
5. Do not use an ointment with cortisone.
6. Give much vitamin A.

Other treatment

The skin eruption of measles does not need special treatment. Tell the mother to keep the child clean. She may give him a bath if he needs it. We have no special medicine to make the rash go away.

Do not give antibiotics to every child with measles. Give an antibiotic only to those children with measles who have a bacterial infection.

Isolation

Measles is a contagious disease. Keep other children who have not had measles away from the child with measles. This is very important, especially for children with malnutrition. Send a report of each case to the government health authorities.

Prevention

We have a vaccine to prevent measles. We give this to every child at the age of 9 months. If you vaccinate every child in your area against measles at the age of 9 months, measles will disappear from your area.

Some health services vaccinate children against measles at the age of 6 months. If you do this, you must vaccinate each one again at the age of 15 months.

Keep the vaccine in the refrigerator, or in a cold thermos box, until the time for the injection. Give only 1 injection to each child. Give 0.5 ml in the subcutaneous tissue.

Follow the instructions that come with the vaccine about the preparation of the solution of vaccine. BE SURE to keep the vaccine cold and away from the sun until you give the injection. Write the vaccination on the record of each child you vaccinate.

MENINGITIS

Send the patient to hospital

Meningitis is a very serious disease. It can cause death quickly. Send to hospital every patient you think may have meningitis. But first give a big dose of an antibiotic before sending him.

Treatment in a health center

Treat the patient in your health center ONLY:

- If the hospital is very far away, more than one full day's journey, AND
- If you have the medicines necessary for the treatment.

Antibiotic treatment

The antibiotic treatment depends on the age of the patient.

Newborn babies from 0 to 2 months old:

1. Ampicillin IV 50 mg/kg every 6 hours for 2 weeks, plus
2. Gentamycin IM 2 mg/kg IM every 8 hours for 10 days.

Children from 3 months to 7 years of age:

1. Ampicillin IV or orally 50 mg/kg every 4 hours for 2 weeks, plus
2. Chloramphenicol IV or orally 25 mg/kg every 6 hours for 2 weeks.

Children from 8 to 15 years old:

1. Aqueous penicillin IV 2,000,000 u to 5,000,000 u every 6 hours for 2 weeks, or
2. Ampicillin IV or orally 50 mg/kg every 4 hours for 2 weeks.

Adults

1. Aqueous penicillin IV 5,000,000 u every 6 hours for 2 weeks.
2. If the patient cannot take penicillin because of allergy, give chloramphenicol 1 g IV every 6 hours until he can take it by mouth. Then give 1 g orally every 6 hours to complete 2 weeks.

Bed rest

Keep a patient with meningitis in bed and very quiet. Be sure he gets enough liquids. If he cannot drink, give him liquids by infusion. If a patient is in coma, see the strategy on UNCONSCIOUSNESS (COMA) IN A CHILD for the treatment - see page 435. For a small child with fever, give him aspirin and baths in cool water to bring the temperature down below 38 C.

Stopping the treatment

Stop the treatment after 2 weeks if the patient has no more fever or stiffness of the neck. But if the fever or stiffness continue, send the patient to hospital.

Isolation

Meningitis is very contagious. Keep a patient with meningitis away from other persons. Let only one member of the family stay with him to help give the care necessary. You and this person must wash your hands very carefully with soap and water after every care you give the patient. Wash very carefully all equipment you use to care for him. Keep the bed and room very clean.

Report each case

Send a report of each case to the government health authorities.

MENTAL DISEASE

There are many kinds of mental illness. Often they are difficult to treat. Send every patient with serious mental illness to the doctor.

The most important part of the treatment is something you can do. Before you send the patient to the doctor, try to find out the cause of the illness. Ask the patient or a member of the family these questions.

1. Has the patient had a serious problem in his life, his family, or his work?
2. Did he have a serious illness when the mental illness began?
3. Has he had an accident with an injury to the head?
4. Has he had treatment already for this illness?
5. Has he had another serious illness? If so, what was it?
6. Has he had treatment from a traditional healer? If so, what treatment? Did the treatment help?

Ask many questions about the life of the patient. Write a good report for the doctor of all you find out about him. This will help the doctor know how to treat him.

MIGRAINE

Send a patient with migraine to the doctor. He needs special examinations. Often the treatment is difficult. Give him aspirin for symptomatic treatment.

MUMPS

The disease

This is an acute virus infection in children. It is not serious. We have no specific treatment for it. The disease lasts 5 to 7 days.

Treatment

1. If the child has much pain or fever, keep him in bed.
2. Give him aspirin.
3. A hot water bottle on his face and ear can help the pain go away.
4. Do not give penicillin or other antibiotics. They will not help.

Sometimes in older boys or young men, the mumps virus goes to the testicle. This causes much pain and swelling. Keep the patient in bed until the pain and swelling go away. Give him aspirin for the pain.

PREVENTION

We have a vaccine for mumps. If many children in your area get mumps, ask your doctor about this vaccine.

Mumps is a contagious disease. Let the government health authorities know about each case.

MYCOBACTERIUM ULCER

This is a serious chronic ulcer of the skin. It comes often on the leg, but can also come on other places. Antibiotics do not help. See Chapter 3, page 147, for the signs of a mycobacterium ulcer. Send to hospital every patient who may have this ulcer. A surgical operation is necessary to remove it completely before it spreads any further.

NEPHRITIS - Kidney disease

Acute nephritis

This is an acute disease of children and young adults. It causes fever, edema, back pain, red blood cells and protein in the urine, and sometimes high blood pressure.

Send the patient to hospital. If this is impossible, treat him in your health center. The treatment to give is:

1. Bed rest until all fever, edema, and back pain are gone.
2. Penicillin IM or penicillin V for 10 days.
3. Much liquid to drink.
4. Food with much protein.
5. No salt in the food until all edema is gone.

The patient must go to hospital if:

1. The symptoms and signs of the disease do not go away in 2 or 3 weeks.
2. There are still many red blood cells or much protein in the urine after 2 or 3 weeks.

Chronic nephritis

This is a chronic disease of the kidneys. There is no specific treatment for it. If the patient has no symptoms, no treatment is necessary. If the patient has many serious symptoms like edema, anemia, high blood pressure, signs of heart failure, or convulsions, send him to hospital.

A nephritis patient with edema must not eat salt. Diuretic medicines will not help. If he has high blood pressure, treat it - see page 641. If he has anemia, give him iron. But if the hemoglobin is below 6 g, send him to hospital for a transfusion.

NEPHROSIS

This is a serious chronic disease, most often in children. Nephrosis causes much edema. The patient has very much protein in his urine. The cause is unknown. The treatment is long and difficult. Send a patient who has nephrosis to hospital.

NEURITIS

The disease

This comes during other diseases like diabetes or leprosy. It can also come in patients receiving INH for tuberculosis.

Treatment

1. Treat the main disease.
2. Give the patient aspirin for pain if necessary.
3. Vitamin B-1 can sometimes help the pain go away.
4. If the patient is taking INH, stop the INH. Give vitamin B-6, 25 mg tablets, 1 tablet 2 times a day.

Bell's palsy

This is a special neuritis which causes a paralysis of one side of the face. We call this "Bell's palsy." On that side of the face, the patient cannot lift his eyebrow, close his eye tightly, or smile.

1. Be sure the patient has no other serious illness. If he has signs of a serious illness, or other signs of a disease of the brain, send him immediately to hospital.

2. If the paralysis has just come, send the patient immediately to the doctor. The doctor may have other medicines that can help him.

3. If the paralysis has been present for some days or weeks, there is no specific treatment. If the patient has pain, give him aspirin. Give him also vitamin B-1. In many cases the paralysis will go away slowly.

4. If he cannot close his eye, put ointment in the eye each day. Cover the eye with a dressing to keep it closed.

Trigeminal neuralgia

Another neuritis of the face causes very strong pain on one side of the face, but no paralysis. We call this "trigeminal neuralgia" because it affects the trigeminal nerve.

1. Give the patient aspirin for pain.

2. Give him phenytoin 100 mg 3 or 4 times a day to keep the pain from coming. He must take this for many months.

NERVOUSNESS - Neurosis

The patient is very nervous, cannot work well, and usually is not happy. He may have pains in different parts of the body as well as in the head.

Ask him many questions about his life, family, and work. Try to find out the cause of the neurosis. Then try to help him find solutions to the problems causing the neurosis.

There are no good medicines for nervousness or neurosis. Diazepam and other medicines like this do not cure it. The neurosis will go away only when the problems causing it go away. Send a patient who has a severe neurosis to the doctor.

NOSE BLEED - see EPISTAXIS on page 621

OBESITY

In most cases this is not a disease. But obesity can cause other problems such as arthritis, high blood pressure, even heart failure. Obesity comes when the person eats much food. Two things are important to help the obesity go away.

Instructions about food

Give these instructions to an obese person.

1. Eat less food.
2. Do not drink much alcoholic or sugar drinks.
3. Do not eat candy or much sugar.
4. Eat much fruit and green vegetables.
5. Drink much water, especially during meals.

Instructions about work and exercise

An obese person must do more physical work or exercise. In this way the body will use more of the food he eats. The body will also begin to use some of the extra fat. Give these instructions to each obese person:

1. Do hard physical work each day, such as work in the garden.
2. If possible, play sports like football, volleyball, or swimming.
3. Do regular exercises in the morning and evening.
4. Take long walks, walking fast, not slowly.

OBSTRUCTION OF THE STOMACH

Send every patient with obstruction of the stomach to hospital immediately. An operation is probably necessary. If the abdomen of the patient is very full, or if there is much pain, pass a naso-gastric tube into the stomach. Remove the liquid in the stomach before sending the patient to hospital.

ONCHOCERCIASIS - see FILARIASIS on page 623

ORCHITIS

This is a very painful swelling of the testicle. The cause is a virus or an injury. We have no specific treatment for it. Put the patient in bed. Give him aspirin for pain. Put a pillow under his scrotum to keep it elevated. He must stay in bed with his scrotum elevated until the pain is gone.

If the swelling and pain do not go away after 1 week, send him to hospital. He may have a more serious disease.

OSTEOMYELITIS

Acute osteomyelitis

The disease

In acute osteomyelitis the patient has severe pain in the bone, with fever and often a tender swelling. If you think a patient may have acute osteomyelitis, give a big dose of penicillin or ampicillin. Then send him immediately to hospital.

If he cannot go to hospital, treat him in your health center.

Bed rest

Put the patient in bed. Put the painful arm or leg at complete rest. For the arm, use a bandage to tie the arm to his chest. For a leg, use a splint to keep the leg from moving.

Antibiotics

Give him an antibiotic: penicillin, ampicillin, or nafcillin for one month. If he has sickle cell anemia with osteomyelitis, give him chloramphenicol for 1 month. Do a white blood cell count every week. If the white blood cell count is below 4,000/mm3, stop the chloramphenicol. Give him ampicillin instead.

Refer to hospital

If the pain and swelling do not go away in 1 week after the start of the treatment, find a way to send the patient to hospital. He needs an X ray and perhaps an operation.

Chronic osteomyelitis

A patient with chronic osteomyelitis often has a hole in the skin over the bone. Pus comes from this hole. Often there is a swelling of the bone. Usually the patient has no fever.

Always send a patient with chronic osteomyelitis to hospital. He needs an X-ray. He may also need an operation. Do not give him an antibiotic before he goes. The doctor will decide which antibiotic to give him after examining him.

OTITIS - see EAR INFECTION on page 618

PELVIC INFECTION

Refer to hospital

Send immediately to hospital a woman with pelvic infection who has one of the following symptoms or signs.

1. A high fever.
2. Much pain and tenderness in the lower abdomen.
3. Much pus or a bad odor coming from the vagina.

Treatment

If the woman is not seriously ill, treat her in your health center. The treatment is:

Bed rest

The patient MUST stay in bed for one week, or until all fever and pain are gone. If not, she will not get well. It is impossible to cure pelvic infection in women who continue to walk and move around.

Medicines

Give her an antibiotic: penicillin, ampicillin, chloramphenicol, or tetracycline for 7 days.

Give her aspirin or paracetamol for pain. A hot water bottle on the lower abdomen helps the pain go away.

If the fever or pain do not go away after 1 week of treatment, the woman must go to hospital.

PEPTIC ULCER

Treatment

It is often difficult to know if a patient has a peptic ulcer or only gastritis. Give treatment for gastritis to all patients who have severe heart burn or other symptoms of gastritis. See page 628 for this treatment. Instructions about food, the patient's life, and his emotions are very important. Take time with each patient to explain these things carefully.

There are two good medicines for the treatment of peptic ulcer. They are cimetidine and ranitidine. Only the doctor can prescribe them. They cost much money, but they can help peptic ulcers to heal quickly.

Complications of peptic ulcers

Severe complications can come from a peptic ulcer. These are:

1. Bleeding in the stomach.
2. Perforation of the ulcer into the peritoneal cavity.
3. Obstruction of the stomach, with chronic vomiting.
4. Development of a tumor in the stomach.

Bleeding in the stomach

The patient will vomit blood, or will pass blood in the stools. Often the stools become very dark, almost black. This is an emergency. Send the patient immediately to hospital. If he has signs of shock, start an infusion before he goes.

Perforation of the ulcer

There is now a hole in the wall of the stomach in the middle of the ulcer. The contents of the stomach go out into the abdominal cavity. This causes acute peritonitis. The patient suddenly has very severe pain in the abdomen. He will have signs of peritonitis, but no signs of infection.

Send such a patient immediately to hospital for an operation. First start an infusion. Pass a naso-gastric tube and take out the liquid from the stomach. Send the patient to hospital with the infusion and the naso-gastric tube. If the hospital is far away, give him 50 to 75 mg of pethidine IM for pain.

Obstruction of the stomach

The patient vomits much or all of the food he eats. The vomiting continues for many days or weeks. He loses much weight. Send him immediately to hospital. But first pass a naso-gastric tube. Take out all the liquid from the stomach. This will make him more comfortable for the journey.

Tumor of the stomach

The patient loses much weight. Often you can palpate a mass in the upper abdomen. Send any patient immediately to hospital who has symptoms of gastritis or a peptic ulcer and:

- Has lost much weight.
- Has a mass in the abdomen.

PERITONITIS

Peritonitis is a very serious disease. It can cause death quickly. Often an operation is necessary. Send immediately to hospital every patient you think may have peritonitis.

Before sending the patient, do these things:

1. Start an infusion of physiologic saline IV.
2. Give a big dose of an antibiotic IV: ampicillin or chloramphenicol.
3. Pass a naso-gastric tube and take out the liquid from the stomach.
4. Do not give an enema.
5. Send the patient to hospital with the infusion and the naso-gastric tube.

PINWORMS - Enterobiasis: see WORMS on page 707

PNEUMONIA

Acute pneumonia

1. Bed rest. The patient may be more comfortable with the head raised.
2. Give the patient an antibiotic for 7 days.
   - Penicillin.
   - Erythromycin.
   - Ampicillin.
3. Give good nursing care.
   - Much liquid to drink.
   - A small bottle or can in which to put sputum.
   - An expectorant - see page 257.

Severe pneumonia

If the attack of pneumonia is severe, with much dyspnea, give the patient the following treatment.

1. Aqueous penicillin IV 2,000,000 to 5,000,000 u for one dose.

2. Then give one of the antibiotics for acute pneumonia, but 2 times the usual dose.

3. If the dyspnea and fever do not start to go away after 2 days, send the patient to hospital. He needs an X-ray and other exams.

Chronic pneumonia

The disease

In older persons the lungs sometimes do not work well. This is especially true in persons who smoke many cigarettes, who have asthma, or who have had many lung infections. These patients have a chronic cough and often dyspnea.

Treatment

1. If the patient has sputum, do 3 sputum exams to look for TB bacilli.

2. If he has a fever or crackles in the lungs with no other signs of heart failure, give him penicillin or penicillin V for 14 days.

3. Give him also an expectorant - see page 257.

4. If he has no fever, just give treatment for bronchitis - see page 606.

Breathing exercises

Talk to these patients about exercises for the lungs. Tell the patient to do these things.

1. Take 20 or more very deep breaths, one right after the other. Do this 3 times a day.

2. Lie down on each side for 15 minutes, then cough deeply. This will help bring up sputum from the bottom of the lungs. That helps the infection go away. Do this 2 times a day.

3. Drink much water every day. This will keep the secretions liquid and easy to bring up.

Refer to hospital

If the cough, fever, or crackles do not go away after 2 weeks of treatment, send the patient to hospital.

POISONING

General treatment

Many poisons can cause death quickly. Often there is no specific treatment. Try to find out:

1. What did the patient take: fuel oil, an acid or strong alkali, a medicine, a chemical or another substance, spoiled food or poison gases?
2. How long ago did he take this?
3. How much did he take?

   - If the patient is in shock, follow the instructions on pages 507.
   - If he has much vomiting, follow the instructions on page 311.
   - If he is in a coma, follow the instructions on page 440.

Swallowing fuel oil

Fuel oils, like petrol (gasoline) or paraffin (kerosene), are not toxic for the body. They cause disease only when the patient aspirates them into the lungs. They can then cause a severe pneumonia. This is how to treat a child or an adult who has swallowed fuel oil.

1. Put the patient in bed.
2. Do not make him vomit, and do not pass a naso-gastric tube.
3. Let him drink water, tea, or milk.
4. Examine his lungs carefully for crackles. If he has crackles or trouble breathing, give him penicillin for 7 days. See the treatment for acute pneumonia, page 676.
5. If he has no signs of pneumonia after 24 hours and he is eating, let him go home.

Swallowing an acid or a strong alkali

1. Put the patient in bed.
2. Do not make him vomit. Do not pass a naso-gastric tube.
3. Make him drink very much water, physiologic saline or milk to dilute the acid or alkali.
4. If he has signs of a burn or wounds in the mouth or throat, give him antibiotics for 7 days.
5. Send him immediately to hospital if:
   - He cannot swallow.
   - He has signs of shock.
   - He has signs of peritonitis or a severe infection.

Poisoning by medicine, chemicals, or spoiled food

1. Do a complete physical examination.
2. If the patient is conscious and has taken the poison only a few hours ago, try to make him vomit.
3. If he does not vomit or is unconscious, pass a naso-gastric tube. Wash out the stomach by passing through the tube 200 ml of water, then taking it back out. Do this several times.
4. Send him to hospital if he is in shock, is unconscious, or has signs of serious infection.

Poisoning by breathing a toxic gas

1. Take the patient immediately away from the poison gas.
2. If he is not breathing, give him artificial respiration.
3. Give oxygen if possible.
4. Put him in a well-ventilated place.
5. Encourage him to breathe deeply.
6. Send him to hospital if he is in shock, is unconscious, or has signs of a severe infection.

Prevention of poisoning

In children

Most cases of poisoning come in small children. Talk to parents in your preschool clinics about this. Give them these instructions.

1. Keep all medicines and other harmful substances out of the reach of your children.
2. Keep all fuel oil bottles and cans closed very tightly and out of the reach of your children.
3. If you give medicines to your children, be sure to give the correct dose. If you do not know the dose, do not give the medicine.
4. Never give any medicine from a bottle or can which has no label.

Motor fumes

Tell people never to stay in a closed building when a fuel motor is running.

Insecticides

They must be very careful when using insecticides. Some insecticides are very poisonous if we breathe them. One should always wear a cloth mask when using these insecticides and follow the directions carefully.

Spoiled food

Mothers must be very careful about the food they serve. They should not keep foods which spoil quickly. They should never use food from a can if the can is swollen or gives gas or a bad odor when opened. If a food is spoiled and smells bad, they must throw it away.

POLIO

The disease

This is a serious acute disease. It comes most often in babies and small children. A virus causes it. We have no specific treatment for it.

Treatment

If a child with fever develops paralysis of one or both legs or of another part of the body, put the child in bed.

1. If the child has pain in the legs or paralyzed parts, give him aspirin.
2. Put hot compresses on the paralyzed muscles. Be sure they are not hot enough to burn the skin.
3. Move the paralyzed arms or legs many times each day.
4. Give him much liquid to drink.
5. If he has trouble breathing, send him immediately to hospital.

Isolation

Polio is a contagious disease. Keep all other children away from a child who has just gotten polio. Keep them away for 2 weeks. Send a report of each case of acute polio to the government health authorities.

Rehabilitation

If the paralysis has been present for a week or more, the only treatment is instructions to the parents about exercises for the paralyzed limbs. Tell them to do these things.

1. Move all the joints of the paralyzed limb or limbs in the full range of movement. Show them how to do this.
2. They must do this 20 times each time and do it 3 times a day. This will keep the joints strong and prevent them from becoming stiff.
3. Take the child to the doctor. The doctor may be able to do more things to help the paralyzed limbs become strong again.

Prevention

We have a vaccine against polio. We give this vaccine by mouth.

1. Put 2 drops in the mouth of the baby or young child.
2. Give him the first dose on the day of birth.
3. Then, starting at the age of 6 weeks, give him 2 drops 1 time a month for 3 doses.

Children who receive 3 doses of polio vaccine with 1 month or more between doses will not get polio. If you vaccinate all the babies in your area, there will be no more polio. Talk to your doctor about this.

DISEASES OF PREGNANCY

Anemia of pregnancy

1. Follow the strategy on "ANEMIA" to look for all possible causes of anemia. Give the woman treatment for every cause you find. See page 474.
2. Give her iron, 200 mg 2 or 3 times a day.
3. Give her folic acid 5 mg 1 or 2 times a day until the end of the pregnancy.

Ectopic pregnancy

The disease

This causes much bleeding inside the abdomen. The woman has signs of peritonitis but no fever. She also has signs of anemia. She may have signs of shock.

You must think about the diagnosis of ectopic pregnancy in EVERY woman who has severe pain in the abdomen.

Treatment

1. Send immediately to hospital any woman you think may have an ectopic pregnancy.
2. If there are signs of shock, start an infusion of physiologic saline before sending her.

Toxemia of pregnancy

If the signs of toxemia are severe, send the woman to hospital. If they are not severe, treat her in your health center. But she must go to hospital for the delivery.

Rest

She must get much rest. Tell her not to do hard work. Tell her to rest one hour in the morning and one hour in the afternoon.

No salt

She must not put salt in her food, or eat foods with much salt. She must not take medicines with sodium, like sodium bicarbonate or sodium salicylate.

Diuretics

If she has much edema, give hydrochlorthiazide 50 mg each morning for 7 days.

Regular examinations

Check the blood pressure at least 1 time a week. Send the woman to hospital:

1. If her blood pressure goes above 140/90.
2. If she has much dizziness or strong headache.
3. If she has a convulsion.

Vomiting of pregnancy

Vomiting comes often during the first 3 months. Tell the woman to eat some food early in the morning. Tell her to eat 3 small meals a day and not to put strong spices into her food. Give her vitamins. The vomiting will probably stop at the end of the third month.

If the vomiting becomes severe, or the vomiting continues into the fourth month, send her to hospital.

PREMATURITY

Babies with a birth weight under 2 kilos are "premature." Send all premature babies to hospital. They need special care. If this is not possible, help the mother care for her premature baby in her home. Premature babies need these things.

Breast milk

The mother should give the baby breast milk in small quantities every 2 hours. If the baby cannot suck, the mother must squeeze breast milk out of her breast. She can then give this to her baby by a medicine dropper or a small spoon.

Warmth

Premature babies cannot stand cool temperatures. Tell the mother to keep the baby close to her body at all times. She can wrap a big cloth around her body with the baby inside. The warmth of the mother's body will keep the baby warm. The mother must be sure he can breathe well.

Protection from infections

Tell the mother to keep all the baby's cloths very clean. She must wash all cloths that get dirty. She should give the baby a bath each day in warm water. She must not give him powdered milk in a baby bottle.

Follow the weight

Weigh the baby each day or as often as possible. If the baby gains a little weight each day, that is a good sign. If he does not gain weight for several days, or loses weight, the mother must take him to hospital.

PROSTATITIS

Acute prostatitis

The treatment for acute prostatitis is:
1. Bed rest.
2. Trimethoprim-sulfamethoxazole or ampicillin for 7 days.
3. Much water to drink.
4. Aspirin for pain if necessary.

Chronic prostatitis

The treatment for chronic prostatitis is:
1. An antibiotic like trimethoprim-sulfamethoxazole, ampicillin, or tetracycline for 2 to 4 weeks.
2. A massage of the prostate by rectal exam 1 time a week to help the infected liquid come out of the prostate through the urethra.
3. Much water to drink.

PYELONEPHRITIS

The disease

A patient with pyelonephritis has:

1. Protein in the urine.

2. Many white blood cells in the urine and sometimes red blood cells.

3. Often granular cylinders or "casts" in the urine.

4. He may also have high blood pressure, anemia, or heart failure.

Treatment

Send a patient with pyelonephritis to hospital. He needs special examinations and careful treatment for many weeks. But if this is not possible, treat him in your health center. This is the treatment to give.

1. Give him an antibiotic for 4 weeks: ampicillin, tetracycline, or tri-methoprim-sulfamethoxazole.

2. Tell him to drink much water every day. Do a urine exam every week to see if the urine is becoming normal. Check his general condition every week: blood pressure, hydration, edema, signs of heart failure, hemoglobin. If he is not getting better, he MUST go to hospital.

3. If the urine is not clear at the end of the 4 weeks of treatment, the patient must go to hospital. He may have a serious problem in the urinary system that needs special treatment or an operation.

PYOMYOSITIS

This is an abscess deep in the muscles. The treatment is an incision and drainage of the abscess. This requires anesthesia. Send every patient with pyomyositis to hospital for the incision and drainage.

RABIES

Treatment

We have no treatment for rabies. A patient who gets rabies will die quickly. There is no need to send the patient to hospital.

Prevention

It is very important to prevent rabies. A patient bitten by a dog, cat, or other animal with rabies must have rabies vaccination. This will keep the patient from getting rabies.

Vaccinate against rabies a person bitten by a dog or a cat:

1. If the animal dies.
2. If someone has killed the animal.
3. If the animal cannot be found.

A person bitten by a dog or cat does not need the vaccination if the animal is still alive ten days after the bite. Therefore, if a dog or cat bites someone, tell the owner of the animal to keep it in a safe place for 10 days. The owner must give it food and water. If the animal dies for any reason, the person bitten must receive the rabies vaccination.

After 10 days, if the animal is well, the owner can set it free. Then the bitten person does not need the vaccination. It is very important to observe the animal for 10 days. Rabies vaccination can be dangerous and it costs very much money. So we do not vaccinate a person unless the animal dies, is killed, or runs away.

Send to hospital any person who needs rabies vaccination.

Preventing rabies in animals

Talk to the people in your area about the importance of rabies vaccination for their dogs and cats. The local veterinarian probably has rabies vaccine for animals. Every dog and cat should get a vaccination every two years. In this way, rabies will disappear from your area.

We do not use the rabies vaccine for animals to prevent rabies in people. Animal vaccine is different from human vaccine.

SCABIES

Medicines for scabies.

Give one of these medicines to a patient who has scabies.

1. Benzyl benzoate liquid.
2. Hexachlorocyclohexane 1% (*Lindane or *Kwell), liquid or cream.
3. Sulfur, 5% in vaseline.

Instructions to the patient.

1. First take a good bath in water with soap.
2. Apply the medicine to your whole body from your chin to your feet.
3. Do not apply it to your face or head. Scabies usually does not affect the face or head.
4. Leave the medicine on the skin for 24 hours. Then take another bath.
5. Repeat the treatment every day for three days.
6. Wash all your clothes and bed linens at the same time.

Treat the whole family

Treat at the same time all who live in the same house. Talk to the whole family about the importance of keeping clean and keeping clothes clean.

SCHISTOSOMIASIS

The disease

It is not necessary to treat every person who has schistosome eggs in the stools or urine. Treat only those who have symptoms of the disease.

Send to hospital a patient with schistosomiasis who has one of the following symptoms or signs.

1. Severe bleeding from the rectum or in the urine.
2. Signs of liver or heart disease.
3. Much loss of weight.

For a patient who is not very ill, use one of the following medicines.

Medicines for schistosomiasis

1. Niridazole (*Ambilhar), for Schistosoma mansoni or Schistosoma hematobium.
   - Tablets of 100 or of 500 mg.
   - Give 25 mg/kg per day, divided in 2 doses, after eating.
   - Give this every day for 5 to 7 days.
   - Do not give it during pregnancy or to a patient who has severe liver disease, mental disease, or epilepsy.

- It makes the urine dark, but this is normal.
- If signs of nervous disease come, stop the treatment.

2. Metrifonate (*Bilarcil), for Schistosoma hematobium.
   - Tablets of 100 mg.
   - Give 7.5 mg/kg one time every 2 weeks for 3 doses.
3. Oxamniquine (*Vansil), for Schistosoma mansoni.
   - Capsules of 250 mg, or syrup with 50 mg/ml.
   - Give 10 to 15 mg/kg 2 times a day for 2 days.
   - The urine may become red.
   - This medicine costs much money.
4. Praziquantel, for both S. hematobium and S. mansoni.
   - Give 30 to 45 mg/kg in one dose, by mouth.
   - It is very good, but it costs much money. Often it is not available.

Other measures of treatment.

1. A patient with schistosomiasis must drink much water during the treatment.
2. He also needs food with much protein.

Prevention

Talk to people in your communities about how to keep from getting schistosomiasis. Tell them these rules.
1. You must have a good latrine.
2. Use it every time for passing stools and for passing urine.
3. NEVER pass stools or urine in or near water.
4. If possible, stay out of water that can carry schistosomiasis. If you must work in water, wear rubber boots.

SCIATICA

The disease

This causes severe pain in the buttocks and the back of one or both legs. The pain is worse when the patient sits down or bends forward.

1. Complete rest in bed is necessary for 3 weeks. The patient must lie only on his back or on one side. He must not sit up. If he has pain, give him aspirin 4 times a day.

2. After 3 weeks, he can stand up and begin to walk around. But he still must not sit down for another 3 weeks.

3. After 3 more weeks he can sit, stand, and walk.

Exercises

A patient with sciatica must do exercises to make the back strong. Explain this exercise to him.

1. Lie flat on your stomach on your bed or on the floor.

2. Then lift your head and feet off the bed or floor and hold them there for 10 seconds.

3. Do this 20 times each time.

4. Do this 3 times a day.

Swimming is also very good exercise. Kick your legs strongly in the water while swimming.

These exercises will make the back muscles strong. This will help the pain of sciatica to go away and not come back.

SEPTICEMIA

This is a very serious infection of the whole body. It can cause death quickly. Start an infusion of physiologic saline or 5% glucose. Give a big dose of an antibiotic: aqueous penicillin IV 5,000,000 u with ampicillin 1 g IV, or chloramphenicol 1 g IV. Send the patient immediately to hospital.

SICKLE CELL ANEMIA - SCA

The disease

The child is born with sickle cell anemia. It is a hemolytic anemia. During a crisis many red blood cells die quickly. This causes a severe anemia and often jaundice. It can cause death. We have no specific treatment for this disease.

Prevention of attacks of anemia is the most important part of the treatment. Talk to the parents of the child about this. They must understand the disease. They must know what they can do to help their child grow well and keep from having many crises.

Prevention of attacks

Medical care

Give the following things to every child with sickle cell anemia.

1. All of the regular vaccinations.
2. Chloroquine 5 mg/kg 1 time a week to protect the child from malaria. Do not use pyrimethamine (*Daraprim).
3. Folic acid, 5 mg 1 time a day every day.
4. Benzathine penicillin G, 2,400,000 u 1 time a month to help prevent infections.
5. Do not give iron.

Instructions to the parents

The parents must do these things for their child.

1. Give him food with much protein.
2. Bring him to the health center quickly when a fever comes, or when he has severe pain somewhere in the body.

There are two kinds of crises that can come in sickle cell anemia.

Hemolytic crisis

The hemoglobin drops very quickly to 3 or 4 g. In this case, send the child immediately to hospital. A transfusion is necessary quickly. But if the hemoglobin is 5 g or more, treat the child in your health center with:

1. Bed rest.
2. Much liquid to drink.
3. Chloroquine if the thick blood film is positive for malaria.
4. Penicillin if the child has signs of an infection like pneumonia, an ear infection, or infection elsewhere.

If the child has signs of osteomyelitis, send to hospital.

Painful crisis

This gives sudden severe pain in the abdomen, in the arms or legs, or in the head. The hemoglobin usually does not go down much. If the pain is severe, send the child to hospital. A transfusion is probably necessary. If the pain is not severe, or if the hospital is far away, treat the child in your health center with:

1. Bed rest.
2. Much liquid to drink, or an infusion if necessary. The child should receive 120 ml/kg every 24 hours.
3. Aspirin or paracetamol every 4 hours.

SINUSITIS

Acute sinusitis

1. Give an antibiotic for 10 to 14 days: penicillin, ampicillin, or erythromycin.
2. The patient also needs:
   - Bed rest.
   - Much liquid to drink.
   - Aspirin for pain.
   - Nose drops, such as ephedrine 0.5% or phenylephrine 0.25%.
   - Hot compresses to the painful place on the face or forehead.

Chronic sinusitis

1. Give the patient one of the above antibiotics for two weeks.
2. Give also:
   - A medicine to help open the nasal passages.
   - Aspirin for pain.
   - Much liquid to drink.
3. If the patient does not get better after 2 weeks, send him to hospital.

SNAKE BITE

History

Take a good history. Find out exactly when the snake bit the patient.

Identify the snake

Try to find out the kind of snake that bit the patient. If someone killed the snake and brought it with the patient, look in the mouth of the snake. Use instruments to open the mouth of the snake and not your fingers. Look for long teeth, or "fangs."

Cobra

If the snake has two long fangs in front, fixed in the upper jaw, it is a very dangerous cobra. Send the patient immediately to hospital. Do not put a tourniquet on the arm or leg. This can cause much damage to the arm or leg.

Viper

If the snake has two fangs turned back under the upper lip but which can come down when you pull on them, the snake is a viper. In this case, examine the patient well. Send him immediately to hospital if he has signs of snake poisoning, such as:

● Much swelling around the bite.

● Much pain around the bite.

● A fast pulse.

Non-poisonous snake

If the snake has no fangs, it is not poisonous.

Treatment

Treat the patient in your health center if:

● The snake has no fangs.

● You do not know the kind of snake that bit the patient AND the patient has no signs of poisoning or only a very little swelling.

1. Keep the patient in bed.

2. Look at the patient every hour.

3. If no swelling comes in 24 hours, the patient can go home.

4. If swelling does come, send the patient to hospital.

Anti-snake serum

If you have anti-snake serum in your health center, give this to a patient who shows signs of snake poisoning.

1. First do a skin test for sensitivity. See page 695.
2. If the skin test is positive, do not give the anti-snake serum.
3. If the skin test is negative, inject 1 ampoule of the serum in the tissue around the snake bite.
4. Give another ampoule IM in the upper part of the arm or leg that the snake bit.
5. If the patient has important signs of snake poisoning, send him to hospital after you have given him the anti-snake serum.

SORE THROAT

Bacterial infection

Look at the throat and tonsils carefully. If the patient has white spots on the tonsils or on the back of the throat, give him this treatment:

1. Penicillin, erythromycin, or ampicillin for 7 days.
2. Keep him in bed until the pain and fever are gone.
3. Tell him to drink much water.
4. Give him aspirin for pain.

Virus infection

If the throat is red, but with no white spots, the cause is a virus. Antibiotics will not help. Give the patient aspirin for pain. Tell him to:

1. Drink much water.
2. Gargle. Wash out the throat with water and then spit it out.
3. Take a small spoonful of honey in the morning and in the evening. Swallow the honey slowly, letting it stay in the mouth and throat as long as possible.

SPRAIN

1. Make sure there are NO signs of a fracture.
2. Put the sprained limb at rest.
   - An arm, wrist, or hand: put the arm in a sling.
   - A knee or ankle: put the patient in bed with the leg raised a bit.
3. Give him aspirin for pain.
4. He can start using the sprained limb when all pain and swelling are gone.
5. If the pain and swelling do not go away in 3 or 4 days, send him to hospital for an X-ray.

TETANUS

Prevention

Vaccinate every baby against tetanus.

1. This requires 3 injections of 0.5 ml IM of DPT or triple vaccine.
2. Start at 6 weeks of age, and leave one or more months between each injection.
3. Give a booster dose of tetanus toxoid 0.5 ml IM every 10 years.

Vaccinate pregnant mothers

Every pregnant mother should have 2 injections of tetanus toxoid one or more months apart during the pregnancy. This will protect her and the newborn baby from tetanus. One injection of toxoid is sufficient for her during the following pregnancies.

Vaccinate adults

Many older children and adults have not had the 3 injections of DPT as a baby or 3 injections of tetanus toxoid. They should now receive 3 injections of tetanus toxoid with 1 month or more between them. A booster dose every 10 years is sufficient.

Treatment of wounds

After every deep wound, you must protect the patient from tetanus.

Treatment of the wound

1. Wash the wound very carefully with clean water or physiologic saline.
2. Take out all dirt.
3. Cut off all dead tissue.
4. If the wound is very big or dirty, send the patient to hospital.

Tetanus toxoid

If the patient has had tetanus toxoid during the last 10 years, one booster dose of 0.5 ml IM of toxoid is sufficient.

Tetanus antitoxin

If the patient has not had tetanus toxoid during the last 10 years, give 1,500 units of tetanus antitoxin SC. Before doing this, do a sensitivity test.

1. Inject 0.1 ml of antitoxin into the skin to make a small bump.
2. Wait 20 minutes.
3. If swelling or itching comes around the bump, do not give the antitoxin.
4. If no swelling or itching develops, give the antitoxin to the patient.

Treatment of tetanus

Send every case of tetanus immediately to hospital. Tetanus is a very serious disease and can quickly cause death. If it is ABSOLUTELY impossible to send the patient, treat him in your health center. A patient who has tetanus needs the following.

1. Bed rest in a very quiet place, with no noise and very little light.
2. Tetanus antitoxin, 10,000 IM units after a negative sensitivity test. 10,000 units is sufficient.
3. Procaine penicillin, 1 time a day for 10 days.
4. Careful cleaning of the wound where the tetanus bacilli are.
5. Medicine to stop the muscle spasms. Use either:
   - Diazepam, 0.2 mg/kg IM every 4 hours, or
   - Chlorpromazine, 1 mg/kg IM every 4 hours.
   - Continue giving this until all the spasms are gone.

6. Very good nursing care.
   - Put a good mattress and clean sheets on the bed.
   - Turn the patient gently from one side to the other every 3 hours.
   - Give him much liquid. If he can drink, give liquids by mouth. If not, give him liquids either by rectal infusion, nasogastric tube or IV infusion. He needs 3 liters/day, or 100 ml/kg/day for a child.
   - Protection against skin ulcers.
7. Treatment of any other infections that come.

THROMBOPHLEBITIS

1. Bed rest until pain and swelling go away.
2. Penicillin or ampicillin for 7 days.
3. The patient should drink much water.
4. Send him to hospital if the pain and swelling do not go away.

TOOTHACHE

1. Give the patient aspirin for pain.
2. If he has signs of infection, such as fever, much tenderness, or a high white blood cell count, give him penicillin or ampicillin for 7 days.
3. If the toothache continues, send him to hospital.

TRYPANOSOMIASIS - "African sleeping sickness"

This disease exists only in Central and West Africa.

Diagnosis

We make the diagnosis by finding trypanosomes:
- In a thick blood film.
- In liquid taken by aspiration from a lymph node in the neck.
- In spinal fluid.

Treatment

The treatment is difficult and dangerous. It is impossible to give this treatment in a health center. Send to hospital every patient who has trypanosomiasis. Send also any patient you think may have trypanosomiasis but in whom you cannot find the trypanosomes.

Prevention

Early diagnosis

Try to make the diagnosis of trypanosomiasis when the disease is just starting. Send each patient quickly for treatment. If we can find and treat every case of trypanosomiasis, the disease will disappear.

The danger for the community is to have many people with trypanosomes who are not taking treatment. The tse-tse fly can then take trypanosomes from them and give them to other persons. So early diagnosis and treatment are very important.

Examine everyone in each of your communities 1 or more times a year. Look for persons:

1. Who have a fever every day.
2. Who have lost weight.
3. Who have a chronic headache, trouble sleeping, or trouble thinking clearly.
4. Who have big lymph nodes in the neck. Do an aspiration of one node on everyone who has big nodes in the neck.

Education

Talk to your people about the symptoms and signs of the disease.

1. Tell them to come quickly to the health center if they get any of the symptoms or signs of trypanosomiasis.
2. Tell them to send to the health center any of their friends who has any of these symptoms or signs.
3. Send to hospital every case you find and every person who you think may have trypanosomiasis.

The fight against tse-tse flies

Try to get rid of tse-tse flies by doing these things:

1. Cut down the trees and bushes near water sources or places where people take baths.

2. Make traps to catch and kill the flies.

3. Keep big animals like cows and pigs away from where people live.

4. We have no good insecticides to kill tse-tse flies.

TUBERCULOSIS

Diagnosis

We make the diagnosis of tuberculosis by examining the sputum of patients. Patients who have TB bacilli in their sputum have tuberculosis. Patients who do not have TB bacilli in their sputum may not have tuberculosis. They may have another disease. We do not treat them for tuberculosis. Send to hospital any patient you think has tuberculosis but who has a negative sputum exam.

If you find TB bacilli in the sputum of a patient, consult with your doctor. The doctor may tell you to treat this patient in your health center. But send to hospital all tuberculosis patients who have:

● Much dyspnea.

● Much blood in the sputum.

● Much weakness or weight loss.

Principles of treatment

1. Always give 2 or 3 tuberculostatic medicines at the same time. Never give just one. If you do, this will cause the TB bacilli to develop resistance to the medicines.

2. Use streptomycin for the treatment of tuberculosis ONLY. Do not use it for any other infection or disease.

3. The treatment lasts a very long time. One year is the minimum. 18 to 24 months may be necessary.

4. The treatment is ambulatory for most patients. A patient can live at home. It is not necessary to take him away from his family. He has already been with his family. So he has already exposed his family to the disease.

5. He must come regularly to the health center for his medicine and for a control of his progress.

6. He must follow the treatment regularly without stopping the medicine even for a short time.

7. He must finish the full treatment. If a patient stops the treatment before the end, the disease may come back. The bacilli may then resist the treatment.

8. Keep a "visit calendar" to know the date each patient must come back for treatment and control.

9. Stopping the treatment even for a few weeks is dangerous for the patient and for his family. So look for any patient who fails to come for treatment on the expected day.

10. Consult with your doctor regularly about every patient you are treating.

11. Stop the treatment only when the doctor tells you to do so.

12. Keep a good record of the treatment and progress of every patient.

Control visits

Weigh each patient at each visit. Ask him about his symptoms.

Examine him for signs of the disease. Send to the doctor a patient who has one of the following conditions.

1. He is losing weight.

2. He continues to have much cough and sputum, or dyspnea.

3. He still has lung signs of the disease.

Tuberculostatic medicines

Isoniazide (INH or *Rimifon), tablets of 50 or 100 mg

1. The dose is 10 mg/kg in one dose each day, or 300 mg/day for an adult.

2. INH can cause pain in the legs: neuritis. In case of INH neuritis, stop giving the INH. Give vitamin B-6 (pyridoxine), 50 mg each day.

3. INH can also cause jaundice. If jaundice comes, stop the INH immediately. Send the patient to the doctor.

Thiacetazone

1. The dose is 5 mg/kg in one dose each day.
2. This can cause heartburn, vomiting, or dizziness. The patient should take the medicine with meals. The evening meal is best.
3. This can also cause a very severe skin eruption. Tell the patient that, if severe itching starts, he must stop taking the medicine immediately and come to the clinic. Send the patient immediately to hospital.

Combination of INH and thiacetazone in one pill

1. INH 300 mg + thiacetazone 150 mg, or INH 100 mg + thiacetazone 50 mg.
2. The dose for adults is 1 tablet per day of INH 300 mg + thiacetazone 50 mg.
3. The dose for children is 10 mg/kg of INH and 5 mg/kg of thiacetazone per day.

Streptomycin, in vials of 1 g or 5 g

1. The dose is 20 mg/kg 1 time a day, or 1 g/day for a normal adult.
2. We give streptomycin every day for 30 to 60 days at the beginning of the treatment.
3. Streptomycin can cause dizziness, much noise in the ears, or loss of hearing. Sometimes it is necessary to give only half the normal dose because of this toxicity. In case of diminished hearing, stop the streptomycin completely.

The usual treatment for tuberculosis

1. Streptomycin, 20 mg/kg 1 time a day for 30 to 60 days.
2. INH 10 mg/kg + thiacetazone 5 mg/kg 1 time a day for one year or even longer.
3. For children under 15 kg, give only streptomycin and INH.

Other medicines

We have other medicines for tuberculosis: rifampicin, ethambutol, pyrazinamide. Only a doctor can prescribe these medicines.

Other aspects of the treatment

Instructions.

Be sure each patient and the family understand what tuberculosis is like. Be sure they understand these principles.

1. You must continue the treatment for at least one year.
2. It is dangerous to stop the treatment even for a short time.
3. Come regularly for medicines and for a control of the progress of the disease.
4. You can work again as soon as you feel strong.

Good food.

Good food is necessary for the patient to get well. He must eat foods with much protein. This will help him become strong quickly.

Treat other diseases

Examine each new patient for other diseases like malaria, intestinal worms, anemia, and other infections. Treat any disease you find.

Transmission of the disease

Tuberculosis is contagious. The TB bacilli come out in the sputum and in the air breathed out from the lungs. The bacilli can then go into another person. People living in the same house with the patient can get tuberculosis easily. People who work close to a tuberculosis patient can also get the disease easily.

Tell these rules to every tuberculosis patient:

1. When coughing, cover your mouth with a cloth.
2. Do not spit on the ground.
3. Put your sputum in a small cup with a cover, or in a bottle or can.
4. Throw the bottle or can in the latrine or in a hole at the end of the day.
5. Or else, throw the sputum in the latrine and wash the cup very carefully in water and soap at the end of the day.

Prevention

The most important measures to prevent tuberculosis are these:

1. Examine for signs of tuberculosis every member of the patient's family and every person who lives or works close to the patient. Send to the doctor all persons you think may have tuberculosis.

2. Teach people about eating foods with much protein. People who are well nourished usually do not get tuberculosis.

3. BCG vaccination may give some protection. But this is not certain. Talk with your doctor about this.

4. Send a report of each new case to the government health authorities.

TYPHOID FEVER

The disease

Typhoid fever is a very serious infection in the intestines. It causes many complications such as perforation of the intestine causing peritonitis, severe bleeding in the intestines, or septicemia.

Diagnosis

It is not possible to make the diagnosis of typhoid fever in a health center. But you must suspect typhoid fever in every patient who has:

1. A high fever that does not go away after treatment with chloroquine.

2. A high fever and a severe headache.

3. A high fever and much delirium.

4. A high fever and a pulse below 100/minute.

5. Fever and much pain in the abdomen. The patient may have signs of peritonitis. Often he has tenderness only and no signs of peritonitis.

6. Fever and a low white blood cell count: 4,000/mm3 or less.

Treatment

Send immediately to hospital every patient you think may have typhoid fever.

Before sending the patient

If the hospital is far away:

1. Give the patient a big dose of chloramphenicol, 1 g to an adult, or 25 mg/kg to a child.

2. If he is dehydrated, start an infusion.

3. If he has signs of peritonitis, pass a nasogastric tube.

4. Send him to hospital with the infusion and the nasogastric tube.

Prevention

Typhoid fever goes from one person to another by food or water that has typhoid bacilli. Teach your people what to do to keep from getting typhoid fever. Give them these instructions.

1. Drink only clean potable water. Be sure the water source or the well has good protection around it. No latrine must be near the source or the well.

2. Every house should have a good latrine. Everyone must use the latrine to pass stools or urine.

3. Everyone who prepares food to eat must wash her hands carefully in water with soap before preparing the food.

4. Keep the kitchen very clean. Wash all pots, pans, and dishes after every use. Keep all animals away from the kitchen and places where food is prepared and cooked.

5. We have a vaccine against typhoid fever. If there are many cases of typhoid fever in your area, talk to your doctor about it.

URTICARIA - see ALLERGY on page 596

VARICOCELE

This means big veins in the spermatic cord. There is no need to treat it.

VARICOSE VEINS

These are big veins under the skin of the legs. They can cause pain and swelling in the legs. The treatment is:

An elastic bandage to wrap around the leg

1. Start wrapping the bandage around the foot just above the toes.
2. Be sure to cover the heel.
3. Keep wrapping the leg up to above the knee.
4. Show the patient how to do this.
5. He must take off the bandage each night and put it on again in the morning.

Protection of the leg against wounds and sores

These do not heal well because the circulation is not good. They often become infected. Tell the patient about this. If the patient is a man, tell him to wear long pants. An elastic bandage will also protect the leg or legs.

Tell the patient not to sit with his leg or legs hanging down. When sitting, he should put his leg or legs on another chair or on something else to keep them up.

Give the patient aspirin if he has much pain.

Send him to hospital if he has:

1. Much pain in the leg and the pain does not go away.
2. Much swelling of the leg because of the varicose veins.
3. An ulcer of the skin that will not heal.
4. The doctor will probably do an operation to take out the varicose veins.

WHOOPING COUGH

Treatment

Antibiotics do not help whooping cough. Give penicillin only if the child has much dyspnea, crackles in the lungs, a high fever that does not come from malaria, or another infection.

Give an expectorant - see page 257. This will not stop the cough. But it will make the secretions more liquid.

Rehydration

Dehydration makes whooping cough much worse. Tell the mother to give the child much liquid to drink. A small baby must continue to get breast milk. The mother must also give the baby or child much water and other liquids to drink. If he is very ill and cannot drink, give him liquids by a naso-gastric tube, by an infusion, or by rectum.

Food

Good nutrition is very important. Talk to the mother about this. The child must get much food with protein. Tell the mother to give him frequent small feedings. See the treatment for malnutrition on page 658.

Other infections

Examine the child each day for signs of other infections. Look for signs of pneumonia, an ear infection, or malaria. Treat any infection you find. Do a stool exam to look for worms. Give worm medicine if the child has worms.

Convulsions

If the child has convulsions, give diazepam, 0.2 mg/kg IM. Then send the child immediately to hospital. Convulsions in a child with whooping cough are a sign of very serious disease.

Prevention

Vaccinate every baby against whooping cough. The whooping cough vaccine comes together with tetanus and diphtheria vaccines. We call it DPT, or triple, vaccine. The baby needs 3 injections one or more months apart.

1. Give the first injection when the baby is 6 weeks old.
2. Give 0.5 ml IM.
3. Give the second injection 1 month later.
4. Give the third injection 1 month after that.
5. If possible, give a fourth injection, or booster dose, when the child is 18 months old.

If every child in your area receives 3 DPT injections, whooping cough will disappear from your area.

Send a report of each case to the government health authorities.

WORMS

Medicines

These are the important medicines for treating intestinal worms.

Bephenium hydroxynaphthoate (*Alcopar)

It comes in packets of 5 g of powder. It is safe for small children, during pregnancy, and for patients who have serious anemia or liver disease.

1. For adults and older children, give 1 packet of 5 g before eating in the morning and in the evening.
2. Put the powder in a glass of water.
3. For children under 10 kg, give one half a packet morning and evening.

Levamisole (*Decaris or *Ketrax)

It comes in tablets of 40, 50 or 150 mg.

1. For adults, give 1 dose of 150 mg.
2. For children, give 2.5 mg/kg in 1 dose.
3. Do not give a purge.

Mebendazole (*Vermox)

It comes in tablets of 100 mg.

1. For children and adults, give 100 mg morning and evening for 3 days.
2. It is safe and not toxic.
3. But do not give it to pregnant mothers.

Niclosamide (*Niclocide, *Yomesan)

It comes in tablets of 0.5 g. The dose is:

1. For adults, 4 tablets in 1 dose 2 hours before eating.
2. For children from 34 to 50 kg, 3 tablets in 1 dose before eating.
3. For children from 11 to 33 kg, 2 tablets in 1 dose before eating.
4. Tell the patient to chew the pills well before swallowing them. No purge is necessary.

Piperazine (*Antepar)

It comes in tablets of 300 or 500 mg, or liquid of 10% (100 mg/ml). It is safe and not toxic.

Pyrantel pamoate (*Antiminth, *Combantrin)

It comes in tablets of 125 mg, or liquid with 50 mg/ml. The dose is 11 mg/kg up to 1 g.

Tetrachlorethylene

It comes as liquid or in gelatin capsules of 0.2, 1 or 5 ml. It is quite safe, but it can cause dizziness and sometimes vomiting. Do not use it during the first 3 months of pregnancy, or in patients with severe liver disease.

1. The dose is 0.1 ml/kg up to 5 ml.
2. Give it in the morning before eating.
3. The patient must not eat for 4 hours after taking the medicine.
4. The patient must not take alcohol or fatty foods for 24 hours before or after.
5. Do not give a purge.

Thiabendazole (*Mintezol)

It comes in tablets of 0.5 g or in liquid with 100 mg/ml.

1. Give 25 mg/kg 2 times a day for 2 or 3 days.
2. Give it with meals.
3. When giving tablets, tell the patient to chew the tablets well before swallowing.

Treatment of worm infections

For each infection, give one of the following medicines.

Hookworm - Ankylostomiasis

1. Tetrachlorethylene, 1 dose. Repeat each day for 3 days if the patient has many eggs or larva in the stools.
2. Pyrantel pamoate, 1 dose. Repeat each day for 3 days if the patient has many eggs or larva in the stools.

3. Mebendazole, 100 mg 2 times a day for 3 days.

4. Bephenium, 2 times a day for 1 day. If there are many worm eggs in the stools, repeat the dose the second and the third day.

Pinworm - Enterobiasis

1. Pyrantel pamoate, 1 dose, repeated after 2 weeks and then 2 weeks later.

2. Mebendazole, 100 mg in 1 dose, repeated after 2 weeks, then 2 weeks later.

3. Pinworm goes easily from one person to another, especially to children. Treat all members of the family at the same time. They should wash all their clothes and bed linens at the time of the treatment.

Roundworm - Ascariasis

1. Piperazine, 75 mg/kg up to 4 g 1 time a day for 2 days for adults, or 150 mg/kg 1 time a day for 2 days for children. Do not give a purge.

2. Pyrantel pamoate, a single dose.

3. Mebendazole, 100 mg 2 times a day for 3 days.

4. Levamisole, a single dose.

Strongyloidiasis

1. Thiabendazole, 25 mg/kg 2 times a day.

2. Give this for 2 or 3 days.

Tapeworm

1. Niclosamide, a single dose.

2. Mebendazole, 300 mg 2 times a day for 3 days.

Whipworm - Trichuriasis

1. Mebendazole, 100 mg 2 times a day for 3 days.

2. Thiabendazole does not work well.

Prevention

Talk to your patients and their families about how to keep from getting intestinal worms. These are the things they must do.

1. Every house must have a good latrine.

2. Every person must use the latrine every time for passing stools or urine.

3. Latrines must be 50 or more meters away from the well or water source.

4. Protect the well or water source from all contamination. If it is not protected, tell them what to do to protect it.

5. If the well or water source is not protected, boil all water for drinking and cooking.

6. Wash hands with soap and water:

   - Before eating.
   - Before preparing food to eat.
   - After using the latrine.

7. Wear shoes and socks if possible. This is to keep from getting hookworm.

8. Keep the kitchen clean. Keep all animals away from the kitchen and from where food is prepared. Prepare food on a table and cook it on a stove. Do not prepare food or cook it on the ground.

9. Wash all dishes and cooking pots and utensils after every use.

10. Protect all food from flies.

Appendix

Table 8: Frequently used medicines

Medicine	Dose	Dangers
Antibiotics		
penicillin – procaine IM 400,000 u/ml	1 or 2 ml 1 time per day for 7 to 10 days	rare anaphylactic shock sometimes urticaria
– benzathine IM 600,000 u/ml	1 time a week, or 1 time a month	as above
– benzyl (aqueous)	1,000,000 u to 5,000,000 u IV every 4 hours	as above

– phenoxymethyl –
  *Penicillin V
  tabs: 125 or 250 mg
  syrup: 25 mg/ml
	125 or 250 mg
	4 times a day
	for 7 to 10 days
		as above

ampicillin
  tabs: 250 to 500 mg
  syrup: 25 mg/ml
	250 or 500 mg
	4 times a day
	for 7 to 10 days
		rare anaphylactic shock
		sometimes urticaria

amoxycillin **tabs**: 250 mg	250 to 500 mg 4 times a day for 7 to 10 days	sometimes urticaria
erythromycin **tabs**: 250 mg	250 or 500 mg, or 10-20 mg/Kg 4 times a day for 7 to 10 days	sometimes urticaria
tetracycline **tabs**: 250 mg	250 to 500 mg 4 times a day for 1 to 4 weeks	not for children below 8 years of age or for pregnant mothers

chloramphenicol
    tabs: 250 mg
    syrup: 25 mg/ml
	250 to 500 mg
	or 25 mg/kg
	4 times a day for 7 days
		not for newborn or
		   premature babies
		can cause anemia or loss of
		   white blood cells
		Do not use for more than one week.

trimethoprim +
   sulfamethoxazole
   *****Bactrim, *Septra**
     tabs: 80 mg
       trimethoprim + 400 mg
       sulfamethoxazole
	2 tabs every 12 hrs
	for 7 to 14 days
	Children: 1/2 tab
	1 or 2 times a day
	for 7 to 14 days
		nausea, vomiting
		drug rash, urticaria.

nitrofurantoin
   *****Furadantin**
     tabs: 50 or 100 mg
	50 or 100 mg, or
	1-2 mg/kg 4 times a day
	for 7 to 14 days
		nausea, vomiting, diarrhea
		cough, chest pain, dyspnea
		drug rash, urticaria

Anti-malaria drugs

chloroquine
   *****Nivaquine**
   *****Resochin**
   *****Avlochlor**
     tabs: 100 or 150 mg
     syrup: see label
     injection: see label
	5 mg/kg 2 times a day
	for 2 days, then
	5 mg/kg the third day
		overdose: convulsions, death
		Give by injection **only** if patient
		   is unconscious or is
		   vomiting severely.
		can cause itching

quinine
   tabs: 200, 325, or
     500 mg
   Injection: 300 mg/ml
   20% sol.: 10 mg/drop
	10 mg/kg 3 times a day
	for 7 days
		noise in the ears
		dizziness
		nausea, vomiting
		Do not use for prevention.

sulfadoxine +
   pyrimethamine
   *****Fansidar**
     tabs: 500 mg sulfa +
       25 mg pyrimethamine
	3 tabs in one dose
	Children: 1/2 to 2
	tabs in one dose
		severe drug rash
		urticaria
		Do not use for prevention.

Gastrointestinal Drugs

Antacids **magnesium trisilicate**	2 tabs chewed every 4 to 6 hours	
aluminium hydroxide	2 tabs chewed every 4 to 6 hours	
Antispasmodics **belladonna tincture**	10 drops 3 times a day	dry mouth urine retention trouble seeing
belladonna extract	1 or 2 tabs 3 times a day	dry mouth urine retention trouble seeing

propantheline
  *Probanthine
    tabs: 15 mg
	1 tab 3 times a day	dry mouth

Diuretics

hydrochlorthiazide
  *Esidrix
    tabs: 25 or 50 mg
	1 or 2 tabs each morning	causes loss of much urine
		lowers blood pressure
		Patient needs potassium from fruits

furosemide
  *Lasix
    tabs: 40 mg
    injection: 10 mg/ml
	1 or 2 tabs each day
	Children: 1-4 mg/kg
	each day
		strong diuretic
		Use only in severe edema or in
		  severe heart failure

Anti-ameba drugs - see page 597

Anti-leprosy drugs - see page 646

Anti-tuberculosis drugs - see page 699

Analgesics

aspirin **tabs**: 100 or 500 mg	1 tab 3 or 4 times a day **Children**: 10 mg/kg 3 or 4 times a day	heart burn peptic ulcer

paracetamol
    tabs: 500 mg
	1 tab 3 or 4 times a day
	Children: 10 mg/kg
	3 or 4 times a day
		severe liver damage
		  with jaundice

pethidine
    injection: 50 or
        100 mg\ml
	1 mg/kg IM every 6 hrs
	only for severe pain
		vomiting, slow breathing
		constipation
		drug abuse

morphine **injection**: 10 mg/ml	0.1 mg/kg IM every 6 hrs only for severe pain	vomiting, slow breathing constipation drug abuse

Anticonvulsants

phenobarbital
    tabs: 30 or 100 mg
    syrup: 3 mg/ml
    Injection: 100 or
        200 mg/ml
	4 mg/kg 3 or 4 times
	a day to stop convulsions
		sleepiness
		slow breathing
		can cause drug abuse

phenytoin
    *Epanutin
    *Dilantin
    tabs: 100 mg
	1 tab 1 to 3 times a day	bleeding gums
		drug rash

diazepam
    *Valium
    tabs: 5 mg
    injection: 5 mg/ml
	1 tab 1 to 3 times a day
	10-20 mg/dose IM or
	IV every 6 hrs
	Children: 1 mg/kg/dose
		sleepiness
		slow breathing

Antihistamines

promethazine
  *Phenergan
    tabs: 25 mg
    syrup: 1 mg/ml
    Injection: 25 mg/ml
	25 mg 1 to 3 times a day
	Children: 1 mg/kg
	1 to 3 times a day
		sleepiness

chlorpheniramine
  *Piriton
    tabs: 4 mg
    syrup: 2 mg/5 ml
    Injection: 10 mg/ml
	1 tab 1 to 4 times a day
	Children: 0.1 mg/kg
	3 to 4 times a day
		some sleepiness

Vitamins and Minerals

ferrous sulfate
  or gluconate
  *Iron
    tabs: 200 or 300 mg
    syrup: see label
	1 tab 2 or 3 times a day
	Children: 10 mg/kg/day
		for certain kinds of anemia

folic acid
    tabs: 5 mg
	1 or 2 tabs daily	for anemia of pregnancy
		  and sickle cell anemia

multivitamins	1 tab 1 to 3 times a day	
vitamin A	1 to 3 tabs daily, or 1 to 3 ml IM daily	
thiamine *Vitamin B-1	1 or 2 tabs daily **tabs**: see label	
riboflavin *Vitamin B-2	25 to 100 mg daily **tabs**: see label	

pyridoxine *Vitamin B-6	1 or 2 tabs daily tabs: 50 mg
ascorbic acid *Vitamin C	500 to 1000 mg daily tabs: see label
nicotinamide *Niacin	20 mg daily tabs: see label

phytomenadione
  *Vitamin K
    tabs: 5 or 10 mg
    injection: 1 mg/ml
	5-10 mg daily orally
	or 1 mg IM daily

For an excellent book on current medicines, see:

Guidelines to Drug Usage, by G. Upunda, J. Yudkin, and G.V. Brown
Macmillan Education Publications, London, 1980.
available from: TALC, Box 49, St. Albans, Hertfordshire, AL1 4AX, England
             and: AMREF, Wilson Airport, P.O. Box 30125, Nairobi, Kenya.

Word List

Abortion: the uterus pushes the fetus out of the uterus during the first five months of the pregnancy.

Abscess: a collection of pus in the tissues.

Acute: of short duration, from one day to one month.

AIDS: Acquired Immune Deficiency Syndrome, a chronic viral infection transmitted by blood and by sexual contact.

Allergy: a reaction of the body against certain foreign substances.

Alveoli: tiny spaces filled with air in the lungs. Oxygen from the air goes from them into the blood.

Ameba: a very small parasite of the intestines that can cause blood in the stools or dysentery.

Amebiasis: an infection of ameba.

Amenorrhea: the absence of menstrual periods. This comes during a pregnancy, during nursing, before puberty, after the menopause, and during certain illnesses.

Anaphylactic shock: sudden shock coming after an injection or an insect bite. Unless treated quickly, it is often fatal.

Anemia: a diminution of hemoglobin in the blood.

Anesthesia: the loss of feeling in a part of the body.

Ankylostomiasis: hookworm infection. The worms are in the small intestine.

Anorexia: loss of appetite.

Appendicitis: an inflammation of the appendix. This is a serious disease and needs an operation immediately to remove it.

Appendix: a short tubular organ attached to the cecum.

Arthritis: inflammation of a joint.

Acacias: roundworm infection. The ascaris worms are in the intestines.

Ascites: the accumulation of edema liquid inside the abdomen.

Asthma: a disease of the lungs. The patient has trouble pushing air out of the lungs.

Auscultation: listening to the breathing, the heart, or the intestinal sounds through a stethoscope.

Axillary: refers to the armpit.

Bacillus: a long bacteria.

Bacteria: microscopic organisms. Some can cause infections.

BCG: the vaccination against tuberculosis.

Bile: a yellow-green bitter liquid made by the liver. It goes into the intestines and helps with the digestion of food.

Bilharzia: the disease caused by Schistosomes.

Bilirubin: hemoglobin in the blood serum that has turned yellow.

Biopsy: a surgical operation to take out a small piece of tissue to examine under the microscope.

Bronchial tubes: tubes in the lungs that let air go in and out and that connect the trachea to the lungs.

Bronchitis: inflammation in the bronchial tubes.

Cancer: a malignant tumor, usually fatal.

Cardiac: refers to the heart.

Cataract: a thickening of the lens of the eye causing blindness in the eye.

Cecum: the beginning of the large intestine. It is in the right lower quadrant of the abdomen.

Cellulitis: an acute infection of the subcutaneous tissues.

Cerebral malaria: malaria in the brain.

Cerebro-spinal fluid: the liquid surrounding the brain and spinal cord.

Chancre: a sore or ulcer on a genital organ transmitted by sexual contact.

Chicken pox: a contagious viral infection of children causing vesicles and pustules on the skin.

Chronic: of long duration: several weeks, months, or years.

Cirrhosis: chronic inflammation of the liver.

Clonus: an abnormal jerking up and down of the foot when bent up strongly.

Colic: intermittent pain that comes and goes every few minutes.

Coma: being unconscious because of a severe disease or injury.

Congenital: a condition with which a baby is born.

Conjunctiva: the membrane that lines the inside of the eyelids and part of the globe of the eye.

Conjunctivitis: an infection of the conjunctiva.

Contagious: a disease that goes from one person to another.

Contusion: injury to the soft tissues of the body, such as the muscles, with no wound.

Cornea: the front transparent part of the eye.

Crackles: soft crackling sounds in the lungs made by liquid in the alveoli. They are a sign of disease of the lungs or of the heart.

Crepitations: the scraping of the broken ends of a fractured bone.

Croup: an acute severe infection of the larynx and vocal cords.

CSF: Cerebro-Spinal Fluid.

Cyanosis: a blue color of the skin or mucous membranes. It comes when there is little oxygen in the blood.

Cystocele: the front wall of the vagina comes out of the vagina.

Definite diagnosis: when the diagnosis is certain.

Dehydration: too little water in the tissues.

Delirium: mental confusion. The patient cannot think or talk clearly.

Diabetes: a chronic disease in which the patient has much sugar in the body and passes sugar in the urine. The patient has too little insulin.

Diaphragm: the big muscle between the chest and the abdomen. It is the important muscle for breathing.

Diarrhea: frequent liquid stools.

Diastolic: the lower pressure of the blood.

Differential diagnosis: a list of all the possible causes of the illness of a patient.

Dislocation: the bone has come out of the joint.

Dullness: the sound of percussion over a solid part of the body or a part that contains liquid.

Duodenum: the first part of the small intestine. It comes right after the stomach.

Dysentery: an acute or chronic infectious diarrhea.

Dysmenorrhea: pain just before, during, or right after the menstrual period.

Dyspareunia: pain in a woman during sexual intercourse.

Dyspnea: difficulty breathing.

Dysuria: pain when urinating.

Ecchymosis: a dark color of the skin due to blood in the skin or subcutaneous tissues.

Eclampsia: toxemia of pregnancy with convulsions.

Ectopic pregnancy: a pregnancy outside of the uterus, usually in the uterine (fallopian) tube.

Eczema: an acute infection of the skin.

Edema: swelling of the tissues because of the accumulation of liquid.

Elephantiasis: chronic swelling of the skin and subcutaneous tissues. The part of the body affected becomes very big and heavy, like an elephant.

Empyema: a collection of pus in the chest in the space around a lung.

Epididymitis: an infection of the spermatic cord.

Epigastric: refers to the upper middle part of the abdomen below the sternum.

Epistaxis: bleeding from the nose.

Expectorant: a medicine that makes bronchial secretions more liquid and more easy to cough out.

Expiration: the action of breathing air out of the lungs.

Extension: the action of making a joint or a limb straight or bending it back.

Febrile: with fever.

Fecal: refers to the stools.

Femoral: refers to the upper medial part of the thigh or upper leg.

Fetus: a baby before birth, still inside the uterus.

Fever: an elevated temperature of the body.

Filaria: a parasitic worm living in the skin, the lymph nodes, or the blood.

Filariasis: an infection with filaria worms.

Fissure: a small painful crack in the skin or a mucous membrane.

Fistula: an abnormal passage between two organs or an organ and the skin.

Flank: the side of the abdomen below the ribs and above the hip.

Flexion: the action of bending a joint or a limb.

Fontanel: a space between the bones of the skull in a small infant. The fontanel disappears at about 15 months of age.

Fracture: a broken bone.

Frequency: passing urine very often, every few minutes.

Fungus: a plant microbe that can cause infections.

Gall bladder: a small organ below the middle of the liver. It stores bile coming from the liver.

Gastric: refers to the stomach.

Gastritis: an inflammation of the stomach

Generic: the real name of a medicine.

Genital: refers to the male or female organs of reproduction.

Goiter: an increase in the size of the thyroid gland.

Gonorrhea: an infection of the genital organs transmitted by sexual contact.

Heart murmur: an abnormal sound between the heart beats.

Hematuria: blood in the urine.

Hemiplegia: paralysis of one side of the body.

Hemoglobin: the red substance in the blood that carries oxygen to the tissues.

Hemoglobinometer: an instrument to measure the amount of hemoglobin in the blood.

Hemolytic: something that destroys the red blood cells.

Hemoptysis: blood in the sputum.

Hemorrhage: bleeding.

Hemorrhoids: swellings around the anus.

Hepatitis: an infection of the liver caused by a virus, usually accompanied by jaundice.

Hereditary: passed from parents to children.

Hernia: a small sack of peritoneum that comes out through the muscles of the abdomen.

Herpes: a virus that causes small sores in the mouth or the vagina.

Hg: a short way to write hemoglobin.

History: the story of the illness of the patient.

Homan's sign: pain in the back of the leg on strong dorsi-flexion of the foot.

Hydrocele: an accumulation of liquid around the testicle.

Hypertension: high blood pressure.

Hypertrophy: becoming more big than normal.

Ileus: no waves of peristalsis in the intestines. The abdomen is silent.

Iliac: refers to the lower quadrants of the abdomen.

Impetigo: an acute bacterial infection in the skin.

Infection: a disease caused by microbes or by parasites.

Inflammation: a reaction of the tissues characterized by pain, swelling, heat, and redness.

Inguinal: refers to where the upper leg joins the abdomen.

Insomnia: inability to sleep well.

Inspiration: breathing air into the lungs.

Insulin: a hormone made by the pancreas that helps the body use sugar properly. Too little insulin causes diabetes.

Intestine: the digestive tube from the stomach to the anus.

Intoxication: a poisoning of the body by a certain substance.

Iris: the thin membrane in the eye around the pupil.

Jaundice: a yellow color of the mucous membranes, the eyes, and the skin.

Leprosy: a chronic infection of the nerves and skin causing anesthesia and spots on the skin.

Leucorrhea: liquid coming from the vagina.

Leukemia: a malignant tumor of the white blood cells.

Lice: a small insect that lives in the hair of the head, the body, or the pubic region. It causes much itching.

Ligament: a band of strong tissue holding bones and joints together.

Lipoma: a soft benign fatty tumor in the subcutaneous tissue.

LP: a short way to write Lumbar Puncture.

Lumbar puncture: removing a small amount of cerebro-spinal fluid through a needle in the lumbar region.

Lumbar region: the low part of the back.

Lymph: a clear liquid that circulates between cells in the tissues.

Lymph node: a small mass of tissue through which the lymph passes on its way back to the heart. Lymph nodes act as filters to remove bacteria and foreign bodies from the lymph.

Lymphadenitis: an acute infection of the lymph nodes.

Lymphatic: having to do with the channels for lymph.

Macula: a small thin flat spot on the skin.

Malaria: an acute infection, with fever, caused by parasites in the blood called plasmodium. Mosquitoes transmit these parasites.

Malnutrition: a chronic disease caused by a lack of protein in the food. The tissues become weak and resistance to infections diminishes.

Marasmus: a state of malnutrition caused by insufficient food of all kinds.

Measles: an acute viral infection of small children. It makes an eruption on the skin.

Melena: blood in the stools.

Meningitis: a serious acute infection of the membranes surrounding the brain and the spinal cord. It is often fatal.

Menopause: the end of the reproductive period of a woman. She no longer has her monthly menstrual periods.

Menorrhagia: much bleeding during the menstrual periods.

Menstrual period: the monthly loss of blood from the uterus in a woman.

Metrorrhagia: vaginal bleeding not during the menstrual periods.

Microbes: very small living organisms that we cannot see with our eyes. We can see them only through a microscope. Some microbes cause infections.

Microscope: a machine that enables us to see very small objects.

Microscopic: too small to be seen with our eyes. We can see it only through a microscope.

Migraine: a severe headache on one side of the head.

Mucous: refers to mucus.

Mucous membrane: membranes that line the inside of the mouth, the nose, the vagina, and the digestive and urinary organs.

Mucus: the thick liquid produced by the mucous membranes.

Mycobacterium ulcerans: a bacteria that causes a special deep ulcer of the skin and subcutaneous tissues.

Nausea: the desire to vomit.

Nephritis: an inflammation of the kidneys.

Nephrosis: a chronic disease of the kidneys causing much swelling and much protein in the urine.
Nodule: a big hard lump in the skin or subcutaneous tissue.

Obesity: over weight because of too much fat.
Observation: looking closely at something to see what it is like.
Onchocerciasis: a filarial infection caused by Onchocercus volvulus.
Orchitis: an infection of the testicle.
Orthopnea: difficulty breathing when lying flat in bed. The patient must sit up in order to breathe easily.
Osteoarthritis: an inflammation of the joints because of old age.
Osteomyelitis: an infection in a bone.
Otitis: an infection in the ear.
Otoscope: a special flashlight for examining the ears.
Ovary: the reproductive organ of women that produces the ovule that becomes an egg. It is in the lower abdomen (the pelvis).
Ovulation: when an ovum leaves and ovary to start its journey to the uterus.
Oxyuris: pinworms. These tiny worms live in the large intestine.

Palpation: the act of feeling parts of the body with the hands in order to find signs of disease.
Pancreas: a digestive organ in the epigastric region of the abdomen.
Papule: a small raised bump in the skin.
Paralysis: a diminution or loss of power in one or more muscles.
Parasites: a very small animal that gets into the body and causes a disease.
PE: a short way to write Physical Examination.
Pelvic: refers to the pelvis.
Pelvis: the bottom part of the abdominal cavity. It is surrounded by the pelvic bone.
Penis: the male external sexual organ.
Peptic: refers to the stomach.
Percussion: the act of tapping on the chest or abdomen to hear the sound produced. This can show certain signs of disease.
Peristalsis: waves of regular contractions that pass along the stomach and intestines to push food along the digestive tube.
Peritoneum: the membrane lining the inside of the abdomen.
Peritonitis: inflammation, usually infection, of the peritoneum.
Pharyngitis: inflammation of the pharynx.
Pharynx: the throat, or the back part of the mouth.

Placenta: a soft organ that attaches the fetus to the inside of the uterus. The air and food that the baby needs go through the placenta. The placenta comes out right after the baby comes out of the uterus.

Placenta previa: the placenta comes out ahead of the baby. This causes much bleeding and requires transfusions and an immediate operation.

Plaque: a big flat spot on the skin.

Plasmodium: the parasite that causes malaria.

Pleura: the membrane covering the lungs and the inside of the chest.

Pleural cavity: the space between the lungs and the inside of the chest.

Pneumonia: an infection of the lungs.

Polio: a viral infection of the nerves. It can cause a permanent paralysis.

Polyneuritis: painful inflammation of many nerves.

Polyuria: urinating large amounts of urine.

Pott's disease: tuberculosis of the bones of the back.

Probable abortion: the uterus is trying to push the fetus out. There is pain and bleeding from the vagina.

Prolapse: the uterus comes down and hangs outside of the vagina.

Prostate: a small organ below the bladder of a man. It produces the semen, the sexual secretions of a man.

Prostatitis: an infection of the prostate.

Pterygium: a small membrane of conjunctiva that grows out over the cornea.

Pulse: the beating of the heart that sends blood through the arteries.

Pupil: the black hole in the center of the eye. It lets light pass inside the eye.

Purulent: filled with pus.

Pus: thick liquid coming from an infection. It has dead bacteria and dead white blood cells.

Pustule: a small bump on the skin filled with pus.

Pyelonephritis: an infection of one or both kidneys.

Pylorus: the opening at the far end of the stomach, between the stomach and the duodenum.

Pyomyositis: a purulent infection in the muscles.

Pyuria: pus in the urine.

Quadrant: a part (one quarter) of the abdomen.

Rales: another name for crackles in the lungs.

RBC: a short way to write Red Blood Cells.

Rebound tenderness: strong pain in the abdomen when you push on it and then take away the hand quickly. It is a sign of peritonitis, appendicitis, or bleeding inside the abdomen.

Rectocele: the back wall of the vagina comes down and out of the vagina.

Rectum: the last part of the large intestine. It opens through the anus.

Renal: refers to the kidneys.

Resonance: a sound like a drum produced by percussion on a part of the body full of air or gas.

Respiration: breathing, or the act of taking air into the lungs and pushing it out again.

Retention: difficulty or inability to pass urine.

Rheumatoid: a form of arthritis with much pain and inflammation of the joints.

Rhonchi: loud lung sounds made by liquid in the bronchial tubes.

Saliva: liquid in the mouth that helps with eating and digestion.

Scabies: an infection of the skin by very small insects that cause much itching.

Schistosome: a worm that lives near the liver and causes bleeding in the stools or in the urine. It can also cause liver disease.

Schistosomiasis: the disease caused by schistosomes.

Sciatic nerve: the big nerve going down the back of the leg.

Sciatica: painful inflammation of the sciatic nerve.

Scrotum: the sack of skin containing the testicles and the spermatic cord.

Sed rate: a short way to write blood sedimentation rate.

Septic: caused by a bacterial infection, often with pus.

Septicemia: a bacterial infection of the blood, affecting the whole body.

Shock: a collapse of the circulation. The pulse and blood pressure disappear from the arms.

Sickle cell anemia: a hereditary anemia. The red blood cells are easily destroyed in the body.

Sigmoid: the lower part of the large intestine just above the rectum.

Sign of disease: a change made in the body by a disease.

Sinus: a hole in the skin from which liquid or pus comes.

Sinusitis: infection of one or more sinuses of the face or head.

Sleeping sickness: see Trypanosomiasis.

Spermatic cord: the cord going from the testicle to the penis to take the spermatozoa to the urethra.

Sphincter: a circle of muscle that closes and opens an opening such as the eye, the mouth, the anus, or the urethra.

Sprain: an injury to a joint. Some ligaments are torn.

Sputum: liquid coming from the lungs and bronchial tubes after a cough.

Sternomastoid: the muscle in the neck going from the back of the ear to the top of the sternum.

Sternum: the bone in the middle of the front of the chest.

Strangulated hernia: a hernia that cannot be reduced. It requires an immediate operation.

Stricture: a scar that closes or almost closes the urethra or rectum.

Suppressant: a medicine that diminishes coughing.

Supraclavicular: just above the clavicle, in the low part of the neck.

Symptom: an unpleasant feeling a patient has when he is ill.

Syphilis: an infection transmitted by sexual contact.

Systolic: the upper blood pressure. It comes during each pulse beat.

TB: a short way to write tuberculosis.

Tenderness: pain caused by palpation on a part of the body.

Tenesmus: desire to urinate or pass stools even when the bladder or the rectum are empty.

Tetanus: a severe infection causing painful muscle contractions.

Threatened abortion: the uterus is trying to push out the fetus. The woman has pain but no bleeding.

Thrill: a vibration of the chest wall because of a serious disease in a valve of the heart.

Thrombophlebitis: inflammation of the veins of the leg.

Tonsil: a small collection of lymphatic tissue at each side of the pharynx.

Tonsillitis: infection of the tonsils.

Toxemia: a disease during the last three months of pregnancy. The mother has edema, protein in the urine, and high blood pressure.

Trachea: the big air tube in the neck. It goes from the pharynx down into the lungs to join with the bronchial tubes.

Trachoma: a serious infection of the conjunctiva of the eye.

Trichomonas: a microscopic parasite that lives in the vagina or urethra. It causes itching.

Trichuris: whipworms. They live in the large intestine.

Trismus: inability to open the mouth because of strong spasms in the muscles of the lower jaw.

Trypanosomiasis: a severe chronic infection caused by a parasite. The parasites get into the blood, the lymph nodes, and the brain.

Tubercle bacillus: the microbe causing tuberculosis.

Tuberculosis: a chronic infection of the lungs and other organs caused by a bacillus.

Tumor: an abnormal growth of tissue in a certain organ.

Typhoid fever: a severe acute infection with high fever and delirium.

Ulcer: a hole in the skin or inside the mouth, stomach, or duodenum.

Umbilicus: the scar in the middle of the abdomen where the umbilical cord of the fetus was attached.

Ureter: the tube from the kidney to the bladder that carries urine to the bladder.

Urethra: the tube carrying urine from the bladder through the penis to the outside.

Urticaria: an allergic skin eruption of big bumps that itch.

Vaccination: giving a special medicine, or vaccine, to protect the person against a specific infectious disease.

Varicocele: swollen veins in the spermatic cord.

Varicose veins: swollen veins in the legs.

Vertebra: the bones of the back, in the spinal column.

Vesicle: a bump on the skin filled with liquid.

Virus: a very small microbe causing infections. It is too small to see even with a microscope.

Vulva: the external genital organs of a woman.

WBC: a short way to write White Blood Cells.

Wheezing: a sound made while pushing air out of the lungs. It is a sign of asthma.

Whooping cough: an infection of small children. It makes long spasms of coughing followed by a loud sound or "whoop."

Index